NUTRITION and HEART DISEASE

Causation and Prevention

NUTRITION and HEART DISEASE

Causation and Prevention

EDITED BY

Ronald Ross Watson & Victor R. Preedy

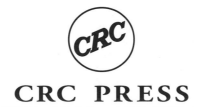

CRC PRESS

Boca Raton   London   New York   Washington, D.C.

Library of Congress Cataloging-in-Publication Data

Nutrition and heart disease : causation and prevention / edited by Ronald R. Watson, Victor R. Preedy.
    p. cm.
    Includes bibliographical references and index.
    ISBN 0-8493-1674-X (alk. paper)
    1. Heart—Disease—Nutritional aspects—Handbooks, manuals, etc. I. Watson, Ronald R. (Ronald Ross) II. Preedy, Victor R.

RC682.N873 2003
616.1′2071—dc22   2003055581

Visit the CRC Press Web site at www.crcpress.com

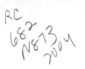

Preface

Heart disease is the primary cause of death and disability in Western countries. Coronary artery disease is the most prevalent cause of death and stroke is high on the list. For those reasons, sufficient understanding of prevention measures is vital. Nutrition and diet play key roles in preventing many types of heart damage and dysfunction. Poor nutrition and diet can cause the same heart diseases that efficacious nutrition can prevent. Dilated cardiomyopathy and associated symptoms of congestive heart failure are diagnosed with increasing frequency. The importance of nutrition and diet in preventing and possibly treating or ameliorating these conditions is discussed in this book.

Dietary agents such as fat and alcohol can under certain circumstances increase or reduce the risks of cardiovascular disease. For example, chronic alcohol abuse is clearly associated with hypertension, heart failure, bleeding disorders, fibrillation, and stroke but moderate consumption of nonalcoholic materials in alcoholic beverages can benefit cardiovascular health. Water and beverages play important roles in heart disease. Some special diets are known to increase risks while others reduce risks in unique populations. This book is intended to serve as a desk reference for nutrition and cardiovascular researchers, primary care physicians, and dieticians. It will support research and help educate health-oriented lay persons, scientists, and health care professionals.

Editors

Ronald Ross Watson, Ph.D., is an internationally recognized nutritionist and immunologist. He directs several biomedical grants funded by the National Institutes of Health (NIH) relating to the causes of heart disease. Dr. Watson has studied the importance of fats in the diet for 20 years. His model studies have involved dietary deficiencies and excesses. Dr. Watson has edited 54 biomedical books, including a recent book: *Alcohol and Heart Disease*. He contributed several chapters to this book based on research from his four grants from the National Heart, Lung, and Blood Institute to study cardiovascular disease.

Dr. Watson initiated and directed the National Institute of Alcohol Abuse and Alcoholism (NIAAA) Alcohol Research Center at the University of Arizona College of Medicine. The main goal of the center was to understand the role of ethanol-induced immunosuppression on immune function and disease resistance in animals.

Dr. Watson attended the University of Idaho and graduated from Brigham Young University in Provo, Utah, with a degree in chemistry in 1966. He completed his Ph.D. program in biochemistry at Michigan State University in 1971. His postdoctoral schooling in nutrition and microbiology was completed at the Harvard University School of Public Health and included two years of postdoctoral research experience in immunology. Dr. Watson is a member of several national and international nutrition, immunology, and cancer societies and research societies on alcoholism.

Victor R. Preedy, Ph.D., is a professor in the Department of Nutrition and Dietetics at King's College in London. He directs studies regarding protein turnover, cardiology, nutrition, and the biochemical aspects of alcoholism, in particular. Dr. Preedy graduated in 1974 from the University of Aston with a combined honors degree in biology, physiology, and pharmacology. He earned a Ph.D. in 1981 in the fields of nutrition and metabolism, specializing in protein turnover. In 1992, he gained membership in the Royal College of Pathologists based on his published works, and in 1993 he was awarded a D.Sc. for his outstanding contributions to protein and metabolism research. He was one of the university's youngest recipients of this distinguished award.

Dr. Preedy was elected a fellow of the Royal College of Pathologists in 2000. He has published over 450 articles including over 134 peer-reviewed manuscripts based on original research and 70 reviews. His current major research interests include protein turnover with reference to alcohol's role in enteral nutrition, messenger, transfer, and ribosomal RNA degradation products, and the molecular mechanisms responsible for alcoholic heart muscle damage.

Contributors

Maria Assunta Ancora, D. Biol.
CNR Institute of Clinical Physiology
Lecce, Italy

Susan Appt, D.V.M.
Wake Forest University School
 of Medicine
Comparative Medicine Clinical
 Research Center
Winston-Salem, North Carolina

Pauline Ashfield-Watt, Ph.D.
Institute of Food Nutrition and Human
 Health
Massey University
Auckland, New Zealand

Henrique Barros, M.D., Ph.D.
Serviço de Higiene e Epidemiologia
Faculdade de Medicine
Universidade do Porto
Porto, Portugal

Wanda J.E. Bemelmans, Ph.D.
National Institute for Public Health
 and the Environment
Centre for Prevention and Health
 Services Research
Bilthoven, the Netherlands

Michel Beylot, M.D., Ph.D.
INSERM
Faculte Laennec
Lyon, France

Simin Bolourchi-Vaghefi, Ph.D.
Department of Public Health
College of Health
University of North Florida
Jacksonville, Florida

Michael Burr, M.D., D.Sc., FFPHM
University of Wales
College of Medicine
Cardiff, Wales

**Maria Annunziata Carluccio,
D. Biol., Ph.D.**
CNR Institute of Clinical Physiology
Lecce, Italy

Susana Casal, Ph.D.
REQIMTE
Serviço de Bromatologia
Faculdade de Farmacia
Universidade do Porto
Porto, Portugal

Raffaele De Caterina, M.D., Ph.D.
Chair of Cardiology
Gabriele d' Annunzio University
Chieti, Italy

Andrew L. Clark, M.A., M.D., MRCP
Academic Cardiology
Castle Hill Hospital
Cottingham, Hull, England

Thomas B. Clarkson, D.V.M.
Wake Forest University School
 of Medicine
Comparative Medicine Clinical
 Research Center
Winston-Salem, North Carolina

Lee Hooper, B.Sc., SRD
University of Manchester
University Hospital NHS Trust
Manchester, England

Douglas F. Larson, Ph.D.
Sarver Heart Center
University of Arizona College
  of Medicine
Tucson, Arizona

Carla Lopes, Ph.D.
Serviço de Higiene e Epidemiologia
Faculdade de Medicine
Universidade do Porto
Porto, Portugal

Michel de Lorgeril, M.D.
Laboratoire du Stress Cardiovasculaire
  et Pathologies Associees
UFR de Medecine et Pharmacie
Grenoble, France

**Ian McDowell, Senior Lecturer,
M.D., FRCP, FRCPath**
University Hospital of Wales
Cardiff, Wales

**Cynthia Mlakar, B.S.,
M.A. (Educ.)**
Science Department
Tortolita Middle School
Marana Unified District
Tuscon, Arizona

Marika Massaro, D. Biol., Ph.D.
CNR Institute of Clinical Physiology
Lecce, Italy

Ronald P. Mensink, Ph.D.
Department of Human Biology
Maastricht University
Maastricht, the Netherlands

Elke Naumann, M.Sc.
Department of Human Biology
Maastricht University
Maastricht, the Netherlands

Beatriz Oliveira, Ph.D., Pharm D.
REQIMTE
Serviço de Bromatologia
Faculdade de Farmacia
Universidade do Porto
Porto, Portugal

J. Michael Overton, Ph.D.
Department of Nutrition, Food,
  and Exercise Science and
Program in Neuroscience
Florida State University
Tallahassee, Florida

Jogchum Plat, Ph.D.
Department of Human Biology
Maastricht University
Maastricht, the Netherlands

Patricia Salen, B.Sc.
Laboratoire du Stress Cardiovasculaire
  et Pathologies Associees
UFR de Medecine et Pharmacie
Grenoble, France

Egeria Scoditti, D. Biol.
CNR Institute of Clinical Physiology
Lecce, Italy

Katrina Simpson, B.S.
University of Arizona
Tucson, Arizona

Steven J. Swoap, Ph.D.
Department of Biology
Williams College
Williamstown, Massachusetts

**Poothirikovil Venugopalan, M.D.
(Pediatrics), FRCP, FRCPCH**
Consultant Pediatrician
  and Pediatric Cardiologist
Sultan Qaboos University Hospital
Muscat, Sultanate of Oman

A.R.P. Walker, Ph.D.
National Health Laboratory Service
Braamfontein, Johannesburg,
  South Africa

Ronald R. Watson, Ph.D.
Sarver Heart Center
University of Arizona College
  of Medicine and College
  of Public Health
Tucson, Arizona

Klaus K.A. Witte, M.B., MRCP
Academic Cardiology
Castle Hill Hospital
Cottingham, Hull, England

Bo Yang, M.D., Ph.D.
Sarver Heart Center
University of Arizona College
  of Medicine
Tucson, Arizona

Jian-Min Yuan, M.D., Ph.D.
Department of Preventive Medicine
Keck School of Medicine
University of Southern California
Los Angeles, California

Contents

Section I

Diet and Heart Disease Prevention

1 The Role of the Dietitian in Reducing Cardiovascular Risk: An Evidence-Based Approach

Lee Hooper

CONTENTS

1.1 WHAT DIETITIANS OFFER

Dietitians work to encourage and support the eating of food that promotes health. In the words of the American Dietetic Association, dietitians serve the public by promoting optimal nutrition and well-being:

> Dietitians are professionals who provide reliable, objective nutrition information, separate facts from fads, and translate the latest scientific findings into easy-to-understand nutrition information.[1]

The British Dietetic Association defines the role of dietitians as follows:

They interpret and translate the science of nutrition into practical ways of promoting nutritional well-being, disease treatment, and the prevention of nutrition-related health problems. Their advice is evidence-based.[2]

Two key elements of these descriptions are that the nutrition information or advice provided is (1) based on good strong science (reliable, objective, evidence-based) and (2) provided in a format that real people can understand and use (practical, easy to understand).

It is vital that we do more than give lip service to the idea of evidence-based practice; we must understand it and use it in everyday healthcare. This chapter will explore the evidence on who should provide dietary advice to reduce cardiovascular risk and the best evidence-based advice to help people with cardiovascular diseases alter the foods that they eat every day. It will start with a short introduction to evidence-based practice.

1.2 EVIDENCE-BASED PRACTICE

According to David Sackett, one of the originators of evidence-based medicine terminology, evidence-based practice is

the conscientious, explicit and judicious use of current best evidence in making decisions about the care of individual patients … [it] means integrating individual clinical expertise with the best available external evidence from systematic research.[3]

When we are discussing the effectiveness of an intervention in healthcare (be it the effectiveness of a drug, physical therapy, dietary change, or type of dietary advice), the best available evidence comes from the top of the levels of evidence hierarchy. A good levels of evidence model for effectiveness of an intervention was produced by the Oxford Centre for Evidence-Based Medicine.[4] It is summarized in Table 1.1.

We should thus base our dietary advice on the best evidence — where possible, from systematic reviews (meta-analyses) of randomised controlled trials or individ-

---

TABLE 1.1
Levels of Evidence for a Question about Efficacy of a Dietary Intervention

Best evidence ↑	Level 1a. A systemic review (meta-analysis) of randomised controlled trails (without heterogenity between trials)
	Level 1b. A single randomised controlled trial with a narrow confidence interval
	Level 2a. A systematic review (meta-analysis) of cohort studies (without heterogeneity between study results)
	Level 2b. An individual cohort study, or a low-quality randomised controlled trial
	Level 2c. Ecological studies
	Level 3. Case control studies
	Level 4. Case series
Worst evidence	Level 5. Expert opinion without explicit critical appraisal, or based on physiology, bench research, or "first principles"

Adapted from Centre for Evidence-Based Medicine.[4]

ual high-quality randomised controlled trials. A systematic review is an impartial and unbiased review of *all relevant* research evidence. It is

a review that has been prepared using a systematic approach to minimizing biases and random errors which is documented in a materials and methods section. A systematic review may or may not include a meta-analysis — a statistical analysis of the results from independent studies that generally aims to produce a single estimate of a treatment effect.[5]

Studies of antioxidant vitamins highlight the need to base our dietary interventions on randomised controlled trials or systematic reviews of randomised controlled trials rather than on cohort data. Good evidence from individual cohort studies (and meta-analyses of cohort studies) indicates that people taking more beta-carotene or vitamin E are protected from cardiovascular disease, even after controlling for other lifestyle factors. However, no evidence of a protective effect of either beta-carotene or vitamin E was seen in large long-term randomised controlled trials[6] or in meta-analyses of randomised controlled trials.[7,8] It appears that the clustering of healthy lifestyle traits and socioeconomic advantage is so strong that it is almost impossible to control for these multiple confounding factors when assessing evidence from cohorts. While evidence from cohorts may point out interventions to try in randomised controlled trials, we need to base our understanding of the effectiveness of dietary interventions on good quality randomised studies of interventions.

In addition to choosing the type of study to provide the necessary evidence, we must consider the quality of each individual study chosen (see information about the Critical Appraisal Skills Programme (CASP) Web site in Section 1.6, Useful Contacts) and, equally important, the outcomes measured. For example, a randomised controlled trial may show that eating more of a particular fruit raises levels of specific antioxidant compounds in the blood. However, a randomised controlled trial that assesses disease outcomes would provide better evidence of that fruit's usefulness in protecting against cardiovascular disease. We must have good randomised controlled trial evidence that raising these antioxidant compounds in the blood does indeed reduce cardiovascular disease outcomes to help us interpret the findings.

Evidence-based practice is important and places emphasis on systematic reviews of randomised controlled trials or large high-quality individual randomised controlled trials. For these reasons, most of the evidence presented in this chapter is based on these types of trials.

1.3 WHO SHOULD GIVE DIETARY ADVICE?

What evidence indicates who should give dietary advice to reduce cardiovascular risk? A systematic review of randomised controlled trials addresses this issue.[9,10]

1.3.1 SYSTEMATIC REVIEW EVIDENCE

This systematic review aimed to assess how effective dietary advice provided by a dietitian was, compared with such advice provided by other health professionals and self-help resources, in terms of reducing total serum cholesterol in adults. The reviewers electronically searched the Cochrane Library, MEDLINE, EMBASE, CINAHL, Human Nutrition, the Science Citation Index, and the Social Sciences Index. They also hand-searched conference proceedings and contacted experts to find all of the randomised controlled trials through 1999. Randomised controlled trials that compared the effects of dieticians' advice on serum cholesterol levels with the effects of advice by other health professionals or self-help packages were selected. Decisions on inclusion were duplicated by two independent reviewers and disagreements were resolved by discussion or by a third reviewer. Two reviewers independently extracted the data from included studies and assessed trial quality.

Eleven relevant randomised controlled trials (of twelve comparisons) were found and included in the review. Four studies compared advice from dietitians with advice from doctors, one study compared advice from dietitians with advice from nurses, and seven studies compared advice from dietitians with self-help resources.

These studies were carried out in the U.K., the U.S., and Australia in a variety of settings including general practices, workplaces, and clinics. Some participants had heart disease at baseline; others had slightly or distinctly raised serum cholesterol; and some had risk factors for diabetes. Duration of studies varied from 6 to 104 weeks, and data were used only for participants who did not take or had stopped taking lipid lowering medications (so that the outcomes were not biased by the effects of these medications in some groups). Outcome measures in the trials included total serum cholesterol in all studies, along with low density lipoprotein (LDL) cholesterol, high density lipoprotein (HDL) cholesterol, blood pressure, weight, and patient satisfaction in one or more studies. Participants seen by dietitians tended to be seen more frequently or for longer than those seen by doctors and took part in group sessions and/or individual consultations. Self-help resources were usually simple leaflets.

The quality of included studies was variable, but none reported randomisation procedure in enough detail to enable allocation concealment to be rated as adequate. (Allocation concealment reflects the lack of ability of personnel within the study to accept or reject potential participants according to which intervention they will receive if they enter the trial. It appears to be important in ensuring that two groups entering a study are truly randomised. Where allocation concealment is adequate, effect sizes tend to be smaller and less biased.[11])

Patient follow-up of at least 80% in both groups was achieved for four studies only, but blinded and reliable assessment of blood cholesterol was done for all studies. Most studies ensured that participants in different groups did not meet and compare notes on their treatments (this is termed *adequate protection against contamination*). Several studies revealed significantly different cholesterol levels at baseline between the groups (in four studies the baseline cholesterol levels were higher in the non-dietitian group, whereas in one study the levels were higher in the dietitian group). This is important because it is easier to achieve a fall in cholesterol by starting from a higher baseline. Overall, two studies met five of the six quality criteria, five met four criteria, and four met only two criteria. Studies comparing dietetic input with doctors' advice were of higher quality overall than studies comparing dietetic input with self-help resources.

Meta-analysis (statistically combining the results of all the relevant studies) showed significantly greater falls in total serum cholesterol in participants advised by dietitians instead of doctors (of 0.25 mmol/L, 95% confidence interval [CI] 0.12 to 0.37 mmol/L). This difference was greater in shorter-term studies and declined over time.

However, dieticians' advice did not produce significantly greater falls in total serum cholesterol than self-help resources (greater falls by dietitians of 0.10 mmol/L, 95% CI –0.03 to 0.22 mmol/L) or nurses' advice (greater falls by nurses of 0.08 mmol/L, 95% CI –0.11 to 0.27 mmol/L). Meta-analyses on HDL cholesterol, LDL cholesterol, systolic and diastolic blood pressure, and body weight showed significantly greater falls only in HDL cholesterol when advice was provided by a dietitian (–0.06 mmol/L, 95% CI –0.01 to –0.11) instead of a nurse.

In conclusion, the studies included were not of good quality and analyses were based on limited numbers of trials (and participants). However, the evidence suggests that dietary advice from a dietitian is more effective for lowering total serum cholesterol than is advice from a doctor, but may not be more effective than advice provided by trained nurses or self-help materials.

More high-quality trials would be useful to help elucidate longer-term results, the effects of contact time (the period over which contact takes place), the effects of training other health professionals, the settings that are most effective, and the effects of offering other lifestyle advice in addition to dietary advice. The review set out to address all these issues, but was unable to do so because of the shortage of sizeable trials.

Further relevant studies have been published since 1999 and the *Cochrane Review* will be updated to include these studies in the near future. Access the Cochrane Library (refer to Section 1.6) to see the latest version of the review. These additional studies may begin to further elucidate the effectiveness of different health professionals and self-help resources and unravel issues such as quantity, type, and frequency of dietary advice required to maintain gains and combat risk factors.

1.3.2 TRIAL EVIDENCE

Several randomised controlled trials address the issue of whether dietetic consultation adds anything to a standard consultation with a doctor. Such studies are not included in the systematic review discussed above but are useful because dietary advice is often provided routinely by physicians and it is worth understanding whether additional time spent with a dietitian adds enough to be worth arranging and funding.

A trial by Henkin et al[12] randomised 70 hypercholesterolemic patients to dietary counseling by a physician only and 66 to counseling by a physician and a dietitian. The physician sessions were 30 minutes long and included reevaluation of cardiovascular risk factors, a brief physical examination, and counseling on smoking cessation, physical activity, weight control, and the Step I diet. Those receiving the additional time to discuss dietetic issues were offered 2 to 4 individual counseling sessions within 3 months (as needed), the use of food diaries, and Step II advice where appropriate. After 3 months, some participants in the physician-only group were given dietetic appointments if their LDL cholesterol levels were not ideal. Some participants in the dietitian-plus-physician group moved on to lipid lowering medications.

At 3 months, the mean fall in total serum cholesterol levels was 5 mmol/L in the physician-only group and 9 mmol/L in the dietitian-plus-physician group (a significant difference of 4 mmol/L, 95% CI 1 to 7). LDL cholesterol also fell significantly more in the dietitian-plus-physician group (by 5 mmol/L, 95% CI 1 to 9 mmol/L).

A similar study by Delahanty[13] enrolled 45 participants with hyperlipidemia (not on lipid lowering medication) for primary care physician advice (usual care), and 45 participants for primary care physician advice plus dietetic intervention (based on an NCEP (National Cholesterol Education Program) cholesterol lowering protocol involving 2 to 3 visits in the first 3 months, plus an additional 2 to 3 visits within 6 months if lipids were not in the target range at 3 months). Total serum cholesterol levels dropped from 6.16 to 6.03 mmol/L at 6 months in the usual care group, and from 6.19 to 5.77 mmol/L at 6 months in the dietetic-plus-physician group (a significant difference). LDL cholesterol fell from 4.24 to 4.13 mmol/L in the usual care group compared with 4.29 to 3.98 mmol/L at 6 months in the dietetic-plus-physician group (not a significant difference). No significant differences in HDL cholesterol, triglycerides, or reported activity between the groups were noted at 6 months, but weight fell more in the dietetic-plus-physician group (usual care baseline 83.2 kg remained at 83.2 kg at 6 months; the dietetic-plus-physician group baseline 79.6 kg decreased to 77.7 kg at 6 months).

This study also assessed cost effectiveness of additional dietetic treatment and found that the additional cost of this treatment totaled $217 per participant to achieve a 6% reduction in total cholesterol and $98 per participant to sustain the reduction. Overall this was a cost of $36 per 1% decrease in total cholesterol and LDL levels.

1.4   PROTECTIVE DIETARY CHANGES FOR CARDIOVASCULAR DISEASE PATIENTS

Since dietary support and advice by health professionals and self-help materials are effective at reducing cardiovascular risk, at least in the short term, what actual changes to diet are effective in protecting people from cardiovascular disease? Again considering systematic reviews of randomised controlled trials as the best level of evidence, we are lucky that quite a few have been published in the area of diet and cardiovascular disease. The most important studies show that dietary intervention actually makes a difference to health or mortality.

1.4.1   DIETARY INTERVENTIONS THAT MAY REDUCE ILLNESS AND DEATH

To date, the most effective dietary intervention for people who already have cardiovascular disease is omega-3-rich fish oil. Evidence for this comes from a high-quality systematic review of randomised controlled trials.[14] Advice to increase intakes of long chain omega-3 fats for people with some cardiovascular disease (compared with no such advice) appears to reduce the risk of fatal myocardial infarction (relative risk 0.7, 95% CI 0.6 to 0.8), sudden death (relative risk 0.7, 95% CI 0.6 to 0.9), and overall death (relative risk 0.8, 95% CI 0.7 to 0.9), but not nonfatal myocardial infarction (relative risk 0.8, 95% CI 0.5 to 1.2). The effects of these cardioprotective doses of omega-3 fats appear consistent whether the advice is dietary (eating more oily fish, usually 2 to 3 large portions weekly) or supplemental (taking the equivalent of 0.5 to 1.0 g of a mixture of eicosapentanoic acid (EPA) and docosahexanoic acid (DHA) fatty acids daily).

A further systematic review examined the effects of omega-3 fats in diabetics.[15] Unfortunately, no studies or large subgroups of published studies assess the effects of omega-3 fats on disease endpoints in diabetics. There is no evidence of detrimental effects of cardioprotective doses of omega-3 fats on glycemic control or LDL cholesterol levels (higher levels of supplementation have been used to reduce triglyceride levels; the smaller cardioprotective doses mentioned above may well save lives of diabetics but do not alter triglycerides significantly). More evidence would be useful to clarify this issue.

Several systematic reviews have assessed the effect on morbidity and mortality of reductions in dietary fats.[16–18] A systematic review including 27 studies and over 30,000 person-years of follow-up revealed that a reduction in saturated fat, if followed for at least 2 years, produced a small but potentially important reduction in risk of cardiovascular events.[19] Most of the included studies aimed to replace saturated fats with unsaturated fats, rather than achieving big reductions in total fat intake. This alteration of dietary fat intake had a minimal effect on total mortality (rate ratio 0.98, 95% CI 0.86 to 1.12). Cardiovascular mortality was (nonsignificantly) reduced by 9% (rate ratio 0.91, 95% CI 0.77 to 1.07) and cardiovascular events significantly reduced by 16% (rate ratio 0.84, 95% CI 0.72 to 0.99). Trials with at least 2 years' follow-up provided stronger evidence of protection from cardiovascular events (rate ratio 0.76, 95% CI 0.65 to 0.90).

Although no studies compare the effect of reducing saturated fats to that of increasing omega-3 fats, an indirect comparison suggests that the effect of reducing saturated fats is smaller than the effect of increasing omega-3 fats, takes longer to be seen, but may increase in importance over periods longer than 2 years.

Other systematic reviews suggest no evidence of protective effects of dietary supplements of antioxidant vitamins[20–22] and no evidence of effects of garlic capsules on peripheral arterial occlusive disease.[23]

Evidence for a Mediterranean diet high in omega-3 fats, fruits, and vegetables and low in saturated fats and processed foods comes from only one trial in men who had recovered from myocardial infarctions.[24] While the effects of increasing fruits and vegetables and reducing processed foods appear promising, it is not clear how much of the protective effect seen in this study was due to the rapeseed (canola) margarine supplied to the intervention group (high in omega-3 fats), how much was due to reductions in saturated fats, and how much (if any) was due to fruits and vegetables.

1.4.2 DIETARY INTERVENTIONS THAT MAY ALTER RISK FACTORS

It is, of course, useful to know which dietary interventions affect which risk factors. The problem is that the answers are not always entirely consistent with effects on health. The reason is that altering one dietary component may affect many other dietary components and risk factors. If all of these effects worked in the same direction (to promote health), then the overall effect on health might be much greater than the estimated effect on the risk factor alone. On the other hand, if some effects on risk factors are positive and others are negative, the result might be no overall gain in health or even an overall loss of health even though the effects on the single risk factor measured looked promising. For this reason, understanding the effects of changes in diet on individual risk factors is interesting but not as helpful as understanding overall effects on health.

Unless otherwise specified, all references in this section are to systematic reviews of randomised controlled trials.

1.4.2.1 Dyslipidemia

While dietary advice has a role to play in normalizing abnormal serum lipids in people with cardiovascular disease, aspects of diet that clearly protect against death and disease should be given greater emphasis than lipid reduction in this group. Dietary changes are likely to result in reductions of total cholesterol of about 5%,[25–27] while statin trials reduce total cholesterol by 18 to 28%; therefore, lipid lowering medication is more effective than dietary advice.[25] Metabolic ward studies suggest that replacing 60% of saturated fats by other fats and avoiding 60% of dietary cholesterol would reduce serum total cholesterol by 0.8 mmol/L (about 13%), but it appears difficult to maintain this in a normal lifestyle.[25] Replacing saturated fats with unsaturated fats leads to improved lipid levels[28] and a reduction in cardiovascular events, but it is not clear whether polyunsaturated or monounsaturated fats are more cardioprotective.[29]

Daily use of realistic levels of soluble fiber (found in oats, pectin, psyllium, guar gum) will lower total serum cholesterol by about 2%,[30,31] while large intakes of purified soy protein will lower total cholesterol levels by about 10%.[32] Garlic supplements appear to lower serum cholesterol but trials are of poor quality and may have been biased.[33–37]

1.4.2.2 Weight

Weight can be altered by dietary change, but this appears to be difficult. Trials are often of very short duration and suffer from high drop-out rates, limiting their validity. Several good quality systematic reviews offer insights. A behavioral component improves weight loss in dietary and exercise programs (including very low calorie diets), as do written meal plans, weekly shopping lists, and group (rather than individual) therapy. Weight maintenance strategies (such as support groups) should be integral parts of all weight loss programs.[38] There is little strong evidence that the proportion of dietary fat (as distinct from calories eaten) has an effect on body weight.[38–40] In terms of managing cardiovascular risk, people with hyperlipidemia should receive dietary lipid lowering advice in addition to weight management advice.[41]

1.4.2.3 Elevated Homocysteine Levels

Elevated homocysteine levels can be reduced by supplementation with folic acid, alone or with vitamins B_6 and B_{12},[22,42,43] but it is not yet clear whether the reduction will reduce cardiovascular risk.

1.4.2.4 Blood Pressure

Increased intakes of both potassium[44,45] and calcium[46,47] appear to help reduce blood pressure; reductions in weight[48] and sodium intake[49–56] are also helpful. Salt restriction leads to reductions of 4 to 5 mmHg systolic and 2 to 3 mmHg diastolic in people with high blood pressure. Omega-3 fats do not appear to make much difference to blood pressure (although their effects on mortality are strong and important).[57,58]

The combined beneficial effect of a diet high in fruits, vegetables, and low fat dairy foods including whole grains, poultry, fish, and nuts and containing smaller amounts of red meat, salt, and sweets (the DASH diet, with smaller amounts of total and saturated fat, sodium, and cholesterol and larger amounts of potassium, calcium, magnesium, dietary fiber, and protein) than the typical U.S. diet was investigated in a high-quality randomised controlled trial.[59] Participants were adults with systolic blood pressures of 120 to 159 mmHg and diastolic pressures of 80 to 95 mmHg; more than half the participants were black and more than half were women.

The overall effect on blood pressure of such a diet, compared with a typical U.S. diet, was a fall in systolic blood pressure of approximately 9 mmHg and in diastolic blood pressure of 4.5 mmHg. The trial was very carefully managed and participants were provided with all foods during their three 30-day diet periods. If people can make these dietary changes in real life for long periods, the diet has the potential to effect large blood pressure reductions.

1.5 SUMMARY

The research evidence suggests that dietitians are needed to give dietary advice to those at high risk of cardiovascular disease, in lieu of or in addition to dietary advice from physicians. In what circumstances trained nurses or self-help materials can substitute for a dietitian's role is not clear (more research is needed), but they can serve as useful allies when a dietitian's time is limited.

Dietary advice for people with cardiovascular disease should include advice to increase long-chain omega-3 fats first and foremost. Other useful advice is to replace saturated fats with unsaturated fats and to adopt a Mediterranean-style diet. These steps represent the most important dietary advice known to reduce illness and mortality and should be given before patients receive additional advice to alter specific risk factors in their diets.

1.6 USEFUL CONTACTS

American Dietetic Association
120 South Riverside Plaza, Suite 2000
Chicago, IL 60606-6995
Tel: 312/899 0040
Web site: http://www.eatright.org/

British Dietetic Association
5th Floor, Charles House
148/9 Great Charles Street
Queensway
Birmingham B3 3HT, U.K.
Tel: +44 (0) 121 200 8080
Fax: +44 (0) 121 200 8081
Email: info@bda.uk.com
Web site: http://www.bda.uk.com/

Cochrane Collaboration

The Cochrane Collaboration developed in response to Archie Cochrane's call for systematic, up-to-date reviews of all relevant randomised clinical trials of healthcare. Cochrane's suggestion that the methods used to prepare and maintain reviews of controlled trials in pregnancy and childbirth should be applied more widely was taken up by the Research and Development Programme initiated to support the United Kingdom's National Health Service. Funds were provided to establish a Cochrane Centre to collaborate with other organizations in the U.K. and elsewhere to facilitate systematic reviews of randomised controlled trials across all areas of healthcare. For more information about the Cochrane Collaboration see http://www.cochrane.org/. The sections of the Cochrane Collaboration that relate most specifically to cardiovascular disease include:

- Cochrane Heart Group
  http://www.epi.bris.ac.uk/cochrane/heart.htm
- Cochrane Hypertension Group
  http://www.epi.bris.ac.uk/cochrane/htn/htn.html
- Cochrane Peripheral Vascular Diseases Group
  http://www.link.med.ed.ac.uk/pvd/
- Cochrane Stroke Group
  http://www.dcn.ed.ac.uk/csrg/

Cochrane Library

Information about the Cochrane Library and access to it can be found at http://www.update-software.com/Cochrane/default.HTM or navigate there from the main Cochrane Collaboration site at http://www.cochrane.org/ by clicking on the Cochrane Library logo.

Critical Appraisal Skills Programme (CASP)

CASP provides training and resources for critical appraisal and has very good downloadable critical appraisal checklists for a variety of study types (including randomised controlled trials and systematic reviews). Its Web site URL is http://www.phru.org.uk/~casp/casp.htm

REFERENCES

1. American Dietetic Association, Find a dietitian, http://www.eatright.org/find.html [1-4-2003].
2. British Dietetic Association, Media release: Kids Should Eat 2 B Fit, http://www.bda.uk.com/ [2-14-2003].
3. Sackett, D.L., Rosenberg, W.M.C.R., Gray, M.J.A., Haynes, R.B.Haynes, and Richardson, W.S., 1996, Evidence based medicine: what it is and what it isn't, *BMJ*, 312, 71.
4. Phillips, B., Ball, C., Sackett, D., et al., Levels of evidence and grades of recommendation, Centre for Evidence-Based Medicine, http://www.cebm.net/levels_of_evidence.asp [1-4-2003].
5. Egger, M., Smith, G.D., O'Rourke, K., 2001, Rationale, potentials, and promise of systematic reviews, in *Systematic Reviews in Healthcare: Meta-Analysis in Context*, Egger, M. et al., Eds., BMJ Publishing Group, London, p. 3.
6. Heart Protection Study Collaborative Group, 2002, MRC/BHF Heart Protection Study of antioxidant supplementation in 20,536 high risk individuals: a randomized placebo-controlled trial, *Lancet*, 360, 23.
7. Egger, M., Schneider, M., and Smith, D.G., 1998, Spurious precision? Meta-analysis of observational studies, *BMJ*, 316, 140.
8. Hooper, L., Ness, A. Ness, and Smith, D.G., 2001, Antioxidant strategy for cardiovascular disease, *Lancet*, 357, 1705.
9. Thompson, R.L., Summerbell, C.D., Hooper, L., et al., 2001, Dietary advice given by a dietitian versus other health professional or self-help resources to reduce blood cholesterol, Cochrane Library Issue 2, Update Software, Oxford.
10. Thompson, R.L., Summerbell, C.D., Hooper, L., et al., 2003, Relative efficacy of differential methods of dietary advice: a systematic review, *Am. J. Clin. Nutr.*, 77, 1052S.
11. Schulz, K.F., Chalmers, I., Hayes, R.J., and Altman, D.G., 1995, Empirical evidence of bias: dimensions of methodological quality with estimates of treatment effects in controlled trials, *JAMA*, 273, 408.
12. Henkin, Y., Shai, I., Zuk, R., et al., 2000, Dietary treatment of hypercholesterolemia: do dietitians do it better? A randomized, controlled trial, *Am. J. Med.*, 109, 549.
13. Delahanty, L.M., 2001, Clinical and cost outcomes of medical nutrition therapy for hypercholesterolemia: a controlled trial, *J. Am. Diet. Assn.*, 101, 1012.
14. Bucher, H.C., Hengstler, P., Schindler, C., and Meier, G., 2002, N-3 polyunsaturated fatty acids in coronary heart disease: a meta-analysis of randomized controlled trials, *Am. J. Med.*, 112, 298.
15. Farmer, A., Montori, V., Dineen, S., and Clar, C., 2002, Fish oil in people with type 2 diabetes mellitus, Cochrane Library Issue 4, Update Software, Oxford.
16. Truswell, A.S., 1994, Review of dietary intervention studies: effect on coronary events and on total mortality, *Aust. N.Z. J. Med.*, 24, 98.
17. Ebrahim, S. and Smith, G.D., *Health Promotion in Older People for the Prevention of Coronary Heart Disease and Stroke*, Vol. 1, Health Education Authority, London.
18. Hooper, L., Summerbell, C.D., Higgins, J.T.T., et al., 2001, Dietary fat intake and prevention of cardiovascular disease: systematic review, *BMJ*, 322, 757.
19. Hooper, L., Summerbell, C.D., Higgins, J.T.P., et al., 2000, Reduced or modified dietary fat for prevention of cardiovascular disease, Cochrane Library Issue 2, Update Software, Oxford.

20. Jha, P., Flather, M., Lonn, E., et al., 1995, Antioxidant vitamins and cardiovascular disease: a critical review of epidemiologic and clinical trial data, *Ann. Intern. Med.*, 123, 860.

21. Lonn, E.M. and Yusuf, S., 1997, Is there a role for antioxidant vitamins in the prevention of cardiovascular diseases? An update on epidemiological and clinical trial data, *Can. J. Cardiol.*, 13, 957.

22. Scottish Intercollegiate Guidelines Network (SIGN), 1999, Lipids and the primary prevention of coronary heart disease, Edinburgh.

23. Jepson, R.G., Kleijnen, J., and Leng, G.C., 1999, Garlic for peripheral arterial occlusive disease, Cochrane Library Issue 2, Update Software, Oxford.

24. De Lorgeril, M., Renaud, S., Mamelle, et al., 1994, Mediterranean alpha-linolenic acid-rich diet in secondary prevention of coronary heart disease, *Lancet*, 343, 1454.

25. Clarke, R., Frost, C., Collins, R., et al., 1997, Dietary lipids and blood cholesterol: quantitative meta-analysis of metabolic ward studies, *BMJ*, 314, 112.

26. NHS Centre for Reviews and Dissemination, 1998, Cholesterol and coronary heart disease: screening and treatment, *Effective Healthcare*, 4, 1.

27. Tang, J.L., Armitage, J.M., Lancaster, T., et al., 1998, Systematic review of dietary intervention trials to lower blood total cholesterol in free-living subjects [see comments], *BMJ*, 316, 1213.

28. Mensink, R.P. and Katan, M.B., 1992, Effect of dietary fatty acids on serum lipids and lipoproteins: a meta-analysis of 27 trials, *Arterioscler. Thromb. Vasc. Biol.*, 12, 911.

29. Gardner, C.D. and Kraemer, H.C., 1995, Monounsaturated versus polyunsaturated dietary fat and serum lipids, *Arterioscler. Thromb. Vasc. Biol.*, 15, 1917.

30. Ripsin, C.M., Keenan, J.M., Jacobs, J., et al., 1992, Oat products and lipid lowering: a meta-analysis, *JAMA*, 267, 3317.

31. Brown, L., Rosner, B., Willett, W.W., and Sacks, F.M., 1999, Cholesterol-lowering effects of dietary fiber: a meta-analysis, *Am. J. Clin. Nutr.*, 69, 30.

32. Anderson, J.W., Johnstone, B.M., and Cook-Newell, M.E., 1995, Meta-analysis of the effects of soy protein intake on serum lipids, *New Engl. J. Med.*, 333, 276.

33. Kleijnen, J., Knipschild, P., and Ter Riet, G., 1989, Garlic, onions and cardiovascular risk factors: a review of the evidence from human experiments with emphasis on commercially available preparations, *Br. J. Clin. Pharmacol.*, 28, 535.

34. Warshafsky, S., Kamer, R.S., and Sivak, S.L., 1993, Effect of garlic on total serum cholesterol, *Ann. Int. Med.*, 119, 599.

35. Silagy, C. and Neil, A., 1994, Garlic as a lipid lowering agent: a meta-analysis, *J. Roy. Coll. Phys.*, 28, 39.

36. Stevinson, C., Pittler, M.H., and Ernst, E., 2000, Garlic for treating hypercholesterolaemia: a meta-analysis of randomized clinical trials, *Ann. Int. Med.*, 133, 420.

37. Ackermann, R.T., Mulrow, C.D., Ramierz, C.D., et al., 2001, Garlic shows promise for improving some cardiovascular risk factors, *Arch. Int. Med.*, 161, 813.

38. NHS Centre for Reviews and Dissemination, 1997, The prevention and treatment of obesity, *Effective Healthcare*, 3, 1.

39. Yu-Poth, S., Zhao, G., Etherton, T., et al., 1999, Effects of the National Cholesterol Education Program's Step I and Step II dietary intervention programs on cardiovascular disease risk factors: a meta-analysis, *Am. J. Clin. Nutr.*, 69, 632.

40. Pirozzo, S., Summerbell, C.D., Cameron, C., and Glasziou, P., 2002, Advice on low-fat diets for obesity, Cochrane Library Issue 4, Update Software, Oxford.

41. Scottish Intercollegiate Guidelines Network (SIGN), Obesity in Scotland: integrating prevention with weight management: a national clinical guideline recommended for use in Scotland, 1996, Edinburgh.

42. Booth, G.L., Wang, E.L., and Canadian Task Force on Preventive Healthcare, 2000, Preventive healthcare 2000 update: screening and management of hyperhomocysteinemia for the prevention of coronary artery disease events, *Can. Med. Assn. J.*, 163, 21.

43. Hansrani, M. and Stansby, G., 2002, Homocysteine lowering interventions for peripheral arterial disease and bypass grafts, Cochrane Library Issue 4, Update Software, Oxford.

44. Cappuccio, F.P. and MacGregor, G.A., 1991, Does potassium supplementation lower blood pressure? A meta-analysis of published trials, *J. Hypertens.*, 9, 465.

45. Whelton, P.K., He, J., Cutler, J.A., et al., 1997, Effects of oral potassium on blood pressure: meta-analysis of randomized controlled clinical trials, *JAMA*, 277, 1624.

46. Allender, P.S., Cutler, J.A., Follman, D., et al., 1996, Dietary calcium and blood pressure: a meta-analysis of randomized clinical trials, *Ann. Int. Med.*, 124, 825.

47. Griffith, L.E., Guyatt, G.H., Cook, R.J., et al., 1999, The influence of dietary and non-dietary calcium supplementation on blood pressure: an updated metaanalysis of randomized controlled trials, *Am. J. Hypertens.*, 12, 84.

48. Brand, M.B., Mulrow, C.D., Chiquette, E., et al., 1999, Weight reduction through dieting for control of hypertension in adults, Cochrane Review Issue 2, Update Software, Oxford.

49. Law, M.R., Frost, C.D., and Wald, N.J., 1991, By how much does dietary salt reduction lower blood pressure? III. Analysis of data from trials of salt reduction, *BMJ*, 302, 819.

50. Midgley, J.P., Matthew, A.G., Greenwood, C.M., and Logan, A.G., 1996, Effect of reduced dietary sodium on blood pressure: a meta-analysis of randomized controlled trials, *JAMA*, 275, 1590.

51. Cutler, J.A., Follmann, D., and Allender, P.S., 1997, Randomized trials of sodium reduction: an overview, *Am. J. Clin. Nutr.*, 65, 643S.

52. Graudal, N.A., Galloe, A.M., Anders, M., and Garred, P., 1998, Effects of sodium restriction on blood pressure, renin, aldosterone, catecholamines, cholesterols and triglyceride: a meta-analysis, *JAMA*, 279, 1383.

53. Alam, S. and Johnson, A.G., 1999, A meta-analysis of randomized controlled trials (RCT) among healthy normotensive and essential hypertensive elderly patients to determine the effect of high salt (NaCl) diet on blood pressure, *J. Human Hypertens.*, 13, 367.

54. Hooper, L., Bartlett, C., Smith, G.D., and Ebrahim, S., 2002, Systematic review of long term effects of advice to reduce dietary salt in adults, *BMJ*, 325, 628.

55. He, F.J. and MacGregor, G.A., 2002, Effect of modest salt reduction on blood pressure: a meta-analysis of randomized trials. Implications for public health, *J. Human Hypertens.*, 16, 761.

56. Jürgens, G. and Graudal, N.A., 2003, Effects of low sodium diet versus high sodium diet on blood pressure, renin, aldosterone, catecholamines, cholesterols, and triglyceride, Cochrane Library Issue 1, Update Software, Oxford.

57. Appel, L.J., Miller, E.R., Seidler, A.J., and Whelton, P.K., 1993, Does supplementation of diet with fish oil reduce blood pressure? A meta-analysis of controlled clinical trials, *Arch. Int. Med.*, 153, 1429.

58. Morris, M.C., Sacks, F., and Rosner, B., 1993, Does fish oil lower blood pressure? A meta-analysis of controlled trials, *Circulation*, 88, 523.

59. Sacks, F.M., Svetkey, L.P., Vollmer, W.M., et al., 2001, Effects on blood pressure of reduced dietary sodium and the Dietary Approaches to Stop Hypertension (DASH) diet, *New Engl. J. Med.*, 344, 3.

2 Seafood and Myocardial Infarction in China

Jian-Min Yuan

CONTENTS

2.1 INTRODUCTION

China is a developing country inhabited by a fifth of the world's population. Coronary heart disease (CHD) used to be rare in China[1] but this is no longer true. For example, the proportion of CHD among all types of heart disease has climbed from fifth highest in China between 1948 and 1958, to second highest between 1959 and 1971, and to first from 1972 through 1979.[1] Although part of the explanation lies in longer lifespans, less malnutrition, and fewer infectious diseases, the principal reason is increasing accessibility to the harmful habits of Western society: high fat and high cholesterol diets, cigarette smoking, and decreased physical activity. Despite the increase of CHD in China during the past several decades, people in China still possess much lower risk of developing CHD than those in North America and Europe. In the U.S., age-adjusted mortality rates (per 100,000 person-years) from CHD in men and women aged 35 to 74 years in the mid-1990s were 224 (21% of total mortality) and 92 (14% of total mortality), respectively. The corresponding figures in China were 100 (9% of total mortality) and 69 (10% of total mortality), respectively.[2]

High consumption of fish or long-chain n-3 polyunsaturated fatty acids from seafood (marine n-3 fatty acids) has been linked to low mortality from CHD in Greenland Eskimos.[3] This observation has stimulated considerable research to test the hypothesis that consumption of fish or marine n-3 fatty acids reduces CHD mortality. Most epidemiologic studies of fish intake and cardiovascular disease to date have been conducted in Occidental populations. Intake levels have been generally low in these populations. Only roughly 14% of men in the U.S. eat more than one serving of fish per week,[4] whereas about 50% of Chinese men in Shanghai report similar consumption frequency.

Experimental data suggest that fish oil containing high concentrations of two marine n-3 fatty acids designated ecosapentanoic acid (EPA) and docosahexanoic acid (DHA) may possess antiarrhythmic properties, and thus can reduce vulnerability to life-threatening arrhythmias during cardiac ischemia. In animal experiments, a diet supplemented with tuna fish oil significantly reduced the incidence and severity of arrhythmia and prevented ventricular fibrillation following coronary occlusion and reperfusion in rats.[5] Infusion of marine n-3 fatty acids prevents ischemia-induced ventricular fibrillation in dogs known to be susceptible to cardiac sudden death.[6] Adult marmoset monkeys fed a diet supplemented with tuna fish oil showed statistically significant elevations in their ventricular fibrillation thresholds before or after acute coronary artery occlusion.[7] In human experiments, myocardial infarction (MI) survivors receiving 5.2 g of EPA and DHA daily for 12 weeks demonstrated statistically significantly increased heart rate variabilities relative to their baseline values before treatment and values of control subjects.[8]

Using the database from the Shanghai Cohort Study, we examined the relationships between dietary seafood or marine n-3 fatty acid intake and mortality from acute MI and other cardio- and cerebro-vascular diseases in middle-aged and older Chinese men in Shanghai.

2.2 METHODS

2.2.1 STUDY POPULATION

Shanghai is a metropolitan city located on the southeastern coast of China. It had approximately 7 million permanent residents in the urban area and 5 million people living in the outskirts in the mid-1980s. Between January 1, 1986, and September 30, 1989, we invited all eligible male residents of four small, geographically defined communities from a wide area of the urban city of Shanghai to participate in a prospective epidemiological study of diet and cancer.[9] The eligibility criteria were ages 45 to 64 years and no history of cancer. At recruitment, we interviewed each subject using a structured questionnaire that sought information on level of education, usual occupation, adult height and usual adult weight, history of tobacco and alcohol use, current diet, and medical history. In addition to the interview, we collected a 10-ml non-fasting blood sample and a single-void urine sample from each study participant. Serum specimens were stored at −70°C and −20°C, and urine samples were stored at −20°C only. During the 3-year recruitment period, 18,244 men (about 80% of eligible subjects) enrolled in the study.

2.2.2 DIETARY ASSESSMENT

At recruitment, specially trained nurses conducted in-person interviews. Each subject was asked to indicate the usual intake frequency (in times per day, per week, per month, or per year) with which he consumed each of 45 food groups and/or items in the past 12 months.[10] For seasonal foods, we obtained the frequencies of consumption when the foods were in season. For example, tangerines were available in Shanghai only from September to March in the early 1980s. Thus, we asked the subjects to indicate their consumption frequencies of tangerines from September to March.

The 45 food groups and/or items listed in the questionnaire covered all common foods consumed in Shanghai before the mid-1980s. The food frequency questionnaires were subsequently validated by a series of 24-hour dietary recall interviews conducted in a randomly chosen subgroup (n = 432) of cohort subjects during April and May 1992 (unpublished data). The data from this 24-hour dietary recall substudy were also used to construct standard portion weights for each of the food items listed in the frequency questionnaire. Specifically, the median weight of all recorded servings was taken as the standard portion weight. Daily nutritive and non-nutritive intakes per subject were computed using the Singapore Food Composition Table[11] that provides nutrient values of raw and cooked foods commonly consumed by Chinese, including those in Shanghai.

The food frequency questionnaire listed three seafood items (fresh fish, salted fish, and shellfish). The commonly eaten fresh fish in Shanghai include carp, beam, and pomfret. The common species of salted fish consumed in Shanghai are yellow croaker and hairtail. Similarly, the common shellfish in Shanghai are shrimp and crab. The standard portion weight (without bone) for fresh fish was determined to be 46.8 g. The corresponding figures for salted fish and shellfish were 25.9 g and 43.3 g, respectively. We calculated the average daily intake of fish and shellfish per subject by summing over the three seafood items the cross-products of intake frequency and standard portion weight. The daily intake of n-3 fatty acids from fish and shellfish was estimated by multiplying the daily amount of each seafood item with the corresponding marine n-3 fatty acid content:[11] fresh fish, 0.57 g per 100 g; salted fish, 0.44 g per 100 g; and shellfish, 0.36 g per 100 g. Warm water fish from the South China Sea (available in Shanghai) are comparable in their fat contents, which are low relative to cold water species (such as salmon) commonly consumed in the U.S.[11]

2.2.3 SERUM CHOLESTEROL MEASUREMENTS

Baseline serum cholesterol measurements were performed on subjects who died from CHD and their matched controls. As of September 1, 1998, we identified 187 subjects who died from CHD. For each fatal CHD case, five control subjects matched to the index case by age (within 2 years), month and year of sample collection, and neighborhood of residence at recruitment were randomly chosen among cohort members who were alive on the date of death of the index case.

The serum specimens stored at −20°C were used for cholesterol measurements, which were performed in the lipid laboratory of the Cardiovascular Disease Institute of Shanghai using standard methods.[12] Total cholesterol, high density lipoprotein (HDL) cholesterol, and triglycerides were measured with the enzymatic colorimetric method. Low density lipoprotein (LDL) cholesterol was calculated according to the Friedewald formula.[13]

2.2.4 FOLLOW-UP

The Shanghai Municipality is divided into 12 urban districts (each containing a number of streets). Each district has its own Vital Statistics Unit. Copies of death certificates from men who were residents of the streets covered by our cohort study were routinely ascertained and matched against the cohort master file. In addition, all surviving cohort members were interviewed in person or by telephone on an annual basis. Follow-up in terms of mortality was essentially complete (99%). As of September 1, 1998, only 207 (1%) cohort members were lost to follow-up. Among the 15,903 surviving members, only 223 (1.4%) subjects had moved away from Shanghai and were followed by mail or telephone.

2.2.5 ENDPOINTS

Causes of deaths (abstracted from death certificates) were systematically coded by a retired nurse with special training according to the *International Classification of Diseases, Ninth Revision* (ICD-9). The specific endpoints of this study were deaths from acute MI that included sudden and non-sudden cardiac deaths within 28 days (ICD-9 Code 410), CHD other than acute MI (ICD-9 Codes 411 through 414), and stroke (ICD-9 Codes 430 through 438). The hospital records and other supporting medical documents of all cardiovascular deaths among cohort members were systematically reviewed; we found no evidence of other more probable causes of death in these individuals.

2.2.6 STATISTICAL ANALYSIS

For each subject, follow-up time was counted from the date of recruitment to September 1, 1998, or date of death or loss to follow-up, whichever occurred first. For dietary seafood intake, study subjects were grouped into five categories: <50, 50 to <100, 100 to <150, 150 to <200, and ≥200 g of fish and shellfish consumed per week, which are approximately equivalent to <1, 1, 2, 3, and ≥4 servings of seafood per week, respectively. For intake of marine n-3 fatty acids, study subjects were categorized into equal quintiles of intake: <0.27, 0.27 to 0.43, 0.44 to 0.72, 0.73 to 1.09, and ≥1.10 g per week.

The contingency table and one-way analysis of variance methods were used to examine the associations between fish and shellfish intake and various baseline characteristics of study subjects. Relative risks (RRs) of subgroups of vascular disease mortality were computed for categories of dietary seafood and n-3 fatty acid intakes using the Cox proportional hazards models.[14] Potential confounders included in the multivariate Cox proportional hazards models were age (year), level of education (primary school or less and middle school or higher), body mass index (<18.5, 18.5 to <21.0, 21.0 to <23.5, 23.5 to <26.0, and ≥26.0 kg/m²), current smoker at recruitment (no or yes), number of cigarettes smoked per day (continuous), number of alcoholic drinks per week (none, 1 to 14, 15 to 28, and ≥29), history of diabetes (no or yes), history of hypertension (no or yes), and total energy intake (kcal per day).[10, 15–17] The 95% confidence interval (CI) and two-sided P value were calculated for each RR.

Serum lipid measurements were available only on subjects who died from CHD and their matched control subjects. Standard matched-set methods[18] were used to examine the associations between dietary intake of fish and shellfish (or n-3 fatty acid) and CHD mortality after further adjustment for the ratio of serum total to HDL cholesterols.

Statistical testing for linear trends of various disease mortalities associated with dietary fish and shellfish (or marine n-3 fatty acid) intake was based on ordinal values. Statistical computing was performed using SAS Version 6.12 (SAS Institute Inc., Cary, NC) and Epilog Windows version (Epicenter Software, Pasadena, CA) statistical software packages. All P values quoted are two-sided.

2.3 RESULTS

2.3.1 CHARACTERISTICS AT BASELINE

Of the 18,244 cohort participants, 19% (n = 3,789) subjects reported eating <50 g of fish and shellfish per week, including 143 (0.8%) who ate no seafood at all. Sixteen percent (n = 2,936) subjects consumed ≥200 g (equivalent to about ≥4 servings) of fish and shellfish per week. The average intake level of seafood in all study subjects was 129.1 g per week (Table 2.1). There was no statistically significant difference in age or body mass index (kg/m²) across various categories of fish and shellfish intake. Consumption of fish and shellfish was positively associated with level of education ($P = 0.001$), cigarette smoking ($P = 0.001$), and alcohol drinking ($P = 0.001$). Men with histories of diabetes or hypertension consumed slightly more fish and shellfish (Table 2.1).

2.3.2 TOTAL PERSON-YEARS AND ENDPOINTS OF FOLLOW-UP

As of September 1, 1998, the 18,244 cohort participants contributed 179,466 person-years of follow-up. During the 12 years of follow-up, 2,134 deaths occurred (1,189 per 100,000 person-years). Nine percent of them died from CHD (n = 187; 104 per

TABLE 2.1
Distributions of Selected Characteristics of Cohort Participants at Baseline
According to Dietary Seafood Intake: Shanghai Cohort Study, Shanghai,
China, 1986 through 1998

	Seafood Intake (g/week)					
	<50	50 to <100	100 to <150	150 to <200	≥200	Total Cohort
Mean fish/shellfish intake (g/week)	29.3	76.2	124.2	176.8	321.9	129.1
Mean marine n-3 fatty acid intake (g/week)	0.15	0.38	0.65	0.91	1.66	0.66
Number of men	3,789	5,613	3,300	2,606	2,936	18,244
Age (year, mean)	55.8	55.6	55.6	55.8	56.2	55.8
Body mass index (kg/m², mean)	22.1	22.1	22.2	22.3	22.2	22.2
Level of education (%):						
Primary school or less	34	27	28	26	28	28
Middle school	44	47	47	48	49	47
College or higher	22	26	25	26	23	25
Smoking status (%):						
Current smokers						
<20 cigarettes/day	25	26	25	25	26	25
≥20 cigarettes/day	24	23	26	26	29	25
Past smokers	7	6	7	7	7	7
Never smokers	44	45	43	42	38	43
Consumption of alcohol (%):						
None	65	61	55	54	47	57
1 to 14 drinks/ week	20	23	26	25	26	24
15-28 drinks/week	9	10	12	13	16	12
≥29 drinks/week	6	6	6	8	11	7
Reported diagnosis:						
Diabetes (%)	1.2	1.2	1.2	1.2	1.6	1.3
Hypertension (%)	23.4	24.4	24.7	24.8	26.4	24.6

Adapted from Yuan, J.M. et al., *Am. J. Epidemiol.*, 154, 809, 2001. With permission.

100,000 person-years), 22% from stroke (n = 480; 267 per 100,000 person-years),
and 41% from cancer (n = 865; 482 per 100,000 person-years).

2.3.3 DEATHS FROM ACUTE MYOCARDIAL INFARCTION

One hundred thirteen cohort members died from acute MI during follow-up (63 per
100,000 person-years). Increasing levels of dietary fish and shellfish intake were
statistically significantly associated with reduced risk of fatal MI (*P* for trend = 0.04).

Adjustment for known cardiovascular risk factors did not materially alter this inverse association (P for trend = 0.03). Men who consumed ≥200 g of fish and shellfish per week (≥4 servings per week) experienced 59% reductions in acute MI mortality (adjusted RR = 0.41; 95% CI = 0.22 to 0.78) relative to those who ate <50 g of seafood per week (Table 2.2).

Individuals who ate ≥50 g (≥1 serving) of fish and shellfish per week experienced 44% reductions in fatal MI risk (adjusted RR = 0.56; 95% CI = 0.37 to 0.85) compared with those who ate less. There was no evidence of further reduction in acute MI mortality with intake level of fish and shellfish higher than one serving per week (P = 0.97 for trend in risk between men in the 50 to <100 g to ≥200 g of fish/shellfish intake per week groups).

Among the three seafood items specifically listed in the questionnaire, fresh fish (86.3 g per week) accounted for 67% of total seafood consumption; shellfish (38.6 g per week) and salted fish (4.2 g per day) represented 30% and 3%, respectively. In analyses conducted separately for fish and shellfish, the inverse associations with acute MI were statistically significant for both fresh/salted fish intake and shellfish intake (P for trend = 0.02 in both instances; Table 2.2).

The average intake of marine n-3 fatty acids in this cohort was estimated to be 0.66 g per week (Table 2.1). Table 2.3 presents the associations between intake of marine n-3 fatty acids and categories of cardio- and cerebro-vascular disease mortality. Similar to the relationships with seafood intake, fatal MI was inversely associated with consumption of n-3 fatty acids derived from fish and shellfish. Compared with men in the lowest 20% of marine n-3 fatty acid intake (<0.27 g per week), those who consumed higher levels showed significantly reduced risk of fatal MI (RR = 0.55; 95% CI = 0.37 to 0.83). Adjustment for known cardiovascular disease risk factors did not alter the inverse association (P for trend = 0.02 after adjustment; Table 2.3).

Early symptoms of cardiovascular disease could result in changes in an individual's dietary habits. We repeated all data analyses described above with the exclusion of all deaths and person-year contributions from the cohort during the first 2 years of follow-up. Results were similar (data not shown). Furthermore, we examined whether the protective effect of seafood (or marine n-3 fatty acid) intake on fatal MI is stronger (to support the hypothesis that marine n-3 fatty acids have antiarrhythmic properties) in cohort subjects whose dietary information was obtained relatively close to the occurrence of fatal MI (i.e., recent intake is more relevant than intake years prior to clinical outcome). Indeed, among subjects with fatal MIs occurring within the 5 years of enrollment, the RR was 0.48 (95% CI = 0.25 to 0.91) for men who ate ≥50 g of seafood per week relative to those consuming less. The comparable figure for subjects with fatal MIs occurring more than 5 years post-enrollment was 0.63 (95% CI = 0.36 to 1.07).

We further examined the relationships between seafood or marine n-3 fatty acid intake and mortality from acute MI, taking into consideration the intake levels of red meats, poultry, vegetables, fruits, soy beans and soy products, legumes, carbohydrates, proteins, total fat, saturated, monounsaturated and polyunsaturated other than marine n-3 fatty acids, and cholesterol. Separate inclusion of these dietary variables in multivariate models did not materially alter the associations between fish and shellfish or marine n-3 fatty acid intake and fatal MI.

TABLE 2.2
Relative Risks of Cardiovascular Disease Mortality According to Dietary Seafood Intake: Shanghai Cohort Study, Shanghai, China, 1986 through 1998

Seafood Intake (g/week)	Person-Years	Acute MI (ICD-9 = 410)[a]		Multivariate		Other CHD (ICD-9 = 411–414)[a]		Multivariate		Stroke (ICD-9 = 430–438)[a]		Multivariate	
		No. of Deaths	RR[b]	RR[c]	95% CI	No. of Deaths	RR[b]	RR[c]	95% CI	No. of Deaths	RR[b]	RR[c]	95% CI
Fish/Shellfish													
<50	36,892	33	1.00	1.00		17	1.00	1.00		101	1.00	1.00	
50–<100	55,115	28	0.56[d]	0.55	0.33–0.91	24	0.93	0.87	0.47–1.62	141	0.94	0.93	0.72–1.21
100–<150	32,499	21	0.69	0.65	0.38–1.14	9	0.58	0.54	0.24–1.22	70	0.79	0.79	0.58–1.07
150–<200	25,767	17	0.67	0.66	0.36–1.19	12	0.97	0.92	0.43–1.94	71	0.99	1.01	0.74–1.37
≥200	29,194	14	0.44[d]	0.41	0.22–0.78	12	0.76	0.68	0.32–1.46	97	1.11	1.11	0.83–1.47
P for trend			0.04	0.03			0.51	0.37			0.44	0.42	
Fish Only													
<30	32,550	29	1.00	1.00		13	1.00	1.00		91	1.00	1.00	
30–<60	39,355	30	0.56[d]	0.54	0.32–0.90	28	1.18	1.08	0.56–2.10	142	0.86	0.84	0.64–1.09
60–<100	39,992	28	0.74	0.72	0.42–1.21	15	0.91	0.84	0.40–1.77	99	0.88	0.87	0.65–1.15
100–<150	24,293	16	0.65	0.63	0.34–1.17	6	0.57	0.53	0.20–1.40	68	0.95	0.95	0.69–1.31
≥150	23,277	10	0.39[d]	0.35	0.17–0.72	12	1.10	0.92	0.41–2.06	80	1.12	1.05	0.77–1.43
P for trend			0.048	0.02			0.55	0.34			0.36	0.47	

Shellfish Only		Cases	RR	RR	95% CI	Cases	RR	RR	95% CI	Cases	RR	RR	95% CI
<10	63,301	52	1.00	1.00		30	1.00	1.00		183	1.00	1.00	
10–<30	34,519	18	0.67	0.65	0.38–1.11	10	0.68	0.66	0.32–1.35	80	0.87	0.86	0.66–1.12
30–<60	50,210	28	0.68	0.66	0.42–1.05	17	0.75	0.73	0.40–1.34	128	0.93	0.96	0.77–1.21
60–<100	20,505	11	0.62	0.64	0.33–1.23	14	1.45	1.55	0.81–2.96	59	1.01	1.08	0.81–1.46
≥100	10,932	4	0.39	0.40	0.14–1.12	3	0.56	0.58	0.17–1.92	30	0.93	1.02	0.69–1.51
P for trend			0.02	0.02			0.91	0.99			0.76	0.73	

[a] MI = myocardial infarction; CHD = coronary heart disease; ICD-9 = International Classification of Diseases, 9th Rev.

[b] RR = relative risk adjusted for age (years) and total energy intake (calories per day).

[c] In addition to age (years) and total energy intake (calories per day), the multivariate Cox proportional hazard model included education level (primary school or less, middle school or higher), body mass index (<18.5, 18.5 to <21, 21 to <23.5, 23.5 to <26, ≥26 kg/m²), current smoker at recruitment (no or yes), average number of cigarettes smoked per day (continuous), number of alcoholic drinks per week (none, 1 to 14, 15 to 28, ≥29), history of diabetes (no or yes), and history of hypertension (no or yes); CI = confidence interval.

[d] Two-sided P < 0.05, test for RR = 1.0.

Adapted from Yuan, J.M. et al., *Am. J. Epidemiol.*, 154, 809, 2001. With permission.

TABLE 2.3
Relative Risks of Cardiovascular Disease Mortality According to Dietary Intake of n-3 Fatty Acids from Seafood: Shanghai Cohort Study, Shanghai, China, 1986 through 1998

Intake of Marine n-3 Fatty Acids in Quintiles (g/week)	Acute MI (ICD-9 = 410)[a]			Multivariate		Other CHD (ICD-9 = 411–414)[a]		Multivariate		Stroke (ICD-9 = 430–438)[a]		Multivariate	
	Person-Years	No. of Deaths	RR[b]	RR[c]	95% CI	No. of Deaths	RR[b]	RR[c]	95% CI	No. of Deaths	RR[b]	RR[c]	95% CI
<0.27	35,583	33	1.00	1.00		15	1.00	1.00		106	1.00	1.00	
0.27–0.43	32,076	12	0.39[d]	0.39	0.20–0.75	12	0.86	0.82	0.38–1.75	75	0.78	0.76	0.57–1.03
0.44–0.72	54,769	37	0.70	0.67	0.42–1.08	21	0.89	0.83	0.42–1.61	124	0.76[e]	0.76	0.58–0.98
0.73–1.09	28,613	16	0.54[e]	0.53	0.29–0.97	15	1.17	1.11	0.54–2.30	81	0.92	0.93	0.69–1.24
≥1.10	28,425	15	0.47[e]	0.43	0.23–0.81	11	0.80	0.71	0.32–1.57	94	1.01	1.00	0.75–1.33
P for trend			0.04	0.02			0.88	0.68			0.70	0.36	

[a] MI = myocardial infarction; CHD = coronary heart disease; ICD-9 = International Classification of Diseases, 9th Rev.

[b] RR = relative risk adjusted for age (years) and total energy intake (calories per day).

[c] In addition to age (years) and total energy intake (calories per day), the multivariate Cox proportional hazard model included level of education (primary school or less, middle school or higher), body mass index (<18.5, 18.5 to <21, 21 to <23.5, 23.5 to <26, ≥26 kg/m^2), current smoker at recruitment (no or yes), average number of cigarette smoked per day (continuous), number of alcoholic drinks per week (none, 1 to 14, 15 to 28, ≥29), history of diabetes (no or yes), and history of hypertension (no or yes); CI = confidence interval.

[d] Two-sided $P < 0.01$, test for RR = 1.0.

[e] Two-sided $P < 0.05$, test for RR = 1.0.

Adapted from Yuan, J.M. et al., Am. J. Epidemiol., 154, 809, 2001. With permission.

We re-examined the association between seafood (or n-3 fatty acid) intake and acute MI mortality after adjustment for the ratio of baseline serum total to HDL cholesterols. The baseline serum measurements of total and HDL cholesterols were available only on 99 subjects who died from acute MIs and their 447 matched control subjects. Baseline serum total cholesterol levels of 10% (n = 10) of case patients and 5% (n = 24) of control subjects were greater than 240 mg/dL. Adjustment for the ratio of total to HDL cholesterol did not materially alter the inverse association between seafood (or marine n-3 fatty acid) intake and acute MI mortality.

2.3.4 DEATHS FROM OTHER VASCULAR DISEASES

Seventy-four deaths from CHD other than acute MI were identified during follow-up (41 per 100,000 person-years). In contrast to the inverse relationship with acute MI mortality, neither fish and shellfish nor marine n-3 fatty acid intake was associated with mortality from other forms of CHD (Table 2.2 and Table 2.3). Adjustment for known cardiovascular disease risk factors or the ratio of serum total to HDL cholesterol did not materially change these associations.

Consumption of fish and shellfish was not related to stroke mortality. Men who ate ≥200 g of seafood per week had fatal stroke risk similar to those who ate <50 g of seafood per day (Table 2.2). Similarly, there was no evidence that high intake of marine n-3 fatty acids was associated with stroke mortality (Table 2.3). Adjustment for known cardiovascular disease risk factors did not materially change the associations between seafood or marine n-3 fatty acid intake and stroke mortality.

2.4 DISCUSSION

Our study was the first prospective investigation of the role of dietary fish and shellfish on cardiovascular disease mortality in a Chinese population.[19] We noted that middle-aged or older men in Shanghai who consumed at least one serving of fish and shellfish per week experienced 44% reductions in risk of fatal MI compared to less frequent consumers.

We would like to point out that the relatively fewer food items (n = 45) in our study questionnaire (compared with the usual 120 to 160 food items listed on validated food questionnaires for Western populations) was a reflection of the limited choices available to residents of China until the late 1980s. In fact, protein-rich foods such as meat, fish, eggs, and milk were rationed in China from the 1950s through the 1970s. At the time of our cohort accrual, only warm water fish were commonly available in Shanghai. The three seafood items (fresh fish, salted fish, and shellfish) listed in the study questionnaire encompassed all commonly available seafood in Shanghai in the early 1980s.

2.4.1 STRENGTHS AND WEAKNESSES OF STUDY

The current study has a number of strengths. Among them are (1) the prospective study design that eliminates the possibility of recall bias; (2) adjustment for various known cardiovascular disease risk factors at baseline including serum total to HDL cholesterol ratio, obesity, hypertension, cigarette smoking and alcohol drinking, and other dietary nutrients, thus minimizing potential confounding effects; (3) the virtually complete follow-up achieved (only 1% of cohort members were lost to follow-up), minimizing the possibility of selection bias; (4) the relatively long follow-up period, minimizing the impacts of recent changes in diet due to symptoms of disease; and (5) the distinct dietary habits (eating fish more often but in smaller portions per meal) not seen in Western populations, thus increasing the informativeness of the study database in testing the study hypothesis.

Our study also has several limitations. The principal limitation is reliance on death certificates as the sole diagnostic sources of cardiovascular disease mortality. However, we reviewed hospital records and other supporting medical documents related to all cardiovascular deaths among cohort members and found no evidence of other more probable causes of death in these individuals. Among CHD deaths, 67% of the patients had been hospitalized for the same disease prior to death, and an additional 16% of the patients had their death certificates signed by attending physicians at major medical centers. The corresponding figures for stroke death were 85% and 9%, respectively. Another important limitation was the single measure of fish consumption and consequent inability to account for changes in intake over time. Other limitations of the study include the relatively small sample size of MI deaths resulting in the estimates of RRs with relatively wide confidence intervals and absence of women in the study population.

2.4.2 POTENTIAL CONFOUNDING OF STUDY RESULTS

As with any observational epidemiological study, the inverse association between fish/shellfish consumption and fatal MI could have been due, at least in part, to residual confounding. High consumption of fish and shellfish may be a marker of a healthy lifestyle. We examined the association between dietary fish/shellfish consumption and MI mortality with adjustments for various indices of diet and other lifestyle factors, and no substantial changes were observed. The inverse fish–MI association remained after further adjustment for the ratio of baseline serum total to HDL cholesterols. Actually, in this population, fish intake was higher in subjects with histories of diabetes and hypertension — conditions that are established risk factors for CHD. As expected, adjustment for these two medical conditions in multivariate analyses led to a stronger inverse fish–MI association.

2.4.3 RESULTS OF OBSERVATIONAL EPIDEMIOLOGICAL STUDIES

Bang and coworkers first noted that low CHD mortality rate in Greenland Eskimos might have been due to their high consumption of marine food. The average per capita fish consumption of Eskimos is about 400 g per day.[20] Further studies showed that Eskimos consumed diets containing large quantities of very long chain and highly polyunsaturated fatty acids such as EPA and DHA that are abundant in fish, shellfish, and sea mammals, and are scarce or absent in land animals and plants.[3, 21] Similarly, low death rates from CHD were observed in residents of a coastal fishing village compared with those of an inland farming village in Japan. Residents of the fishing village consumed greater amounts of fresh fish (about 250 g per day) rich in EPA and DHA, and their plasma contained higher levels of EPA and DHA than inhabitants of the farming village who consumed about 40 g of fish per day.[22]

Prospective studies conducted in various populations consistently found an inverse association between fish (or marine n-3 fatty acids) consumption and deaths from CHD, in particular, MI. Results from those prospective studies are summarized below.

Kromhout and coworkers[23] studied the relation between fish consumption and CHD mortality in 825 middle-aged men from the town of Zutphen, the Netherlands. Information about fish consumption was collected from the participants and their wives at baseline interviews. After 20 years of follow-up, 78 men died from CHD. Compared with men who consumed no fish, men who consumed at least 30 g of fish per day experienced approximately 50% reduction in CHD mortality with a dose-response relation between fish consumption and CHD mortality rate. RRs of CHD mortality for men who consumed 1 to 14 g, 15 to 29 g, 30 to 44 g, and 45 g or more of fish per day were 0.64, 0.56, 0.36, and 0.39, respectively, compared with those consuming no fish.[23]

Kromhout and coworkers[24] examined the relation between fish intake and CHD mortality in another group of 272 elderly Dutch men and women (64 to 87 years of age at the time of entry to the study). Information on fish consumption in the 14 days preceding the interview was obtained by the cross-check dietary history method. At baseline, about 60% of study subjects ate fish and 40% did not. After 17 years of follow-up, an inverse association between fish consumption and CHD mortality was observed; fish eaters had a statistically significant 50% lower CHD mortality rate (RR = 0.51; 95% CI = 0.29 to 0.89) than those who consumed no fish.[24]

Dolecek[25] investigated the effects of dietary polyunsaturated fatty acids and cardiovascular disease outcomes among the participants of the Multiple Risk Factor Intervention Trial involving 12,866 U.S. middle-aged men at high risk for CHD. Only data from study subjects assigned to usual care group were included in the present analysis (n = 6250). After 10 years of follow-up, high levels of dietary n-3 fatty acids derived from fish were significantly associated with reduced risk of CHD mortality (p for trend <0.01).[25]

The Health Professionals Follow-Up Study included 44,895 U.S. male health professionals 40 to 75 years of age who were free of known cardiovascular disease at baseline. Information on fish intake was obtained through self-administered dietary questionnaires. During 6 years of follow-up, there were 1543 coronary events: 264 deaths from CHD, 547 nonfatal MIs, and 732 coronary artery bypass or angioplasty procedures. After controlling for age and coronary risk factors, no significant associations between fish intake (or marine n-3 fatty acids) and risk of CHD mortality, nonfatal MI, or other coronary diseases were noted. The risk of death due to CHD among men who ate any amount of fish, as compared with those who ate no fish, was 0.74 (95% CI = 0.44 to 1.23).[26]

The Honolulu Heart Program began in 1965 to follow a cohort of 8006 Japanese-American men aged 45 to 65 years who lived in Hawaii. Information on fish intake was obtained through in-person interviews at baseline. After 23 years of follow-up, an interaction between fish intake and cigarette smoking on risk of CHD was observed. In men who smoked more than 30 cigarettes per day, high fish intake (two or more times per week) was associated with a 50% reduction in CHD mortality

(RR = 0.5; 95% CI = 0.28 to 0.91) compared with those who consumed fish fewer than two times per week. On the other hand, no relation between fish intake and CHD mortality in nonsmokers or light smokers was noted.[27]

Davigalus and coworkers[28] studied the relation between fish intake and CHD mortality in a cohort of 1822 middle-aged male employees of the Western Electric Company in Chicago. Fish consumption was determined from a detailed dietary history and classified as none, 1 to 17, 18 to 34, and 35 or more grams per day. Mortality from CHD was classified as death from MI (sudden or nonsudden) or death from other coronary causes. After 30 years of follow-up, 430 deaths from CHD occurred; 293 were due to MI (196 were sudden, 94 were nonsudden, and 3 were not classifiable). RRs (95% Cl) of CHD and sudden or nonsudden MI were 0.62 (0.40 to 0.94) and 0.56 (0.33 to 0.93), respectively, for men who consumed 35 g or more of fish daily as compared with those who consumed none. Furthermore, there were dose-response relationships between fish consumption and CHD mortality (P for trend = 0.04) or MI death (P for trend = 0.02). No association between fish intake and death from CHD other than MI was found. The protective effect of fish intake on CHD was mainly attributable to nonsudden death from MI (RR = 0.33; 95% CI = 0.12 to 0.91).[28]

Albert and coworkers[29] studied the relation between fish intake and sudden cardiac death in the Physicians' Health Study. The study included 20,551 U.S. male physicians aged 40 to 84 years and free of MI, stroke, and cancer at baseline who completed food frequency questionnaires that provided information on fish intake. Incidence of sudden cardiac death (death within 1 hour of symptom onset) was ascertained through hospital records and reports of next of kin. After 11 years of follow-up, 133 sudden deaths had occurred. After controlling for age and coronary risk factors, fish intake was associated with a reduced risk of sudden death, with an apparent threshold effect at a consumption level of one fish meal per week. For men who consumed fish at least once per week, the RR of sudden death was 0.48 (95% CI = 0.24 to 0.96) compared with men who consumed fish less frequently than monthly. Dietary n-3 fatty acids from seafood also were associated with a reduced risk of sudden death. Neither dietary fish consumption nor n-3 fatty acid intake was associated with a reduced risk of total (fatal and nonfatal) MI, nonsudden cardiac death, or total cardiovascular mortality.[29]

In the Seven Countries Study involving 1088 Finnish, 1097 Italian, and 553 Dutch men 50 to 69 years of age, an inverse association between fish consumption and CHD mortality was noted. Information about consumption of lean, fatty, and canned fish during the 6 to 12 months preceding the interview was obtained through in-person interviews. After 20 years of follow-up, 463 men died from CHD. Men who consumed fatty fish (high contents of n-3 fatty acids) had significantly lower risk of death from CHD (RR = 0.66; 95% CI = 0.49 to 0.90) compared with those who consumed no fatty fish. No association between consumption of lean fish and CHD mortality was observed.[30]

Pietinen and coworkers[31] studied the relation of intakes of specific fatty acids and risk of CHD in a cohort of 21,930 male cigarette smokers aged 50 to 69 years who participated in the Finnish Alpha-Tocopherol–Beta-Carotene Cancer Prevention Study. A detailed and validated dietary questionnaire was used to obtain information on fish consumption at baseline. After 6 years of follow-up, 1399 major coronary events and 635 coronary deaths occurred. High intake of n-3 fatty acids from fish was related to a statistically non-significant 30% increase in risk of CHD death.[31] Fish intake is a major source of exposure to mercury, a highly reactive metal, that may predispose people to atherosclerotic disease by promoting the production of free radicals or inactivating several antioxidant mechanisms through binding to thiol-containing molecules or to selenium.[32,33]

In 1995, Salonen and coworkers[34] studied the relation of the dietary intake of fish and mercury, as well as hair content and urinary excretion of mercury, to the risk of acute MI and death from CHD, cardiovascular disease, and other causes among middle-aged men in eastern Finland who consumed high fish diets and had exceptionally high CHD mortality rates. The study included 1833 men aged 42 to 60 years who were free of clinical CHD, stroke, claudication, and cancer. Fish intake was significantly correlated with both hair mercury and urinary mercury levels. Dietary intakes of fish and mercury were associated with significantly increased risks of acute MI incidence and death from CHD and cardiovascular disease. Men who consumed 30 g or more of fish had a statistically significant 87% increase in risk of acute MI incidence compared with those who consumed less fish. Both dietary and hair mercury levels were positively associated with acute MI risk. These investigators did not examine the relationship between fish and CHD risk after adjustment for dietary mercury intake or hair mercury contents.[34]

Recently, in a case-control study conducted in eight European countries and Israel, Guallar and coworkers[35] evaluated the joint association of DHA levels in adipose tissue (a biomarker of fish intake) and mercury levels in toenail clippings with the risk of acute MI among men 70 years of age or younger. The study included 684 patients with first diagnoses of acute MI and 714 healthy control subjects. After adjustment for DHA level and coronary risk factors, the toenail mercury levels in patients were 15% higher than those in controls (95% CI = 5 to 25%). Guallar noted a weak relation between increasing DHA levels in adipose tissue and decreased risk of acute MI (P for trend = 0.23) before adjustment for the toenail mercury levels. However, adjustment for mercury levels strengthened the inverse DHA–MI association that reached the statistical significance level (P for trend = 0.01).[35] These data indicate that consumption of mercury-contaminated fish may have adverse effect on acute MI. It is possible that the protective effect of marine n-3 fatty acids on acute MI risk is masked by the adverse effect of mercury in fish.

2.4.4 RESULTS OF BIOMARKER STUDIES

One of the challenges in studying the roles of dietary marine n-3 fatty acids in the etiology of CHD and other outcomes is the well recognized difficulty in assessing the intake frequencies and amounts of specific food items in the diet. In addition, the contents of n-3 fatty acids vary among different species of fish. A biomarker approach to assess an individual's exposure to marine n-3 fatty acids circumvents the inherent limitations of dietary recalls. Moreover, this biomarker approach directly evaluates the protective effect of *in vivo* exposure to specific n-3 fatty acids on the development of CHD.

In a case-control study involving 334 patients with primary cardiac arrest and 493 control subjects aged 25 to 74 years in the U.S., Siscovick and coworkers[36] determined red blood cell membrane fatty acid composition, a biomarker of fatty acid intake. They found an inverse relation between red blood cell membrane-combined EPA and DHA levels and the risk of primary cardiac arrest. Compared with the lowest quartile, the RRs (95% CIs) for cardiac arrest were 0.5 (0.4 to 0.8), 0.3 (0.2 to 0.6), and 0.1 (0.1 to 0.4) for the second, third, and fourth quartiles of red blood cell membrane n-3 fatty acid levels, respectively.[36] In another case-control study conducted in eight European countries and Israel mentioned above,[35] DHA levels in adipose tissue were associated with significantly reduced risk of acute MI after adjustment for toenail mercury (P for trend = 0.01).

In retrospective case-control studies, biological specimens (e.g., blood, urine, or adipose tissue) are usually collected from patients after clinical manifestation of the disease under study. Fatty acid contents in post-diagnostic biospecimens may be altered due to the treatment for the disease and/or the patient's change of dietary habit. Thus, the levels of fatty acids of patients may not represent their levels of exposure before the onset of the disease that are relevant to the etiology and primary prevention of disease. Prospective studies, in which biospecimens are collected from patients before they have disease under study, provide unbiased estimates of dietary intake levels. Two prospective studies examined and found an inverse relation between blood n-3 fatty acid levels and CHD risk.[37,38]

Albert and coworkers[37] used the Physicians' Health Study database to test whether high blood levels of n-3 fatty acids predict the lower risk of sudden death. The study included 94 men who died from sudden cardiac arrest and 184 matched control subjects who were alive and remained free of cardiovascular disease at the time of case ascertainment. Nine specific fatty acids in blood including palmitic and stearic acids (saturated); oleic acid (monounsaturated); alpha linolenic acid (short-chain n-3 polyunsaturated); EPA, DHA and docosapentaenoic acids (DPA) (long-chain n-3 polyunsaturated); and linoleic and arachidonic fatty acids (n-6 polyunsaturated) were determined. Cases had statistically significantly lower baseline blood levels of total and individual long-chain n-3 fatty acids than control subjects. As compared with the lowest quartile, the RRs (95% CIs) of sudden death were 0.52 (0.16 to 1.72) in the second quartile, 0.19 (0.05 to 0.69) in the third quartile, and 0.10 (0.02 to 0.48) in the fourth quartile of total long-chain n-3 polyunsaturated fatty acids (P for trend = 0.001). There were no associations of blood levels of saturated, monounsaturated, and other polyunsaturated fatty acids with risk of sudden death.[37]

Lemaitre and coworkers[38] investigated the associations of baseline plasma phospholipid concentrations of EPA and DHA with risk of developing fatal CHD and nonfatal MI among U.S. elderly adults (65 years of age or older). An increase in plasma phospholipid EPA and DHA from 3.3 to 4.1% of total fatty acids (one standard deviation) was associated with a statistically significant 70% reduction in risk of fatal CHD. On the other hand, plasma EPA and DHA levels were not associated with nonfatal MI.[38]

2.4.5 RESULTS OF DIETARY INTERVENTION TRIALS

Three dietary intervention trials conducted in Britain, India, and Italy demonstrated that increased consumption of fish or dietary supplementation with marine n-3 fatty acids significantly reduced the risk of fatal MI.[39-41] The Diet and Reinfarction Trial in Britain randomized 2033 men after a first MI into two groups. One group received advice to eat at least two portions of fatty fish per week and the other did not. At the end of the 2-year study period, total mortality in the intervention group was significantly reduced by 29% (mainly due to reduction in CHD mortality). However, there was no difference in myocardial reinfarction incidence. The authors hypothesized that fish consumption may reduce the risk of fatal arrhythmia and therefore mortality from MI without affecting the incidence of recurrent MI.[39]

In a randomized, placebo-controlled trial in India, 360 patients with suspected acute MI were randomly assigned to receive fish oil (1.08 g per day of EPA and 0.72 g per day of DHA), mustard oil (2.9 g per day of alpha-linolenic acid), or neither (placebo). After 1 year of treatment, the group of patients receiving fish oil had a statistically significant 30% lower incidence of cardiac death and non-fatal reinfarction than the placebo group. The cardiac event incidence was also reduced in patients receiving mustard oil compared with the placebo group, but the magnitude of the reduction was less than that for the fish oil group.[40] In the intervention trial in Italy, 11,324 post-MI patients were randomly assigned to receive EPA and DHA ethyl esters (850 mg per day), vitamin E (300 mg per day), both, or neither and were followed for 3.5 years. Although no statistically significant benefit was observed with vitamin E, patients receiving marine n-3 fatty acids experienced a statistically significant 45% reduction in sudden cardiac death.[41]

2.4.6 ANTIARRHYTHMIC EFFECT OF FISH OIL

Experimental data suggest that fish oil may possess antiarrhythmic properties, and thus can reduce vulnerability to life-threatening arrhythmias during cardiac ischemia. In animal experiments, a diet supplemented with tuna fish oil significantly reduced the incidence and severity of arrhythmia and prevented ventricular fibrillation following coronary occlusion and reperfusion in rats.[5] Infusion of n-3 fatty acids prevented ischemia-induced ventricular fibrillation in dogs known to be susceptible to sudden death.[6] Adult marmoset monkeys fed a diet supplemented with tuna fish oil showed statistically significant elevations in their ventricular fibrillation thresholds before or after acute coronary artery occlusion.[7]

In human experiments, MI survivors receiving 5.2 g of EPA and DHA per day for 12 weeks demonstrated statistically significantly increased heart rate variability relative to their baseline values before treatment and to controls.[8] Consumption of as little as one serving of fish per week, the threshold level for protection in this study, is associated with an increase in heart rate variability,[42] which relates to a lower risk of arrhythmic death after MI.[43] Data from both the current study and the Physicians' Health Study[29] are consistent with the notion that the amounts of n-3 fatty acids (and/or other unidentified constituents) contained in one serving of fish at weekly intervals are sufficient to protect against arrhythmia in individuals at risk for MI, thereby reducing the risk of fatal MI.

2.4.7 FISH INTAKE AND OTHER CARDIOVASCULAR DISEASES

Our study did not show a significant benefit on mortality from CHD other than acute MI. This negative finding is consistent with that from the Western Electric Study,[28] the only study that examined this particular association.

Pedersen and coworkers[44] reported results of an autopsy study in Greenland. Among 30 cases ascertained, 4 died from fatal hemorrhagic strokes. Compared with cases with no findings of cerebral pathology, hemorrhagic stroke cases had statistically significant or borderline significant high levels of total long-chain n-3 fatty acids (2.3 versus 1.5% of total adipose fatty acids, $P = 0.04$), DHA ($P = 0.044$), DPA ($P = 0.058$), and EPA ($P = 0.085$).[44] Although these results were based on a small number of cases, they suggest that while long-chain n-3 fatty acids may protect against thrombogenesis, high levels may have an adverse effect, and thus may be a risk factor for hemorrhagic stroke.

A number of prospective cohort studies have examined the relationship between fish intake and stroke death and results are mixed.[4,45–47] Keli and coworkers[45] examined the relation of fish intake and total stroke incidence in 552 male residents of the town of Zutphen, the Netherlands. After 15 years of follow-up, 42 first strokes occurred among the 552 men 50 to 69 years of age at the beginning of follow-up. Compared with men who consumed 20 g or less per day of fish, men who consumed more than 20 g per day had a 50% reduction in risk of stroke (RR = 0.49; 95% CI = 0.24 to 1.01).[45] Data from the National Health and Nutrition Examination Survey (NHANES I) indicated that fish intake was associated with a reduced risk of stroke death in white women as well as black men and women, but not in white men.[4] The Physicians' Health Study did not show a relationship between fish intake and stroke death.[46]

He and coworkers[47] examined the relations between intakes of fish and marine n-3 fatty acids and risk of stroke in 43,671 U.S. male professionals. After 12 years of follow-up, 608 strokes occurred, including 377 ischemic, 106 hemorrhagic, and 125 unclassified strokes. Compared with men who consumed fish less frequently than once per month, the RR of ischemic stroke was significantly lower among those who ate fish at least once a month (RR = 0.56; 95% CI = 0.38 to 0.83). On the other hand, the corresponding RR for hemorrhagic stroke was 1.36 (95% CI = 0.48 to 3.82). No dose–response relations between high intake of fish (or n-3 fatty acids from fish) and risk of total, ischemic or hemorrhagic stroke was observed.[47] If the protective effect of marine n-3 fatty acids on fatal MI is mediated via antiarrhythmic and anti-atherogenic properties, then lack of an association between fish (or marine n-3 fatty acid) intake and stroke, particularly, hemorrhagic stroke, is not surprising.

2.5 SUMMARY

Observational studies across various populations with different dietary habits support the notion that moderate consumption of fish exerts a protective effect on death from MI or sudden cardiac arrest. Dietary intervention trials demonstrate the efficacy of marine n-3 fatty acids on acute MI death in patients at high risk of or previously diagnosed with MI. Experimental studies in animals and biomarker studies in humans have indicated that the protective effect of fish on acute MI mortality is likely due to the marine n-3 fatty acids in seafood through their anti-arrhythmic properties. If the observed protection of moderate fish consumption on MI mortality is real, the public health implication of such an intervention could be substantial. In 1998, approximately 456,000 deaths in the U.S. were due to acute MI.[48] At present, only about 15% of adult Americans eat more than one serving of fish per week.[4] Our findings suggest that if this percentage of fish consumption increases to 50% in adult Americans, the result could be approximately 55,000 fewer deaths from acute MI alone in the U.S. annually.

REFERENCES

1. Cheng, T.O., Cardiovascular disease in China, *Nat. Med.*, 4, 1209, 1998.
2. American Heart Association, *1999 Heart and Stroke Statistical Update*, Dallas, TX, 1998.
3. Bang, H.O., Dyerberg, J., and Sinclair, H.M., The composition of the Eskimo food in northwestern Greenland, *Am. J. Clin. Nutr.*, 33, 2657, 1980.
4. Gillum, R.F., Mussolino, M.E., and Madans, J.H., The relationship between fish consumption and stroke incidence: the NHANES I Epidemiologic Follow-up Study (National Health and Nutrition Examination Survey), *Arch. Intern. Med.*, 156, 537, 1996.
5. McLennan, P.L., Abeywardena, M.Y., and Charnock, J.S., Dietary fish oil prevents ventricular fibrillation following coronary artery occlusion and reperfusion, *Am. Heart J.*, 116, 709, 1988.
6. Billman, G.E., Kang, J.X., and Leaf, A., Prevention of sudden cardiac death by dietary pure omega-3 polyunsaturated fatty acids in dogs, *Circulation*, 99, 2452, 1999.
7. McLennan, P.L. et al., Dietary lipid modulation of ventricular fibrillation threshold in the marmoset monkey, *Am. Heart J.*, 123, 1555, 1992.
8. Christensen, J.H. et al., Effect of fish oil on heart rate variability in survivors of myocardial infarction: a double blind randomised controlled trial, *BMJ*, 312, 677, 1996.
9. Ross, R.K. et al., Urinary aflatoxin biomarkers and risk of hepatocellular carcinoma, *Lancet*, 339, 943, 1992.
10. Ross, R.K. et al., Prospective evaluation of dietary and other predictors of fatal stroke in Shanghai, China, *Circulation*, 96, 50, 1997.
11. Hankin, J.H. et al., Singapore Chinese Health Study: development, validation, and calibration of the quantitative food frequency questionnaire, *Nutr. Cancer*, 39, 187, 2001.
12. Mackness, B.I. and Durrington, P.N., Lipoprotein separation and analysis for clinical studies, in *Lipoprotein Analysis: A Practical Approach,* Converse, C.A. and Skinner, E.R., eds., Oxford University Press, Oxford, 1992, 1.
13. Friedewald, W.T., Levy, R.I., and Fredrickson, D.S., Estimation of the concentration of low-density lipoprotein cholesterol in plasma, without use of the preparative ultracentrifuge, *Clin. Chem.*, 18, 499, 1972.
14. Cox, D.R., Regression models and life tables, *J. Roy. Stat. Soc. (B)*, 34, 187, 1972.
15. Yuan, J.M. et al., Morbidity and mortality in relation to cigarette smoking in Shanghai, China: a prospective male cohort study, *JAMA*, 275, 1646, 1996.

16. Yuan, J.M. et al., Follow-up study of moderate alcohol intake and mortality among middle aged men in Shanghai, China, *BMJ*, 314, 18, 1997.

17. Yuan, J.M. et al., Body weight and mortality: a prospective evaluation in a cohort of middle-aged men in Shanghai, China, *Int. J. Epidemiol.*, 27, 824, 1998.

18. Breslow, N.E. and Day, N.E., *Statistical Methods in Cancer Research, Vol. 1: The Analysis of Case-Control Studies*, IARC Scientific Publications, Lyon, 1980, 192.

19. Yuan, J.M. et al., Fish and shellfish consumption in relation to death from myocardial infarction among men in Shanghai, China, *Am. J. Epidemiol.*, 154, 809, 2001.

20. Bang, H.O., Dyerberg, J., and Hjoorne, N., The composition of food consumed by Greenland Eskimos, *Acta Med. Scand.*, 200, 69, 1976.

21. Dyerberg, J. and Bang, H.O., Haemostatic function and platelet polyunsaturated fatty acids in Eskimos, *Lancet*, 2, 433, 1979.

22. Hirai, A. et al., Eicosapentaenoic acid and adult diseases in Japan: epidemiological and clinical aspects, *J. Intern. Med. Suppl.*, 225, 69, 1989.

23. Kromhout, D., Bosschieter, E.B., and de Lezenne Coulander, C., The inverse relation between fish consumption and 20-year mortality from coronary heart disease, *New Engl. J. Med.*, 312, 1205, 1985.

24. Kromhout, D., Feskens, E.J., and Bowles, C.H., The protective effect of a small amount of fish on coronary heart disease mortality in an elderly population, *Int. J. Epidemiol.*, 24, 340, 1995.

25. Dolecek, T.A., Epidemiological evidence of relationships between dietary polyunsaturated fatty acids and mortality in the multiple risk factor intervention trial, *Proc. Soc. Exp. Biol. Med.*, 200, 177, 1992.

26. Ascherio, A. et al., Dietary intake of marine n-3 fatty acids, fish intake, and the risk of coronary disease among men, *New Engl. J. Med.*, 332, 977, 1995.

27. Rodriguez, B.L. et al., Fish intake may limit the increase in risk of coronary heart disease morbidity and mortality among heavy smokers: the Honolulu Heart Program, *Circulation*, 94, 952, 1996.

28. Daviglus, M.L. et al., Fish consumption and the 30-year risk of fatal myocardial infarction, *New Engl. J. Med.*, 336, 1046, 1997.

29. Albert, C.M. et al., Fish consumption and risk of sudden cardiac death, *JAMA*, 279, 23, 1998.

30. Oomen, C.M. et al., Fish consumption and coronary heart disease mortality in Finland, Italy, and The Netherlands, *Am. J. Epidemiol.*, 151, 999, 2000.

31. Pietinen, P. et al., Intake of fatty acids and risk of coronary heart disease in a cohort of Finnish men: the Alpha-Tocopherol, Beta-Carotene Cancer Prevention Study, *Am. J. Epidemiol.*, 145, 876, 1997.

32. Jansson, G. and Harms-Ringdahl, M., Stimulating effects of mercuric and silver ions on the superoxide anion production in human polymorphonuclear leukocytes, *Free Radic. Res. Commun.*, 18, 87, 1993.

33. Clarkson, T.W., The toxicology of mercury, *Crit. Rev. Clin. Lab. Sci.*, 34, 369, 1997.

34. Salonen, J.T. et al., Intake of mercury from fish, lipid peroxidation, and the risk of myocardial infarction and coronary, cardiovascular, and any death in eastern Finnish men, *Circulation*, 91, 645, 1995.

35. Guallar, E. et al., Mercury, fish oils, and the risk of myocardial infarction [comment], *New Engl. J. Med.*, 347, 1747, 2002.

36. Siscovick, D.S. et al., Dietary intake and cell membrane levels of long-chain n-3 polyunsaturated fatty acids and the risk of primary cardiac arrest, *JAMA*, 274, 1363, 1995.

37. Albert, C.M. et al., Blood levels of long-chain n-3 fatty acids and the risk of sudden death [comment], *New Engl. J. Med.*, 346, 1113, 2002.
38. Lemaitre, R.N. et al., n-3 Polyunsaturated fatty acids, fatal ischemic heart disease, and nonfatal myocardial infarction in older adults: the Cardiovascular Health Study, *Am. J. Clin. Nutr.*, 77, 319, 2003.
39. Burr, M.L. et al., Effects of changes in fat, fish, and fibre intakes on death and myocardial reinfarction: diet and reinfarction trial (DART), *Lancet*, 2, 757, 1989.
40. Singh, R.B. et al., Randomized, double-blind, placebo-controlled trial of fish oil and mustard oil in patients with suspected acute myocardial infarction: the Indian experiment of infarct survival 4, *Cardiovasc. Drugs Ther.*, 11, 485, 1997.
41. GISSI Prevenzione Investigators, Dietary supplementation with n-3 polyunsaturated fatty acids and vitamin E after myocardial infarction: results of the GISSI Prevenzione trial (Gruppo Italiano per lo Studio della Sopravvivenza nell'Infarto miocardico), *Lancet*, 354, 447, 1999.
42. Christensen, J.H. et al., Fish consumption, n-3 fatty acids in cell membranes, and heart rate variability in survivors of myocardial infarction with left ventricular dysfunction, *Am. J. Cardiol.*, 79, 1670, 1997.
43. Task Force of the European Society of Cardiology and North American Society of Pacing and Electrophysiology, Heart rate variability: standards of measurement, physiological interpretation and clinical use, *Circulation*, 93, 1043, 1996.
44. Pedersen, H.S. et al., N-3 fatty acids as a risk factor for haemorrhagic stroke, *Lancet*, 353, 812, 1999.
45. Keli, S.O. et al., Dietary flavonoids, antioxidant vitamins, and incidence of stroke: the Zutphen study, *Arch. Intern. Med.*, 156, 637, 1996.
46. Morris, M.C. et al., Fish consumption and cardiovascular disease in the physicians' health study: a prospective study, *Am. J. Epidemiol.*, 142, 166, 1995.
47. He, K. et al., Fish consumption and risk of stroke in men, *JAMA*, 288, 3130, 2002.
48. Zheng, Z.J. et al., Sudden cardiac death in the United States, 1989 to 1998 [comment], *Circulation*, 104, 2158, 2001.

3 Low Occurrence of CHD in Sub-Saharan African Populations

A.R.P. Walker

CONTENTS

3.1 SUMMARY

In sub-Saharan African countries, coronary heart disease (CHD) remains near absent in rural areas. Moreover, even in those urban areas where large proportions of Africans are in advanced stages of transition respecting changes in diet and other aspects of lifestyle, the disease continues to be very uncommon.

In South Africa, perhaps the country with the best socioeconomic conditions in sub-Saharan Africa, the plant food diets high in cereals and legumes consumed by African town dwellers have changed. Intake of energy, fat, and foods of animal origin has increased; simultaneously, intake of fibre-containing foods has decreased. Smoking has risen considerably in males, although far less in females. Levels of physical activity have greatly diminished, especially among better-situated urban dwellers. Among those urban dwellers experiencing major lifestyle changes, mean serum cholesterol levels, although still lower than those of juxtaposed white populations, are now far higher — roughly 50% higher — than those of rural African populations who still live largely traditionally. Obesity in females, but not in males, has risen enormously to levels much higher than those in white women. The prevalence of hypertension in blacks has reached that of the white population. Remarkably, diabetes has increased in prevalence to the point where it now exceeds prevalence in whites.

0-8493-1674-X/04/$0.00+$1.50
© 2004 by CRC Press LLC

Notwithstanding these major rises in risk factors, mortality rates from CHD in black town dwellers remain very low —about a tenth of the rates in the white population. Undoubtedly, CHD incidence will increase over time due to ongoing increases in risk factors. Currently, however, the low mortality rate from the disease among urban Africans stands in gross contrast to the rates of African Americans, whose current proneness to the disease now equals that of white Americans. While the lower than expected prevalence of CHD in urban sub-Saharan Africans remains unexplained, it must be appreciated, in fairness, that incident rates of CHD are widely divergent even in developed populations and are far from being explicable from known risk factors.

As to the future for Africans in Africa, efforts toward prevention and control of risk factors are non-starters. As long as African populations remain relatively impoverished, a situation that largely prevails in most countries, major rises in CHD are unlikely. The recent advent of the catastrophic HIV/AIDS pandemic, especially in southern African populations, has caused considerably heightened mortality, particularly among the young and middle aged, with enormous falls in survival time. However, limited rises in CHD are likely to continue to occur in the less affected upper middle aged and elderly populations.

3.2 EPIDEMIOLOGY OF CHD IN SUB-SAHARAN AFRICAN POPULATIONS

Numerous publications have emphasized the rarity of CHD in sub-Saharan African populations. In 1960, CHD was considered extremely rare in Uganda.[1] A general review in 1977 noted that Africans were regarded as "virtually free of hypertension and CHD."[2] In the same year at Enugu, Nigeria, not 1 patient among 348 with cardiac disorders over a 4-year period had CHD.[3] As to international appreciation, a leading article titled "British and African Hearts" published in 1983 in the U.K. emphasized the tremendous contrast between the experiences of CHD in the two types of populations.[4] In 1993, a rural hospital in Tanzania reported a low prevalence of CHD risk factors and the absence of the disease.[5] The latter phenomenon was also noted in rural Nigeria.[6] In a rural hospital at Gelukspan in the Northwest Province of South Africa, none of the 2593 adult admissions in 1994 arose from CHD.[7] Around the same time, the same observation related to 2010 admissions was noted at the rural Manguzi Hospital in Kwa-Zulu Natal, South Africa.[8]

While the rarity described applies particularly to rural dwellers, CHD remains uncommon even in urban populations. In 1976 in Durban, a major city in Kwa-Zulu Natal, about 10 cases were seen annually at King Edward VIII Hospital from a catchment population of about 2 million.[9] Angiographic and other studies done in Durban in 1980 reaffirmed that CHD was rare in the black population.[10] In 1992, despite rises in risk factors, CHD remained uncommon, [11] as indicated from data noted in 2000.[12] In Soweto, a city adjacent to Johannesburg, Gauteng Province, the population of about a million is perhaps the most advanced in a state of transition of African urban populations in sub-Saharan Africa. At Baragwanath Hospital (3200 beds at this writing), according to records of the Department of Cardiology, 35

Africans were diagnosed with CHD in 1992,[13] 51 in 1993, and 65 in 1994.[14] However, of the 65 diagnosed in 1994, only 36 were Sowetans; the rest lived elsewhere. In 2000, the hospital treated 50 Sowetan CHD patients. This is still a very low annual incidence rate of approximately 5.0 per 100,000 population.[15] At urban Pirenyatwa Hospital, the main referral center for neighboring Zimbabwe, six African patients on average were diagnosed annually with acute myocardial infarction from 1988 to 1993.[16] In 1996 in Nigeria, a comprehensive review concluded, "CHD is still rare ... despite increased incidence in recent years."[17] Clearly, CHD remains uncommon among urban Africans in South Africa and other sub-Saharan African countries.[13,18]

Regarding a perspective on the epidemiological situation described, one important question is: how does the uncommonness of CHD in Africans compare in magnitude with its high frequency in socioeconomically better placed Western populations? In Soweto, sick Africans usually attend Baragwanath Hospital. If we assume that all of the 50 CHD patients mentioned earlier ultimately died from CHD, then CHD would be responsible for only about 1% of the roughly 5000 deaths occurring annually in that city,[19] thereby underlining the low proportion dying from CHD, even when allowing for uncertainties. As to comparisons with proportions in Western countries, in the recently reported Seven Countries Study covering populations in Mediterranean areas and those residing inland, the age-standardized 25-year CHD mortality rate percentages were 4.7 and 7.7%, respectively.[20] However, the proportions reported for countries in Northern Europe and the U.S. were far higher, namely 16.0 and 20.3%, respectively. These comparisons further demonstrate the relative rarity of CHD in urban Africans.

3.3　EPIDEMIOLOGY OF CHD IN AFRICAN AMERICAN AND WHITE POPULATIONS

To provide additional perspective regarding the continuing low rates of CHD in sub-Saharan African populations, it is valuable to consider both some past and present international epidemiological data. In 1979, an analysis was made of 6414 emergency visits in 3 hospitals in St. Louis, MO.[21] Although African Americans were involved in half of all visits, myocardial infarction was found to be 15 times more common in the white population. Thus, roughly a generation or so ago, CHD was very uncommon in African Americans. What a tremendous contrast to the present situation. In 1998, in populations aged 35 years and over, following increases in risk factors, the mortality rate in African American men rose to be only slightly lower than that in white men, namely 321 versus 440 per 100,000 population. Moreover, the rate in African American women compared with white women was higher: 264 versus 202 per 100,000.[22]

Regarding the rapid changes in the incidence of CHD in African Americans described above, it is imperative to stress that the rise in CHD even in white populations is also of relatively recent origin. This fact is insufficiently appreciated. As evidence from the U.K., the 1912 edition of Sir William Osler's *Principles and Practice of Medicine* described angina pectoris as a "rare disease ... a case a year is about average, even in the large metropolitan hospitals." Prior to World War I, the pathology department of the London Hospital performed one or two necropsies per year after recent coronary thrombosis and/or acute myocardial infarction.[23] However, catastrophic rises in rates of occurrence of CHD appeared after the 1920s. While CHD was responsible historically for less than 1% of all mortality,[24] its incidence in some white populations rose to the extent that it caused almost a third of total deaths in the 1970;[25] yet mortality rates for CHD have fallen in recent decades. The decreases appear maximal in the U.S., where the age-adjusted CHD mortality rate has fallen by 50%.[26] The falls in most other countries have been smaller and despite these falls, the incidence of the disease has decreased little. Clearly, there has been universal reluctance to make the appropriate changes in lifestyle.[27] Despite that, the modern treatment of CHD is strikingly effective.

In brief, in both the African American and white populations, it is evident that the development of CHD is of comparatively recent origin. The major increases in incidences and mortality rates from CHD in white populations began about three generations ago and a generation ago in the case of African Americans. In sub-Saharan populations as a whole, meaningful rises in the disease have hardly commenced.

3.4 RISK FACTORS

Numerous studies on developed populations indicate that dietary risk factors include increased intakes of energy and fats.[28–31] Studies indicate that energy levels derived from fats should be 30% or less, not the current 40% or so. Non-dietary risk factors include cigarette smoking and low levels of physical activity. Pathological sequelae of high risk factors include obesity, hypercholesterolemia, hypertension, and diabetes.

As to the risk factors in predominantly rural African populations in southern Africa, the principal dietary sources of energy were in the past and still are to an extent cereals (maize and kaffir corn or sorghum) and their products, wild spinaches, and a variety of legumes (cowpeas, sugar beans, Jugo beans), along with relatively low intakes of most vegetables and fruits and infrequent consumption of small quantities of milk and meat. Fat supplied about 17% of energy to urban Africans such as those residing in Cape Town in 1953.[32] More recently, fats supplied mean energy of 27%.[33] While consumption of cereal products has fallen, consumption of bread, especially white bread, has increased. Serum cholesterol levels of rural Africans in the past ranged from about 3.0 to 3.5 mmol/l[34] and remain low. The range of mean serum cholesterol levels of urban Africans was 3.5 to 4.40 mmol/l[35] and later increased to 4.0 to 5.0 mmol/l.[36] The level for the upper class segment of this population is about 5.0 mmol/l. Interestingly this level is about the same as those in some Mediterranean populations,[37] known for their relatively lower incidences and mortality rates from CHD, compared with rates for other developed populations.

Among more prosperous urban Africans, for example those in South Africa, the prevalence of obesity in women, but not in men, is higher than that in white women.[38] The prevalences of hypertension and of diabetes approach, exceed in the latter, such in white populations.[39,40] Smoking rates have increased, with the rise far more evident in men than in women.[41] Alcohol consumption too has risen, again far more so in men than in women.[42] As already indicated, physical activity, understandably, is progressively decreasing in urban dwellers, especially in the better circumstanced.

In brief, taking into account the rapid CHD promotive changes that have occurred in these factors, as previously emphasized, the continuing low occurrence of CHD in urban Africans cannot be explained. Can anything be learned, in this regard, from the epidemiological experiences, past and present, of developed populations?

3.5 PUZZLING EPIDEMIOLOGICAL SITUATIONS

Regarding comparisons with the situations in African populations, we must recognize that many markedly diverse CHD epidemiological situations that are not explicable on the basis of known risk factors exist, and this emphasizes the limitations of present knowledge. In the PRIME Study in the U.K., classical risk factors did not explain the several-fold differences in CHD mortality rate between France and Northern Ireland, clearly indicating the operation of additional factors.[43]

In the recent MONICA study, data on the trends of change were collected from 38 populations of subjects between 35 and 64 years of age. Factors studied included CHD mortality rates, 28-day case fatalities, and the prevalence of smoking, blood pressure anomalies, cholesterol, and obesity.[44] The scatter plots of the 38 groups showed unexpectedly weak relations between the size of the decline in mortality rate and risk factor scores. For example, the mortality rate in Poland arose from conventional heart risk factors. To demonstrate the extent of variability, the age-adjusted mortality rates of populations in some U.S. states in 1998 were reported to be far higher than those in others. The rates in New York, Oklahoma, and Mississippi were *double* the rates in Utah, Colorado, Montana, and Minnesota, namely 410 to 440 versus 210 to 230 per 100,000 population.[22]

Certain emerging populations have puzzlingly *high* rates, for example, the aborigine in Australia.[45] Their mortality rate from CHD is *twice* the rate of white Australians (6 to 8 times higher in aborigines aged 25 to 64 years) and the life expectancy of an aborigine is 15 to 20 years less than that of a white Australian. The prevalent risk factors in aboriginal populations are obesity, diabetes, smoking, and low rates of physical activity.

3.6 OUTLOOK FOR SUB-SAHARAN AFRICANS

Many populations in developed countries, especially in the U.S., have demonstrated major decreases in mortality rates from CHD,[46] although more than 70% of the overall decline occurred among patients with the disease.[47] The incidence rate has changed little.[48] Considering the limited attempts to avoid CHD now underway in many developed populations[28,50] and the exceptionally averse sequelae prevailing in one developing population, namely the Australian aborigines,[45] the salient question is: what is the likely outlook for sub-Saharan populations? Important factors to consider are differences in the significances of rises in certain risk factors in both developing and developed populations. As an example, the high levels of obesity in South African women (but not men) appear to exert little or no bearing on their proneness to CHD.[38,51] This principle also applies in some measure to obesity in African Americans.[52] This lack of response to a well-known risk factor stands in contrast to the situation in Asia–Pacific populations. While they have relatively low

CHD mortality rates, the associations of obesity with CHD and with stroke are "steeper" than in corresponding situations in white Australian and New Zealand cohorts.[53]

Returning to the outlook for CHD in sub-Saharan Africans, urban moieties represent a factor, for example in Sowetans who, compared with rural dwellers, are experiencing rising prosperity with consequent changes in dietary and non-dietary habits. The continuing adoption of the habits of the juxtaposed white population by segments of African populations is likely to lead to rises in the incidence of CHD. Over time and with continuing propitious circumstances, CHD incidence in African populations could conceivably approach rates in African Americans. On the other hand, we must understand that most African populations, especially rural dwellers, are likely to remain in poor socioeconomic circumstances. As a result of limited changes in their dietary and non-dietary habits, they face little likelihood of significant rises in CHD in the foreseeable future.

One recent influence is the catastrophic HIV/AIDS pandemic that already affects a quarter of the men in many countries in Southern Africa and women and children to a lesser extent. The consequent increases in early morbidity and mortality[54] have decreased mean survival time in South Africa from 62 to 44 years.[55,56] In neighboring Botswana, half of all deaths are due to the infection.[57] However, the HIV/AIDS situation primarily affects the young and those in early middle age; it will not diminish the likelihood of rises in CHD in the near future in the less affected upper-middle aged and elderly Africans, particularly those in better circumstances.

In summary, the present and likely near-future socioeconomic circumstances of sub-Saharan populations, even urban dwellers, are unlikely to evoke significant rises in the incidence of CHD.

REFERENCES

1. Shaper, A.G. and Williams, A.W., Cardiovascular disorders at an African hospital in Uganda, *Trans. R. Soc. Trop. Med. Hyg.*, 54, 12, 1960.
2. Vaughan, J.P., A brief review of cardiovascular disease in Africans, *Trans. R. Soc. Trop. Med. Hyg.*, 77, 226, 1977.
3. Uzodike, V.O., Anidi, A.I., and Ekpechi, L.V.O., The pattern of heart disease in Enugu, Nigeria, *Nigeria Med.*, 7, 315, 1977.
4. British and African hearts, *Lancet* (leading article), i, 1256, 1983.
5. Swai, A.B.M., McLarty, D.G., and Ketange, H.M. et al., Low prevalence of risk factors for coronary heart disease in rural Tanzania, *Int. Epidemiol.*, 22, 651, 1993.
6. Okesina, A.B., Oparinde, D.P., Akindoyin, K.A., and Erasmus, R.T., Prevalence of some risk factors of coronary heart disease in a rural Nigerian population, *East Afr. Med. J.*, 76, 212, 1999.
7. Kakembo, A.S.L., Walker, B.F., and Walker, A.R.P., Causes of admission of African patients to Gelukspan Hospital, North West Province, South Africa, *East Afr. Med. J.*, 73, 746, 1996.
8. Walker, A.R.P., Coppin, B., and Halse, J.M., Causes of admissions of rural African patients in 1992 to Manguzi Hospital, North Kwa-Zulu Natal, South Africa, unpublished study.

9. Seedat, Y.K., Pillay, N., and Foja, H.M., Rarity of myocardial infarction in African hypertensive patients, *Lancet*, ii, 46, 1976.

10. Thandroyen, F.T., Asmal, A.C., Leary, W.P., and Mitha, A.S., Comparative study of plasma lipids, carbohydrate tolerance and coronary angiography in three racial groups, *S. Afr. Med. J.*, 57, 533, 1980.

11. Seedat, Y.K., Mayet, F.G.H., Latiff, G.H., and Joubert, G., Risk factors and coronary heart disease in Durban blacks: the missing link, *S. Afr. Med. J.*, 82, 251, 1992.

12. Mbewu, A.D., Aorto-iliac occlusive disease in the various population groups of South Africa, *S. Afr. Med. J.*, 90, 746, 2000.

13. Walker, A.R.P. and Sarelli, P., Coronary heart disease outlook for Africa, *J. Roy. Soc. Med.*, 90, 23, 1997.

14. Walker, A.R.P., Coronary heart disease in African patients in Baragwanath Hospital, Soweto, Johannesburg, unpublished data.

15. Walker, A.R.P., The epidemiology of coronary heart disease in South Africa, *Cardiovasc. J. South Afr.*, Suppl. 1, C12, 1999.

16. Hakim, J.G., Odwee, M.G., Siziya, S., Tenough, I., and Metenga, J., Acute myocardial infarction in Zimbabwe: the changing scene of coronary artery disease, *Centr. Afr. J. Med.*, 41, 303, 1995.

17. Bertrand, E., Coronary heart disease in black Africans: an overview, *East Afr. Med. J.*, 72, 37, 1995.

18. Walker, A.R.P., Coronary heart disease in Southern Africa: what of the future? *Cardiovasc. J. South. Afr.*, Suppl. 1, C67, 1999.

19. Medical Officer of the City of Johannesburg, South Africa, *Annual Report*, 2000.9

20. Verschuren, W.M.M., Jacobs, D.R., and Bloemberg, B.P.M. et al., Serum cholesterol and long-term coronary heart disease mortality in different cultures: 25-year follow-up of the Seven Countries Study, *JAMA*, 274, 131, 1995.

21. Perkoff, G.T. and Strand, M., Race and presenting complaints in myocardial infarction, *Am. Heart J.*, 85, 716, 1973.

22. Mortality from coronary heart disease and acute myocardial infarction, United States, 1998, *MMWR*, 5090, 2001.

23. McCrae T., *Osler's Principles and Practice of Medicine*, Appleton, London, 1912, 836.

24. Morris, J.N., Recent history of coronary heart disease, *Lancet*, ii, 1, 1951.

25. National Center for Health Statistics. *Vital Statistics of the United States, 1988, Vol. II: Mortality*, U.S. Department of Health and Human Services, Hyattsville, MD, 1991.

26. Hunink, M.G.M., Goldman, L., and Tosteson, A.N.A. et al., The recent decline in mortality from coronary heart disease 1980–1990, *JAMA*, 277, 535, 1997.

27. Rolland-Cachera, M.F., Bellisle, F., and Deheeger, M., Nutritional status and food intake in adolescents living in Western Europe, *Eur. J. Clin. Nutr.*, Suppl. 1, S41, 2000.

28. Beaglehole R., Global cardiovascular disease prevention: time to get serious. *Lancet*, 358, 661, 2000.

29. Maranhao, M., Tse, T.F., Poole-Wilson, P., and Bayes de Luna A., Global cardiovascular disease prevention, *Lancet*, 358, 16, 2001.

30. Jackson, R.T., Are the new lipid management guidelines good for Australia's health? *Med. J.. Aust.,* 175, 452, 2001.

31. Heart Foundation, Lipid management guidelines, *Med. J. Aust.*, 175, S57, 2001.32.

32. Walker, A.R.P., Nutritional, biochemical and other studies on South African populations, *S. Afr. Med. J.*, 40, 814, 1966.

33. Bourne, L.T., Langenhoven, M.L., Steyn, K., Jooste, P.L. Lauscher, J.A., and Van der Vyver, E., Nutrient intake in the urban African population of the Cape Peninsula, South Africa: the BRISK study, *Centr. Afr. J. Med.*, 39, 238, 1993.

34. Stone, W., The blood chemistry of normal Southern Rhodesian natives, *Trans. R. Soc. Med. Hyg.*, 30, 165, 1936.

35. Walker, A.R.P. and Arvidsson, U.B., Fat intake, serum cholesterol concentrations, and atherosclerosis in the South African Bantu. Part I: Low fat intake and age trend of serum cholesterol concentrations in the South African Bantu, *J. Clin. Invest.*, 33, 1358, 1954.

36. Erasmus, R.T., Uyot, C., and Pakeye, T., Plasma cholesterol distribution in a rural Nigerian population: relationship to age, sex and body mass, *Cent. Afr. J. Med.*, 40, 299, 1994.

37. Grima, S.A., Alegrio, E.E., and Jover, E.P., The prevalence of classic cardiovascular risk factors in a working Mediterranean population of 4996 men, *Rev. Esp. Cardiol.*, 52, 910, 1999.

38. Walker, A.R.P., Epidemiology and health implications of obesity with special reference to African populations, *Ecol. Food Nutr.*, 37, 21, 1998.

39. Erasmus, R.P., Blanco, E., Okeisina, A.B., Matsha, T., and Mesa G.J.A., Prevalence of diabetes mellitus and impaired glucose tolerance in factory workers from Transkei, South Africa, *S. Afr. Med. J.*, 91, 157, 2001.

40. Omar, M.A.K., Seedat, M.A., Motala, A.A., Dyer, R.B., and Becker, P., The prevalence of diabetes mellitus and impaired glucose tolerance in a group of urban South African blacks, *S. Afr. Med. J.*, 83, 641, 1993.

41. Yach, D. and Townsend, G.S., Smoking and health in South Africa, *S. Afr. Med. J.*, 73, 391, 1988.

42. Parry, C., Alcohol and other drug use, in *South African Health Review*, Health Systems Trust, Durban, 2000, 441.

43. Tarnell, J.W.G., The PRIME Study classical risk factors do not explain the severalfold differences in risk of coronary heart disease between France and Northern Ireland, *Q. J. Med.*, 91, 667, 1998.

44. Tunstall-Pedoe, H., Kuulasmaa, K., Mahonen, M., Tolonen, H., Ruokokoski, E., and Amouyel, P., Contribution trends in survival and coronary event rates to changes in coronary heart disease mortality: 10-year results from 37 WHO MONICA Project populations, *Lancet*, 353, 1547, 1999.

45. Annual Scientific Meeting of the Cardiac Society of Australia and New Zealand. Conference report on cardiovascular health in indigenous Australians: a call for action, *Med. J. Aust.*, 175, 351, 2001.

46. Sykowski, P.A., Kannel, W.B., and D'Agostino, R.B., Changes in risk factors and the decline in mortality from cardiovascular disease: the Framingham Heart Study, *New Engl. J. Med.*, 322, 1635, 1990.

47. Hunnink, G.M., Goldman, L., and Tosteson, A.N. et al., The recent decline in mortality from coronary heart disease, 1900–1990, *JAMA*, 277, 535, 1997.

48. Walker, A.R.P., With increasing ageing in western populations, what are the prospects for lowering the incidence of coronary heart disease? *Q. J. Med.*, 94, 107, 2001.

49. EUROSPIRE I and II Groups, Clinical reality of coronary prevention guidelines: a comparison of EUROSPIRE I and II in nine countries, *Lancet*, 357, 995, 2001.

50. Walker, A.R.P. and Wadee, A.A., Preventing cardiovascular disease: a despondent view. *Bull. World Hlth. Org.* 80, 233, 2002.

51. Joffe, B.I., Goldberg, R.B., and Seftel, H.C., Insulin, glucose, and triglyceride relationships in obese African subjects, *Am. J. Clin. Nutr.*, 28, 616, 1975.

52. Van Italie, T.B., Health implications of overweight and obesity in the United States, *Ann. Int. Med.,* 103, 983, 1985.
53. Gill, T.P., Cardiovascular risk in the Asia Pacific region from a nutrition and metabolic point of view: abdominal obesity, *Asia Pacific J. Clin. Nutr.,* 10, 85, 2001.
54. Logie, D., AIDS cuts life expectancy in sub-Saharan Africa by a quarter, *BMJ,* 319, 806, 1999.
55. Kale R., Impressions of health in the new South Africa: a period of convalescence, *BMJ,* 210, 1119, 1995.
56. Ncayiyama, D.J., The MRC/AIDS Mortality Report: South Africa's Apocalypse now, *S. Afr. Med. J.,* 92, 90, 2002.
57. Izindaba, Half Botswana's deaths from AIDS, *S. Afr. Med. J.,* 90, 1170, 2000.

4 Dietary Prevention of CHD: Insights into the Mediterranean Diet

Michel de Lorgeril and Patricia Salen

CONTENTS

4.1 INTRODUCTION

The two main causes of death in patients with coronary heart disease (CHD) are sudden cardiac death (SCD) and heart failure (HF). The main mechanism underlying recurrent cardiac events is myocardial ischemia resulting from atherosclerotic plaque rupture or ulceration. Plaque rupture is usually the consequence of intraplaque inflammation in relation to a high lipid content of the lesion and high concentrations of leukocytes and lipid peroxidation products. Thus, in patients with established CHD, the three main aims of the preventive strategy are to prevent malignant ventricular arrhythmia and the development of severe ventricular dysfunction (and heart failure) and minimize the risk of plaque inflammation and ulceration.

This does not mean that traditional risk factors of CHD should not be measured and, if necessary, corrected. It simply means that because complications such as SCD and associated syndromes are often unpredictable, occur out of hospitals and far from any potential therapeutic resources in the majority of cases, and account for about 50% of cardiac mortality in secondary prevention, they should be the priority of any prevention program. For that reason, we will focus our recommendations and comments specifically on clinical efficacy and not on surrogate efficacy.

4.2 DIETARY PREVENTION OF SUDDEN CARDIAC DEATH

In the absence of a generally accepted definition, SCD is usually defined as death from a cardiac cause occurring within 1 hour from the onset of symptoms.[1] The magnitude of the problem is considerable because SCD is a very common, and often the first, manifestation of CHD and accounts for about 50% of cardiovascular mortality in developed countries.[1] In most cases, SCD occurs outside a hospital and without prodromal symptoms. We shall now examine whether diet (more precisely, certain dietary factors) may prevent (or help prevent) SCD in patients with established CHD. We will focus our analyses on the effects of the different families of fatty acids, antioxidants, and alcohol.[2]

4.2.1 FISH, N-3 FATTY ACIDS, AND SCD

The hypothesis that eating fish may protect against SCD is derived from the results of a secondary prevention trial, the Diet and Reinfarction Trial (DART), which showed a significant reduction in total and cardiovascular mortality (both by about 30%) in patients who ate at least two servings of fatty fish per week.[3] The authors suggested that the protective effect of fish might be explained by a preventive action on ventricular fibrillation (VF), since no benefit was observed on the incidence of nonfatal acute myocardial infarction (AMI). This hypothesis was consistent with experimental evidence suggesting that n-3 polyunsaturated fatty acids (PUFAs), the dominant fatty acids in fish oil and fatty fish, have important effects on the occurrence of VF in the setting of myocardial ischemia and reperfusion in various animal models, both *in vivo* and *in vitro*.[4,5] In the same studies, it was also apparent that saturated fatty acids are proarrhythmic as compared to unsaturated fatty acids.

Using an elegant *in vivo* model of SCD in dogs, Billman and colleagues recently demonstrated a striking reduction of VF after intravenous administration of pure n-3 PUFA, including both the long chain fatty acids present in fish oil and alpha-linolenic acid, their parent n-3 PUFA occurring in some vegetable oils.[6] These authors found the mechanism of this protection to result from the electrophysiological effects of free n-3 PUFAs when they are simply partitioned into the phospholipids of the sarcolemma without covalently bonding to any constituents of the cell membranes. After dietary intake, these fatty acids are preferentially incorporated into membrane phospholipids.[7] Nair and colleagues have also shown that a very important pool of free (nonesterified) fatty acids exists in the normal myocardium and that the amount of n-3 PUFA in this pool is increased by supplementing n-3 PUFA in the diet.[7] They noted a huge increase in n-3 PUFA concentrations, in particular for the nonesterified fraction, in the myocardia of pigs fed fish oil. This illustrates the potential of diet to modify the structures and biochemical compositions of cardiac cells.

In the case of ischemia, phospholipases and lipases quickly release new fatty acids from phospholipids, including n-3 fatty acids in higher amounts than the other fatty acids,[7] further increasing the pool of free n-3 fatty acids that can exert an antiarrhythmic effect. It is important to remember that the lipase lipoprotein is particularly active following the consumption of n-3 PUFA.[8] One hypothesis is that the presence of the free form of the n-3 PUFA in the membrane of every cardiac muscle cell renders the myocardium more resistant to arrhythmias, probably by modulating the conduction of several membrane ion channels.[9] It seems that the very potent inhibitory effects of n-3 PUFA on the fast sodium current (Ina)[10,11] and the L-type calcium current (IcaL)[12] are the major contributors to the antiarrhythmic actions of these fatty acids in ischemia. Briefly, n-3 PUFAs act by shifting the steady-state inactivation potential to more negative values, as was observed in other excitable tissues such as neurons.

Another important aspect of the implications of n-3 PUFAs in SCD is their role in the metabolization of eicosanoids. In competition with n-6 PUFAs, they are the precursors to a broad array of structurally diverse and potent bioactive lipids (including eicosanoids, prostaglandins, and thromboxanes) that are thought to play a role in the occurrence of VF during myocardial ischemia and reperfusion.[13,14]

Other clinical data show suppression (by more than 70%) of ventricular premature complexes in middle-aged patients with frequent ventricular extrasystoles after random assignment of either fish oil or placebo doses.[15] Also, survivors of AMI[16] and healthy men[17] receiving fish oil were shown to improve their measurements of heart rate variability, suggesting other mechanisms by which n-3 PUFA may be antiarrhythmic.

Support for the hypothesis of a clinically significant antiarrhythmic effect of n-3 PUFA in the secondary prevention of CHD, as put forward in DART,[3] came from two randomized trials testing the effects of ethnic dietary patterns (instead of effects of a single food or nutrient), i.e., a Mediterranean type of diet and an Asian vegetarian diet, in the secondary prevention of CHD.[18,19] The two experimental diets included high intake of essential alpha-linolenic acid, the main vegetable n-3 PUFA. While the incidence of SCD was markedly reduced in both trials, the number of cases was very small and the antiarrhythmic effect cannot be entirely attributed to alpha-linolenic because the experimental diets were also high in other nutrients with potential antiarrhythmic properties, including various antioxidants.

These findings were extended by a population-based case-control study conducted by Siscovick and colleagues on the intake of n-3 PUFA among patients with primary cardiac arrest, compared to age- and sex-matched controls.[20] Their data indicated that the intake of about 5 to 6 g of n-3 PUFA per month (an amount provided by consuming fatty fish once or twice a week) was associated with a 50% reduction in the risk of cardiac arrest. In that study, the use of a biomarker, the red blood cell membrane level of n-3 PUFA, considerably enhanced the validity of the findings that were consistent with the results of many (but not all) cohort studies. This suggests that consumption of one to two servings of fish per week is associated with a marked reduction in CHD mortality as compared to no fish intake.[21,22] In most studies, however, the SCD endpoint is not reported.

In a large prospective study (more than 20,000 participants and follow-up of 11 years), Albert et al. examined the specific point that fish has antiarrhythmic properties and may prevent SCD.[23] They found that the risk of SCD was 50% lower for men who consumed fish at least once a week than for those who had fish less than once a month. Interestingly, the consumption of fish was not related to nonsudden cardiac death, suggesting that the main protective effect of fish (or n-3 PUFA) is related to an effect on arrhythmia. These results are consistent with those of DART[3] but differ from those of the Chicago Western Electric Study that noted a significant inverse association between fish consumption and nonsudden cardiac death, but not with SCD.[24] Several methodological factors may explain the discrepancy, especially the way of classifying deaths in the Western Electric Study. This again illustrates the limitations of observational studies and the obvious fact that only randomized trials can definitely provide clear demonstrations of causal relationships.

The GISSI Prevenzione Trial was aimed at helping address the question of the health benefits of foods rich in n-3 PUFA (and also in vitamin E) and their pharmacological substitutes.[25] Patients (n = 11,324) surviving recent AMIs (<3 months) and having been instruct to return to a Mediterranean type of diet were randomly assigned supplements of n-3 PUFA (0.8 g daily), vitamin E (300 mg daily), both, or none (control) for 3.5 years. The primary efficacy endpoint was the combination of death and nonfatal AMI and stroke. Secondary analyses included overall mortality, cardiovascular (CV) mortality, and SCD. Treatment with n-3 PUFA significantly lowered the risk of the primary endpoint (the relative risk decreased by 15%). Secondary analyses provided a clearer profile of the clinical effects of n-3 PUFA. Overall mortality was reduced by 20% and CV mortality by 30%. However, it was the effect on SCD (45% lower) that accounted for most of the benefits seen in the primary combined endpoint and both overall and CV mortality. No difference was noted across the treatment groups for nonfatal CV events — a result comparable to that of DART.[3] Thus, the results obtained in this randomized trial were consistent with previous controlled trials,[3,18,19] large-scale observational studies,[21–24] and experimental studies[4–7] that together strongly support an effect of n-3 PUFA in relation with SCD. An important point is that the protective effect of n-3 PUFA on SCD was greater in the groups of patients who complied more strictly with the Mediterranean diet. This suggests a positive interaction between n-3 PUFA and some components of the Mediterranean diet which is, by definition, not high in n-6 PUFA, low in saturated fats, rich in oleic acid, various antioxidants, and fibre, and associated with a moderate consumption of alcohol.

4.2.2 Alcohol and SCD

The question of the effect of alcohol on heart and vessel diseases has been the subject of intense controversy in recent years. The consensus is now that moderate alcohol drinking is associated with reduced cardiovascular mortality, although the exact mechanism(s) by which alcohol is protective are still unclear. In contrast, chronic heavy drinking has been incriminated in the occurrence of atrial as well as ventricular arrhythmias in humans — an effect called "holiday heart" because it is often associated with binge drinking by healthy people, specifically during weekends. Studies in animals have shown varying and apparently contradictory effects of alcohol on cardiac rhythm and conduction, depending on the species, experimental model, and dose of alcohol. If given acutely to nonalcoholic animals, ethanol may even have antiarrhythmic properties.

Few human studies have specifically investigated the effect of alcohol on SCD. The hyperadrenergic state resulting from binge drinking and from withdrawal in alcoholics seems to be the main mechanism by which alcohol induces arrhythmias. In the British Regional Heart Study, the relative risk of SCD in heavy drinkers (>6 drinks per day) was twice as high as risk in occasional or light drinkers.[26] However, the effect of binge drinking on SCD was more evident in men with no pre-existing CHD than in those with established CHD. In contrast, in the Honolulu Heart Program,[27] the risk of SCD among healthy middle-aged men was positively related to blood pressure, serum cholesterol, smoking, and left ventricular hypertrophy, but inversely related to alcohol intake.

The effect of moderate social drinking on the risk of SCD in nonalcoholic subjects has been addressed in only one study. Investigators of the Physicians' Health Study assessed whether light-to-moderate alcohol drinkers apparently free of CHD at baseline have decreased risks of SCD.[28] After controlling for multiple confounders, men who consumed two to four drinks per week or five to six drinks per week at baseline had significantly reduced risks of SCD by 60 to 80%, as compared with those who rarely or never consumed alcohol. Analyses were repeated after excluding deaths occurring during the first 4 years of follow-up (in order to exclude the possibility that some men who refrained from drinking at baseline did so because of early symptoms of heart diseases), and also using the updated measure of alcohol intake ascertained at year 7 to address potential misclassification in the baseline evaluation of alcohol drinking.[28] These secondary analyses basically provided the same results and confirmed the potential protective effect of moderate drinking on the risk of SCD. Despite limitations (the selected nature of the cohort, an exclusively male study group, and lack of information on beverage types and drinking patterns), this study suggests that a significant part of the cardioprotective effect of moderate drinking is related to the prevention of SCD. Further research should be directed at understanding the mechanism(s) by which moderate alcohol drinking may prevent ventricular arrhythmias and SCD.

Current knowledge suggests that in CHD patients at risk of SCD, there is no reason not to allow moderate alcohol drinking. From a practical point of view, we advise patients to drink one or two drinks per day, preferably wine during the evening meal, and never before driving a car or performing dangerous work.

4.2.3 ANTIOXIDANTS AND SCD

The issue of the effect of dietary antioxidants on the risk of CHD in general and on SCD in particular is more controversial. Regarding vitamin E, for instance, the most widely studied dietary antioxidant, discrepant findings between the expected benefits based on epidemiological observations[29,30] and the results of clinical trials[31,32] were published. In a recent controlled trial, a significant decrease in nonfatal AMI and a nonsignificant increase in cardiovascular mortality (in particular the rate of SCD) were reported with a daily regimen of 400 to 800 mg of vitamin E in patients with established CHD.[33] Because of certain methodological shortcomings (that will not be discussed here), this trial was said to confuse rather than clarify the question of the usefulness of vitamin E supplementation in CHD, and provided no indication of possible links between vitamin E and prevention of SCD.

The GISSI Prevenzione Trial brings new information in this regard. Unlike results from n-3 PUFA, the results of vitamin E supplementation do not support significant effects on the primary endpoint, namely a combination of death and nonfatal AMI and stroke.[25] Secondary analysis provides a clearer view of the clinical effect of vitamin E in CHD patients that cannot be easily dismissed. In fact, among the 193 and 155 cardiac deaths in the control and vitamin E groups, respectively, during the trial (a difference of 38, $p < 0.05$), there were 99 and 65 SCDs (a difference of 34, $p<0.05$). This indicated that the significant decrease in cardiovascular mortality (by 20%) in the vitamin E group was almost entirely due to a decrease in the incidence of SCD (by 35%). In contrast, nonfatal cardiac events and nonsudden cardiac deaths were not influenced.[25] These data suggest that vitamin E may be useful for the primary prevention of SCD in patients with established CHD.

The vitamin E data of the GISSI trial do not stand in isolation. In an *in vivo* dog model of myocardial ischemia,[34] we also reported a protective effect of vitamin E on the incidence of VF (the main mechanism of SCD) with a 16% rate in the vitamin E group and 44% in the placebo group ($p < 0.05$). Also in line with the GISSI results, infarct size (the main determinant of acute heart failure and nonsudden cardiac death) was larger in the supplemented group (58.5% of the ischemic area) than in the placebo group (41.9%, $p < 0.05$). Such ambivalent effects of vitamin E may at least partly explain why its effects were neutral or nonsignificant in many studies, with the negative effects hiding the beneficial ones.

Nevertheless, the GISSI trial showed that cardiovascular mortality and SCD were significantly reduced by vitamin E, and the effect on overall mortality showed a favorable trend ($p = 0.07$). Finally, the recently published HOPE Trial testing the effect of 400 IU of vitamin E daily in patients at high risk of CHD (therefore in primary prevention) and reporting apparent lack of effect of vitamin E does not help us determine whether vitamin E is protective against SCD.[35] It was not clear whether the patients actually took the capsules during meals (a prerequisite for intestinal absorption of vitamin E), whether they were more or less deficient in vitamin E (no blood measurement), and whether some took vitamin supplements (a current practice among certain populations). Further, SCD was apparently not among the predefined endpoints and patients with left ventricular dysfunction, a major determinant of the risk of SCD, were not eligible.

4.3 DIET AND HEART FAILURE

The incidence of chronic heart failure (CHF), the common end-result of most cardiac diseases, is increasing steadily in many countries despite (and probably because of) considerable improvements in the acute and chronic treatment of CHD, which is currently the main cause of CHF in most countries.[36] In recent years, most CHF research effort has focused on drug treatment, and little attention has been paid to nonpharmacological management. Some unidentified factors may indeed contribute to the rise in the prevalence of CHF and should be recognized and corrected if possible. For instance, CHF is now seen also as a metabolic problem with endocrine and immunological disturbances potentially contributing to its progression.[37,38] Only recently has it been also recognized that increased oxidative stress may contribute to the pathogenesis of CHF.[39] The intimate link between diet and oxidative stress is obvious: the major antioxidant defenses of the body are derived from essential nutrients.[40]

The vital importance of micronutrients for health and the fact that several micronutrients have antioxidant properties are now fully recognized. Micronutrients may function as direct antioxidants such as vitamins C and E or as components of antioxidant enzymes such as superoxide dismutase or glutathione peroxidase.[40] It is now widely believed (but still not causally demonstrated) that diet-derived antioxidants may play a role in the development (and thus in the prevention) of CHF. For instance, clinical and experimental studies have suggested that CHF may be associated with increased free radical formation[41] and reduced antioxidant defences[42] and that vitamin C may improve endothelial functions in patients with CHF.[43] In the secondary prevention of CHD, in dietary trials in which the tested diet included high intakes of natural antioxidants, the incidence of new episodes of CHF was reduced in the experimental groups.[18,44] Taken together, these data suggest (but do not demonstrate) that antioxidant nutrients may help prevent CHF in postinfarction patients.

Other nutrients, however, may be also involved in certain cases of CHF. While deficiency in certain micronutrients, whatever the reason, can actually cause CHF and should be corrected (see below), it is important to understand that patients suffering from CHF also have symptoms that can affect their food intake and result in deficiencies, for instance tiredness when strained, breathing difficulties, and gastrointestinal symptoms like nausea, loss of appetite, and early feelings of satiety. Drug therapy can lead to loss of appetite and excess urinary losses in case of diuretic use. All of these are mainly consequences, not causative factors, of CHF. Thus, the basic treatment of CHF should, in theory, improve these nutritional anomalies. However, since the anomalies can contribute to the development and severity of CHF, they should be recognized and corrected as early as possible.

Finally, it has been shown that up to 50% of patients suffering from CHF are malnourished to some degree[45] and CHF is often associated with weight loss. The weight loss may be associated with multiple etiologies,[46] in particular, the lack of activity resulting in loss of muscle bulk and increased resting metabolic rate. Another factor is a shift toward catabolism with insulin resistance and increased catabolic activity relative to anabolic steroids.[47] Tumor necrosis factor (TNF), sometimes called cachectin, is higher in many patients with CHF and may explain their weight losses. Interestingly, there is a positive correlation between TNF and markers of oxidative stress in a failing heart,[48] suggesting a link between TNF and antioxidant defenses in CHF (the potential importance of TNF in CHF is discussed in Section 4.3.2). Finally, cardiac cachexia is a well-recognized complication of CHF. Its prevalence increases as symptoms worsen[49] and it is an independent predictor of mortality in CHF patients. However, the pathophysiological alteration leading to cachexia remains unclear and, at present, it has no specific treatment apart from treatment of the basic illness and correction of the associated biological abnormalities.

4.3.1 DIETARY SELENIUM

Selenium deficiency has been identified as a major factor in the etiology of certain nonischemic CHF syndromes, especially in low-selenium soil areas such as eastern China and West Africa.[50] In Western countries, cases of congestive cardiomyopathy associated with low antioxidant nutrients (vitamins and trace elements) have been reported in malnourished HIV-infected patients and in subjects on chronic parenteral nutrition.[51] Selenium deficiency is also a risk factor for peripartum cardiomyopathy.

In China, an endemic cardiomyopathy called Keshan disease seems to be a direct consequence of selenium deficiency. While the question of the mechanism by which selenium deficiency results in CHF remains open, recent data suggest that selenium may be involved in skeletal and cardiac muscle deconditioning (and in CHF symptoms such as fatigue and low exercise tolerance) rather than in left ventricular dysfunction.[42] Actually, in the Keshan area of China, the selenium status coincided with clinical severity rather than with the degree of left ventricular dysfunction as assessed by echocardiographic studies. When the selenium levels of residents were raised to the typical levels in nonendemic areas, the mortality rate declined significantly but clinically latent cases were still found and the echocardiographic prevalence of the disease remained high.[50] What we learn from Keshan disease and studies conducted elsewhere[42] is that even a mild deficiency of selenium may influence the clinical severity of CHF (tolerance to exercise) in patients with known causes of the disease. These data should serve as a strong incentives for the initiation of studies testing the effects of natural antioxidants on the clinical severity of CHF. In the meantime, however, physicians would be well advised to measure selenium in patients with exercise inabilities disproportionate to their cardiac dysfunctions.

Finally, low whole blood thiamine (vitamin B_1) levels have been documented in CHF patients on loop diuretics and hospitalized elderly patients, and thiamine supplementation induced significant improvements in cardiac function and symptoms.[52]

4.3.2 DIETARY FATTY ACIDS, CYTOKINES, LVH, AND CHF

Beyond the well-known effect of high sodium intake in the clinical course of CHF (and the occurrence of acute episodes of decompensation), another important issue is the role of diet in the development of left ventricular hypertrophy (LVH), a major risk factor for CHF and SCD as well as for cardiovascular and all-cause mortality and morbidity.[53,54]

The cause of LVH is largely unknown. While gender, obesity, heredity, and insulin resistance may explain some of the variance in LVH, hypertension (HBP) is generally regarded as the primary culprit.[55] Thus, the risks associated with LVH and HBP are intimately linked. Recent data also suggest that low dietary intake of polyunsaturated fatty acids and high intake of saturated fatty acids along with HBP and obesity at age 50 predicted the prevalence of LVH 20 years later.[56] Although the source of saturated fatty acids is usually animal fat, the source of unsaturated fatty acids in that specific Scandinavian population and at that time was less clear and no adjustment was made for other potential dietary confounders such as magnesium, potassium, calcium, and sodium. Thus, this study did not provide conclusive data about the dietary lipid determinants of LVH.[56] However, it does suggest that dietary fatty acids may be involved in the development of LVH and that this diet–heart connection may partly explain the harmful effects of animal saturated fatty acids on the heart.

Another diet–heart connection in the context of advanced CHF relates to the recent theory that CHF also is a low-grade chronic inflammatory disease with elevated circulating levels of cytokines and cytokine receptors that are otherwise independent predictors of mortality.[37,47] High-dose angiotensin-converting enzyme (ACE) inhibition with enalapril, a treatment that reduces mechanical overload and shear stress (two stimuli for cytokine production in patients with CHF), was recently shown to decrease both cytokine bioactivity and left ventricular wall thickness.[57] Finally, various anticytokine and immunomodulating agents were shown to have beneficial effects on heart function and clinical functional class in patients with advanced CHF,[58] suggesting a causal relationship between high cytokine production and CHF. This also suggests a potential for CHF therapies that alter cytokine production. In that regard, dietary supplementation with n-3 fatty acids (fish oil or vegetable oil rich in n-3 fatty acid) reduced cytokine production at least in healthy volunteers.[59,60] An inverse exponential relationship between leukocyte n-3 fatty acid content and cytokine production by these cells was found; most of the reduction in cytokine production was seen with eicosapentanoic acid lower than 1% in cell membranes — a level obtained with rather moderate n-3 fatty acid supplementation.[60] Further studies are warranted to test whether (and at what dosage) dietary n-3 fatty acids may influence the clinical course of CHF through an anticytokine effect.

4.4 DIET AND PREVENTION OF PLAQUE INFLAMMATION AND RUPTURE

For several decades, the prevention of CHD (including the prevention of ischemic recurrence after prior AMI) has focused on the reduction of the traditional risk factors: smoking, HBP, and hypercholesterolemia. Priority was given to the prevention (or reversion) of vascular atherosclerotic stenosis. As discussed above, it has become clear that clinical efficiency in secondary prevention primarily needs to prevent fatal complications of CHD such as SCD. This does not mean, however, that we should not try to slow the atherosclerotic process, and in particular, plaque inflammation and rupture. Indeed, it is critical to prevent the occurrence of new episodes of myocardial ischemia whose repetition in a recently injured heart can precipitate SCD or CHF. Myocardial ischemia is usually the consequence of coronary occlusion caused by plaque rupture and subsequent thrombotic obstruction of the artery. Recent progress in the understanding of the cellular and biochemical pathogenesis of atherosclerosis suggests that, in addition to the traditional risk factors of CHD, other important targets of therapy are required to prevent plaque inflammation and rupture. In this regard, the most important question is: how and why does plaque rupture occur?

4.4.1 CHD: An Inflammatory Disease

Most investigators agree that atherosclerosis is a chronic inflammatory disease.[61] Pro-inflammatory factors (free radicals produced by cigarette smoking, hyperhomocysteinemia, diabetes, peroxidized lipids, hypertension, and elevated and modified blood lipids) contribute to injure the vascular endothelium, which results in alterations of its antiatherosclerotic and antithrombotic properties. This is thought to be a major step in the initiation and formation of arterial fibrostenotic lesions.[61] From a clinical point of view, however, an essential distinction should be made between unstable, lipid-rich, and leukocyte-rich lesions and stable, acellular fibrotic lesions poor in lipids, as the propensities of these two types of lesions to rupture into the lumen of an artery, whatever the degree of stenosis and lumen obstruction, are totally different.

In 1987, we proposed that inflammation and leukocytes play roles in the onset of acute CHD events.[62] This has recently been confirmed.[63–66] It is now accepted that one of the main mechanisms underlying the sudden onset of acute CHD syndromes, including unstable angina, myocardial infarction, and SCD, is the erosion or rupture of an atherosclerotic lesion[63,64] that triggers thrombotic complications and considerably enhances the risk of malignant ventricular arrhythmias.[65,66] Leukocytes have been also implicated in the occurrence of ventricular arrhythmias in clinical and experimental settings[67,68] and contribute to myocardial damage during both ischemia and reperfusion.[67] Clinical and pathological studies showed the importance of inflammatory cells and immune mediators in the occurrence of acute CHD events, and prospective epidemiological studies showed a strong and consistent association between acute CHD and systemic inflammation markers. A major question is to know why macrophages and activated lymphocytes[61] are found in atherosclerotic lesions and how they get there. Local inflammation, plaque rupture, and attendant acute CHD complications ensue.

4.4.2 Lipid Oxidation Theory of CHD

Steinberg et al. proposed in 1989 that oxidation of lipoproteins causes accelerated atherogenesis.[69] Elevated plasma levels of low density lipoproteins (LDLs) are major factors of CHD, and reduction of blood LDL levels (for instance by drugs) results in less CHD. However, the mechanism behind the effect of high LDL levels is not fully understood. The concept that LDL oxidation is a key characteristic of unstable lesions is supported by many reports.[61] Two processes have been proposed. First, when LDL particles become trapped in artery walls, they undergo progressive oxidation and are internalized by macrophages, leading to the formation of typical atherosclerotic foam cells. Oxidized LDL is chemotactic for other immune and inflammatory cells and up-regulates the expression of monocyte and endothelial cell genes involved in the inflammatory reaction.[61,69] The inflammatory response can have a profound effect on LDL,[61] creating a vicious circle of LDL oxidation, inflammation, and further LDL oxidation.

Second, oxidized LDL circulates in the plasma sufficiently long to enter and accumulate in the arterial intima, suggesting that the entry of oxidized lipoproteins within the intima may be another mechanism of lesion inflammation, in particular in patients without hyperlipidemia.[70] Elevated plasma levels of oxidized LDL are associated with CHD, and the plasma level of malondialdehyde-modified LDL is higher in patients with unstable CHD syndromes (usually associated with plaque rupture) than in patients with clinically stable CHD.[70]

In the accelerated form of CHD typical of post-transplantation patients, higher levels of lipid peroxidation[71-73] and oxidized LDL[74] were found as compared to the stable form of CHD in non-transplanted patients. Reactive oxygen metabolites and oxidants influence thrombus formation (see Reference 75 for a review), and platelet reactivity is significantly higher in transplanted patients than in non-transplanted CHD patients.[76]

The oxidized LDL theory is not inconsistent with the well established lipid-lowering treatment of CHD. There is a positive correlation between plasma levels of LDL and markers of lipid peroxidation[72,77] and low absolute LDL level results in reduced amounts of LDL available for oxidative modification. LDL levels can be lowered by drugs or by reducing saturated fats in the diet. Reduction of the oxidative susceptibility of LDL was reported after replacing dietary fat with carbohydrates. Pharmacological/quantitative (lowering of cholesterol) and nutritional/qualitative (high antioxidant intake) approaches to prevent CHD are additive and complementary, not mutually exclusive.

An alternative way to reduce LDL concentrations is to replace saturated fats with polyunsaturated fats in the diet. However, diets high in polyunsaturated fatty acids increase the polyunsaturated fatty acid content of LDL particles and render them more susceptible to oxidation, which would argue against use of such diets. As a matter of fact, in the secondary prevention of CHD, such diets failed to improve the prognosis of the patients (see Reference 78 for a review). In that context, a traditional Mediterranean diet with low saturated fat and polyunsaturated fat intake appears the best option. Diets rich in oleic acid increase the resistance of LDL to oxidation independent of the content in antioxidants[79,80] and results in leukocyte inhibition.[81] Thus, oleic acid-rich diets decrease the pro-inflammatory properties of oxidized LDL. Constituents of olive oil other than oleic acid may also inhibit LDL oxidation.[82] Various components of the Mediterranean diet may also affect LDL oxidation. For instance, alpha-tocopherol or vitamin C or a diet combining reduced fat, low-fat dairy products, and a high intake of fruits and vegetables was shown to favorably affect either LDL oxidation and/or the cellular consequences of LDL oxidation.[83,84]

Finally, significant correlation was found between certain dietary fatty acids and the fatty acid composition of human atherosclerotic plaques[85,86] which suggests that dietary fatty acids are rapidly incorporated into the plaques. This implies a direct influence of dietary fatty acids on plaque formation and rupture. It is conceivable that fatty acids that stimulate oxidation of LDL (n-6 fatty acids) induce plaque rupture, whereas those that inhibit LDL oxidation (oleic acid) inhibit leukocyte function (n-3 fatty acids)[87] or prevent endothelial activation and the expression of pro-inflammatory proteins (oleic acid and n-3 fatty acids)[88,89] helps pacify and stabilize the dangerous lesions. It is noteworthy that moderate alcohol consumption, a well-known cardioprotective factor, was recently shown to be associated with low blood levels of systemic markers of inflammation,[90] suggesting a new protective mechanism to explain the inverse relationship between alcohol and CHD rate. In the same line, the potential of dietary n-3 fatty acids to reduce the production of inflammatory cytokines[59,60] by leukocytes (as discussed in the section on dietary fatty acids and CHF) should be noted. As both dietary n-3 fatty acids and moderate alcohol consumption are major characteristics of the Mediterranean diet, it is not surprising to observe that this diet was associated with lower rates of new episodes of CHF in the Lyon Diet Heart Study.[44,91,92]

REFERENCES

1. Zipes, D.P. and Wellens, H.J., Sudden cardiac death, *Circulation*, 98, 2234, 1998.
2. de Lorgeril, M., Salen, P., Defaye, P., Mabo, P, and Paillard, F., Dietary prevention of sudden cardiac death, *Eur. Heart J.*, 23, 277, 2002.
3. Burr, M.L., Fehily, A.M., Gilbert, J.F. et al., Effects of changes in fat, fish, and fibre intakes on death and myocardial reinfarction: Diet and Reinfarction Trial (DART), *Lancet* 2, 757, 1989.
4. McLennan, P.L., Abeywardena, M.Y., and Charnock, J.S., Reversal of arrhythmogenic effects of long term saturated fatty acid intake by dietary n-3 and n-6 polyunsaturated fatty acids, *Am. J. Clin. Nutr.*, 51, 53, 1990.
5. McLennan, P.L., Abeywardena, M.Y., and Charnock, J.S., Dietary fish oil prevents ventricular fibrillation following coronary occlusion and reperfusion, *Am. Heart J.*, 16, 709, 1988.
6. Billman, G.E., Kang, J.X., and Leaf, A., Prevention of sudden cardiac death by dietary pure omega-3 polyunsaturated fatty acids in dogs, *Circulation*, 99, 2452, 1999.
7. Nair, S.D., Leitch, J., Falconer, J. et al., Cardiac (n-3) non-esterified fatty acids are selectively increased in fish oil-fed pigs following myocardial ischemia, *J. Nutr.*, 129, 1518, 1999.
8. Harris, S.W., Lu, G., Rambjor, G.S. et al., Influence of (n-3) fatty acid supplementation on the endogenous activities of plasma lipases, *Am. J. Clin. Nutr.*, 66, 254, 1997.
9. Kang, J.X., Xiao, Y.F., and Leaf, A., Free, long. chain, polyunsaturated fatty acids reduce membrane electrical excitability in neonatal rat cardiomyocyte, *Proc. Natl. Acad. Sci. USA*, 92, 3997, 1995.
10. Xiao, Y.F., Kang, J.X., Morgan, J.P. et al., Blocking effects of polyunsaturated fatty acids on Na channels of neonatal rat ventricular myocytes, *Proc. Natl. Acad. Sci. USA*, 92, 1100, 1995.
11. Xiao, Y.F., Wright, S.N., Wang, G.K. et al., N-3 fatty acids suppress voltage-gated Na currents in HEK293t cells transfected with the alpha. subunit of the human cardiac Na channel, *Proc. Natl. Acad. Sci. USA*, 95, 2680, 1998.
12. Xiao, Y.F., Gomez, A.M., Morgan, J.P. et al., Suppression of voltage-gated L-type Ca currents by polyunsaturated fatty acids in neonatal and adult cardiac myocytes, *Proc. Natl. Acad. Sci. USA*, 94, 4182, 1997.
13. Corr, P.B., Saffitz, J.E., and Sobel, B.E., What is the contribution of altered lipid metabolism to arrhythmogenesis in the ischemic heart? in *Life-Threatening Arrhythmias during Ischema and Infarction*, Hearse, D.J. et al., Eds., Raven Press, New York, 1987, 91.
14. Parratt, J.R., Coker, S.J., and Wainwright, C.L., Eicosanoids and susceptibility to ventricular arrhythmias during myocardial ischemia and reperfusion, *J. Mol. Cell. Cardiol.* (Suppl. 5), 55, 66, 1987.

15. Sellmayer, A., Witzgall, H., Lorenz, R.L. et al., Effects of dietary fish oil on ventricular premature complexes, *Am. J. Cardiol.*, 76, 974, 1995.
16. Christensen, J.H., Gustenhoff, P., Korup, E. et al., Effect of fish oil on heart rate variability in survivors of myocardial infarction: a double blind randomised controlled trial, *BMJ*, 312, 677, 1996.
17. Christensen, J.H., Christensen, M.S., Dyerberg, J. et al., Heart rate variability and fatty acid content of blood cell membranes: a dose-response study with n-3 fatty acids, *Am. J. Clin. Nutr.*, 70, 331, 1999.
18. Singh, R.B., Rastogi, S.S., Verma, R. et al., Randomised controlled trial of cardio-protective diet in patients with recent acute myocardial infarction: results of 1-year follow-up, *BMJ*, 304, 1015, 1992.
19. de Lorgeril, M., Renaud, S., Mamelle, N. et al., Mediterranean alpha-linolenic acid-rich diet in secondary prevention of coronary heart disease, *Lancet*, 343, 1454, 1994.
20. Siscovick, D.S., Raghunathan, T.E., King, I. et al., Dietary intake and cell membrane levels of long chain n-3 polyunsaturated fatty acids and the risk of primary cardiac arrest, *JAMA*, 274, 1363, 1995.
21. Kromhout, D., Bosschieter, E.B., and de Lezenne-Coulander, C., The inverse relation between fish consumption and 20-year mortality from coronary heart disease, *New Engl. J. Med.*, 312, 1205, 1985.
22. Shekelle, R.B., Missel, L., Paul, O. et al., Fish consumption and mortality from coronary heart disease, *New Engl. J. Med.*, 313, 820, 1985.
23. Albert, C.M., Hennekens, C.H., O'Donnel, C.J. et al., Fish consumption and the risk of sudden cardiac death, *JAMA*, 279, 23, 1998.
24. Daviglus, M.L., Stamler, J., Orencia, A.J. et al., Fish consumption and the 30-year risk of fatal myocardial infarction, *New Engl. J. Med.*, 336, 1046, 1997.
25. GISSI Prevenzione Investigators, Dietary supplementation with n-3 polyunsaturated fatty acids and vitamin E after myocardial infarction: results of the GISSI Prevenzione Trial, *Lancet,* 354, 447, 1999.
26. Wannamethee, G. and Shaper, A.G., Alcohol and sudden cardiac death, *Br. Heart J.*, 68, 443, 1992.
27. Kagan, A., Yano, K., Reed, D.M. et al., Predictors of sudden cardiac death among Hawaiian-Japanese men, *Am. J. Epidemiol.*, 130, 268, 1989.
28. Albert, C.M., Manson, J.E., Cook, N.R. et al., Moderate alcohol consumption and the risk of sudden cardiac death among U.S. male physicians, *Circulation*, 100, 944, 1999.
29. Rimm, E.B., Stampfer, M.J., and Ascherio, A. et al., Vitamin E consumption and the risk of coronary heart disease in men, *New Engl. J. Med.*, 328, 1450, 1993.
30. Stampfer, M.J., Hennekens, C.H., Manson, J.E. et al., Vitamin E consumption and the risk of coronary heart disease in women, *New Engl. J. Med.*, 328, 1444, 1993.
31. The Alpha-Tocopherol–Beta-Carotene Cancer Prevention Study Group, The effect of vitamin E and beta-carotene on the incidence of lung cancer and other cancers in male smokers, *New Engl. J. Med.*, 330, 1029, 1994.
32. Rapola, J.M., Virtamo, J., Ripatti, S. et al., Randomised trial of alpha-tocopherol and beta-carotene supplements on incidence of major coronary events in men with previous myocardial infarction, *Lancet*, 349, 1715, 1997.
33. Stephens, N.G., Parsons, A., Schofield, P.M. et al., Randomised controlled trial of vitamin E in patients with coronary heart disease: the Cambridge Heart Antioxidant Study (CHAOS), *Lancet*, 347, 781, 1996.
34. Sebbag, L., Forrat, R., Canet, E. et al., Effect of dietary supplementation with alpha-tocopherol on myocardial infarct size and ventricular arrhythmias in a dog model of ischemia and reperfusion, *J. Am. Coll. Cardiol.*, 24, 1580, 1994.

35. Heart Outcome Prevention Evaluation (HOPE) Study Investigators, Vitamin E supplementation and cardiovascular events in high-risk patients, *New Engl. J. Med.*, 342, 154, 2000.

36. Cowie, M.R., Mostred, A., Wood, D.A. et al., Epidemiology of heart failure, *Eur. Heart J.*, 18, 208, 1997.

37. Levine, B., Kalman, J., Mayer, L., Fillit, H.M., and Packer, M., Elevated circulating levels of tumor necrosis factor in severe chronic heart failure, *New Engl. J. Med.*, 323, 236, 1990.

38. Swan, J.W., Anker, S.D., Walton, C. et al., Insulin resistance in chronic heart failure: relation to severity and etiology of heart failure, *J. Am. Coll. Cardiol.*, 30, 527, 1997.

39. Keith, M., Geranmayegan, A., Sole, M.J. et al., Increased oxidative stress in patients with congestive heart failure, *J. Am. Coll. Cardiol.*, 31, 1352, 1998.

40. Evans, P. and Halliwell, B., Micronutrients: oxidant/antioxidant status, *Br. J. Nutr.*, 85, S67, 2001.

41. Dhalla, A.K., Hill, M., and Singal, P.K., Role of oxidative stress in transition of hypertrophy to heart failure, *J. Am. Coll. Cardiol.*, 28, 506, 1996.

42. de Lorgeril, M., Salen, P., Accominotti, M. et al., Dietary blood antioxidants in patients with chronic heart failure: insights into the potential importance of selenium in heart failure, *Eur. J. Heart Failure*, 3, 661, 2001.

43. Hornig, B., Arakawa, N., Kohler, C., and Drexler, H., Vitamin C improves endothelial function of conduit arteries in patients with chronic heart failure, *Circulation*, 97, 363, 1998.

44. de Lorgeril, M., Salen, P., Martin, J.L. et al., Mediterranean diet, traditional risk factors and the rate of cardiovascular complications after myocardial infarction: final report of the Lyon Diet Heart Study, *Circulation*, 99, 799, 1999.

45. Jacobson, A., Pihl-Lindgren, E., and Fridlund, B., Malnutrition in patients suffering from chronic heart failure: nurse's care, *Eur. J. Heart Failure*, 3, 449, 2001.

46. Pittman, J.G. and Cohen, P., The pathogenesis of cardiac cachexia, *New Engl. J. Med.*, 271, 453, 1964.

47. Anker, S.D., Clark, A.L., Kemp, M. et al., Tumor necrosis factor and steroid metabolism in chronic heart failure: possible relation to muscle wasting, *J. Am. Coll. Cardiol.*, 30, 997, 1997.

48. Tsutamoto, T., Atsuyuki, W., Matsumoto, T. et al., Relationship between tumor necrosis factor alpha and oxidative stress in the failing hearts of patients with dilated cardiomyopathy, *J. Am. Coll. Cardiol.*, 27, 2086, 2001.

49. Anker, S.D., Ponikowski, P., Varney, S. et al., Wasting as independent risk factor for mortality in chronic heart failure, *Lancet*, 349, 1050, 1997.

50. Ge, K. and Yang, G., The epidemiology of selenium deficiency in the etiological study of endemic diseases in China, *Am. J. Clin. Nutr.* (Suppl.), 57, 259S, 1993.

51. Chariot, P., Perchet, H., and Monnet, I., Dilated cardiomyopathy in HIV-infected patients, *New Engl. J. Med.*, 340, 732, 1999.

52. Shimon, I., Shlomo, A., Vered, Z. et al., Improved left ventricular function after thiamine supplementation in patients with congestive heart failure receiving long-term furosemide therapy, *Am. J. Med.*, 98, 485, 1995.

53. Levy, D., Garrison, R.J., Savage, D.D. et al., Prognostic implications of echocardiographically determined left ventricular mass in the Framingham Heart Study, *New Engl. J. Med.*, 322, 1561, 1990.

54. Koren, M.J., Devereux, R.B., Casale, N.B. et al., Relation of left ventricular mass and geometry to morbidity and mortality in uncomplicated essential hypertension, *Ann. Int. Med.*, 114, 345, 1991.

55. Dahlof, B., Pennert, K., and Hansson, L., Reversal of left ventricular hypertrophy in hypertensive patients: a meta-analysis of 109 treatment studies, *Am. J. Hypertens.*, 5, 95, 1992.

56. Sundström, J., Lind, L., Vessby, B. et al., Dyslipidemia and an unfavorable fatty acid profile predict left ventricular hypertrophy 20 years later, *Circulation*, 103, 836, 2001.

57. Gullestad, L., Aukrust, P., Ueland, T. et al., Effect of high versus low dose angiotensin converting enzyme inhibition on cytokine levels in chronic heart failure, *J. Am. Coll. Cardiol.*, 34, 2061, 1999.

58. Bozkurt, B., Torre-Amione, G., Warren, M.S. et al., Results of targeted anti-tumor necrosis factor therapy with etanercept (Enbrel) in patients with advanced heart failure, *Circulation*, 103, 1044, 2001.

59. Endres, S., Ghorbani, R., Kelley, V.E. et al., The effect of dietary supplementation with n-3 polyunsaturated fatty acids on the synthesis of interleukine-1 and tumor necrosis factor by mononuclear cells, *New Engl. J. Med.*, 320, 265, 1989.

60. Caughey, G.E., Mantzioris, E., Gibson, R.A., Cleland, L.G., and James, M.J., The effect on human tumor necrosis factor and interleukine-1 production of diets enriched in n-3 fatty acids from vegetable oil or fish oil, *Am. J. Clin. Nutr.*, 63, 116, 1996.

61. Ross, R., Atherosclerosis: an inflammatory disease, *New Engl. J. Med.*, 340, 115, 1999.

62. de Lorgeril, M. and Latour, J.G., Leukocytes, thrombosis and unstable angina, *New Engl. J. Med.*, 316, 1161, 1987.

63. Moreno, P.R., Falk, E., Palacios, J.F. et al., Macrophage infiltration in acute coronary syndromes: implications for plaque rupture, *Circulation*, 90, 775, 1994.

64. Van der Wal, A.C., Becker, E.C., Van der los, D.S. et al., Site of intimal rupture or erosion of thrombosed coronary atherosclerotic plaques is characterized by an inflammatory process irrespective of the dominant plaque morphology, *Circulation*, 89, 36, 1994.

65. Farb, A., Burk, A.P., Tang, A.L. et al., Coronary plaque erosion without rupture into a lipid core: a frequent cause of coronary thrombosis in sudden coronary death, *Circulation*, 93, 1354, 1996.

66. Davies, M.J. and Thomas, A., Thrombosis and acute coronary artery lesions in sudden cardiac ischemic death, *New Engl. J. Med.*, 310, 1137, 1984.

67. de Lorgeril, M., Basmadjian, A., Lavallée, M. et al., Influence of leukopenia on collateral flow, reperfusion flow, reflow ventricular fibrillation, and infarct size in dogs, *Am. Heart J.*, 117, 523, 1989.

68. Kuzuya, T., Hoshida, S., Suzuki, K. et al., Polymorphonuclear leukocyte activity and ventricular arrhythmia in acute myocardial infarction, *Am. J. Cardiol.*, 62, 868, 1988.

69. Steinberg, D., Parthasarathy, S., Carew, T.E., Khoo, J.C., and Witztum, J.L., Beyond cholesterol: modifications of low density lipoproteins that increase its atherogenicity, *New Engl. J. Med.*, 320, 915, 1989.

70. Hodis, H.N., Kramsch, D.M., Avogaro, P. et al., Biochemical and cytotoxic characteristics of an *in vivo* circulating oxidized low density lipoprotein, *J. Lipid Res.*, 356, 669, 1994.

71. Holvoet, P., Stassen, J.M., Van Cleemput, J., Collen, D., and Vanhaecke, J., Correlation between oxidized low density lipoproteins and coronary artery disease in heart transplant patients, *Arterioscler. Thromb. Vasc. Biol.*, 18, 100, 1998.

72. Chancerelle, Y., de Lorgeril, M., Viret, R. et al., Increased lipid peroxidation in cyclosporin-treated heart transplant recipients, *Am. J. Cardiol.*, 68, 813, 1991.

73. de Lorgeril M., Richard, M.J., Arnaud, J. et al., Lipid peroxides and antioxidant defenses in accelerated transplantation-associated arteriosclerosis, *Am. Heart J.*, 125, 974, 1992.

74. Holvoet, P., Perez, G., Zhao, Z. et al., Malondialdehyde-modified low density lipo-proteins in patients with atherosclerotic disease, *J. Clin. Invest.*, 95, 2611, 1995.
75. Ambrosio, G., Tritto, I., and Golino, P., Reactive oxygen metabolites and arterial thrombosis, *Cardiovasc. Res.*, 34, 445, 1997.
76. de Lorgeril, M., Dureau, G., Boissonnat, P. et al., Platelet function and composition in heart transplant recipients compared with nontransplanted coronary patients, *Arterioscler. Thromb. Vasc. Biol.*, 12, 222, 1992.
77. Zock, P.L. and Katan, M.B., Diet, LDL oxidation and coronary artery disease, *Am. J. Clin. Nutr.*, 68, 759, 1998.
78. de Lorgeril, M., Salen, P., Monjaud, I. et al., The diet heart hypothesis in secondary prevention of coronary heart disease, *Eur. Heart J.*, 18, 14, 1997.
79. Bonamone, A., Pagnan, A., Biffanti, S. et al., Effect of dietary monounsaturated and polyunsaturated fatty acids on the susceptibility of plasma low density lipoproteins to oxidative modification, *Arterioscl. Thromb. Vasc. Biol.*, 12, 529, 1992.
80. Tsimikas, S. and Reaven, P.D., The role of dietary fatty acids in lipoprotein oxidation and atherosclerosis, *Curr. Opin. Lipidol.*, 9, 301, 1998.
81. Mata, P., Alonso, R., Lopez-Farre, A. et al., Effect of dietary fat saturation on LDL and monocyte adhesion to human endothelial cells *in vitro*, *Arterioscler. Thromb. Vasc. Biol.*, 16, 1347, 1996.
82. Visioli, F., Bellomo, G., Montedoro, G. et al., Low density lipoprotein oxidation is inhibited *in vitro* by olive oil constituents, *Atherosclerosis*, 117, 25, 1995.
83. Jialial, I. and Grundy, S.M., Effect of combined supplementation with alpha-toco-pherol, ascorbate and beta-carotene on low density lipoprotein oxidation, *Circulation*, 88, 2780, 1993.
84. Miller, E.R., III, Appel, L.J., and Risby, T.H., Effect of dietary patterns on measures of lipid peroxidation: results of a randomized clinical trial, *Circulation*, 98, 2390, 1998.
85. Felton, C.V., Crook, D., Davies, M.J., and Oliver, M.F., Dietary polyunsaturated fatty acids and composition of human aortic plaques, *Lancet*, 344, 1195, 1994.
86. Rapp, J.H., Connor, W.E., Lin, D.S., and Porter, J.M., Dietary eicosapentanoic acid and docosahexaenoic acid from fish oil: their incorporation into advanced human atherosclerotic plaques, *Arterioscler. Thromb. Vasc. Biol.*, 11, 903, 1991.
87. Lee, T.H., Hoover, R.L., Williams, J.D. et al., Effect of dietary enrichment with eicosapentanoic and docosahexaenoic acids on *in vitro* neutrophil and monocyte leukotriene generation and neutrophile function, *New Engl. J. Med.*, 312, 1217, 1985.
88. De Caterina, R., Cybulsky, M.I., Clinton, S.K., Gimbrone, M.A., and Libby, P., The omega-3 fatty acid docosahexaenoate reduces cytokine-induced expression of proat-herogenic and proinflammatory proteins in human endothelial cells, *Arterioscler. Thromb. Vasc. Biol.*, 14, 1829, 1994.
89. Carluccio, M.A., Massaro, M., Bonfrate, C. et al., Oleic acid inhibits endothelial cell activation, *Arterioscler. Thromb. Vasc. Biol.*, 19, 220, 1999.
90. Imhof, A., Froehlich, M., Brenner, H., Boeing, H., Pepys, M.B., and Koenig, W., Effect of alcohol consumption on systemic markers of inflammation, *Lancet*, 357, 763, 2001.
91. Kris-Etherton P., Eckel, R., Howard, B., St. Jeor, S., and Bazzarre, T., Lyon Diet Heart Study: benefits of a Mediterranean style National Cholesterol Education Pro-gram/American Heart Association Step I Dietary Pattern on cardiovascular disease, *Circulation*, 103, 1823, 2001.
92. Marchioli, R., Valagussa, F., Del Pinto, M. et al., Mediterranean dietary habits and risk of death after myocardial infarction, *Circulation* (Suppl. 2), 102, 379, 2000.

5 Effects of Nutritional Education on Cardiovascular Risk Factors

Wanda J.E. Bemelmans

CONTENTS

5.1 INTRODUCTION

Traditional risk factors for coronary heart disease (CHD) that can be modified by changing dietary intake include hypercholesterolemia, hypertension, being overweight, and diabetes mellitus. Overall, changing dietary habits toward a more healthy diet will decrease incidence and mortality of CHD.[1] Consensus more or less covers the key nutritional messages that effectively prevent CHD. These include limited intake of saturated fat, consumption of many fruits and vegetables, and increased intake of fatty fish.[2]

During the 1990s, secondary prevention studies showed remarkable reductions in CHD and total mortality in the intervention groups who obtained dietary guidelines comparable with current dietary guidelines.[3,4] It should be stressed that the beneficial effect of the dietary therapy was not mediated entirely by effects on established cardiovascular risk factors. For example, in the Lyon Diet Heart Study, serum cholesterol levels dropped by 5% in both intervention and control groups. Hence, it is important to realize that nutritional education can prevent the onset of CHD by mechanistic pathways that are partially independent of effects on traditional CHD risk factors.

0-8493-1674-X/04/$0.00+$1.50

Nevertheless, in usual health care, the effects of nutritional health education are evaluated primarily in terms of their effects on total cholesterol level and blood pressure. According to the guidelines for treating hypercholesterolemia and hypertension, the first step should be providing nutritional advice.[5,6] Some patients are indicated to receive dietary therapy only because prescribing medication is not considered cost effective. However, numerous barriers exist in providing dietary therapy in the course of usual health care, for example limited nutritional knowledge and time of physicians and insufficient dietary compliance by patients. Furthermore, limited data exist on the most effective way of providing nutritional education as part of usual health care,[7]

In the northern region of the Netherlands, we executed a primary prevention project focused on coronary heart disease (the MARGARIN project). Patients included had at least three cardiovascular risk factors. The effects of a nutritional education program including group meetings organized by a dietician (intervention group) were compared to the effects of mailed leaflets containing the usual guidelines (control group) during 3 years of follow-up. The latter intervention is comparable to "care as usual." This chapter describes the results on cardiovascular risk factors and dietary intake. The discussion paragraph explains the results in comparison with other research.

5.2 CHARACTERISTICS OF MARGARIN PROJECT

The study design and characteristics of the MARGARIN project, an acronym of Mediterranean Alpha-linolenic enRiched Groningen dietARy INtervention study, have been described in detail elsewhere.[8] One of the main research questions was to compare the effects of a nutritional education program (intervention group) to the effects of a printed leaflet sent by regular mail to a control group. This chapter describes the results with respect to total cholesterol level, blood pressure, body mass index (BMI), and dietary intake.

The baseline examinations of the MARGARIN project were performed in November 1997 and follow-up investigations were organized after 16 weeks and 1, 2, and 3 years. During examinations, several cardiovascular risk factors were assessed and dietary intake was measured by self-administered semi-quantitative food frequency questionnaires. Participants were eligible for inclusion if they had elevated serum total cholesterol levels (6.0 to 8.0 mmol/l) and at least two of the following cardiovascular risk factors: high blood pressure or use of antihypertensive medication, BMI ≥ 27 kg/m^2, present smoking, and a (family) history of CHD. Exclusion criteria were diabetes mellitus, hypothyroidism, and use of acetylsalicylic acid, anticoagulants, or lipid lowering drugs. At baseline, 266 participants completed the examinations (intervention group n = 103, control group n = 163). During the 3-year study period, 29% of the intervention group and 34% of the control group dropped out for several reasons.

5.3 CONTENT OF NUTRITIONAL
EDUCATION PROGRAM

The intervention group was divided into groups of 10 persons, and all subjects were invited to attend three 2-hour meetings organized in March 1998 (the first year of the project). At least two meetings were attended by 68% of men and 78% of women.

Four booklets with core information were distributed and also sent to participants who did not attend the meeting. In the second year of the project, in March 1999, the research dietician organized a 2-hour meeting that focused on reduction of weight. The meeting started with a brief reinforcement of the prior educational messages. In the third year of the project, every participant was invited to a screening for physical fitness. The intervention group was offered a physical training program (2 hours a week). In addition to the educational meetings, the messages were reinforced by written correspondence once a year. The specific dietary guidelines were daily consumption of 5 to 7 slices of bread, 200 to 400 g of vegetables, two pieces of fruit, two to three dairy products, and fish twice a week at dinner.

During the first year, the control group was sent a leaflet containing standard nutritional guidelines via regular mail. In the third year, the control group was invited to a screening test for physical fitness, but was not offered the opportunity to participate in the organized exercise program. The specific dietary guidelines of the control group differed a little from those of the intervention group because the usual Dutch guidelines at that time did not include specific advice on fish consumption. It should be noted, however, that both intervention and control groups of the MAR-GARIN project had free access to a margarine rich in polyunsaturated fatty acids during the first 2 years of the project. This second intervention of this study is described in more detail elsewhere.[8]

5.4   RESULTS

At baseline, the intervention group (IG) included fewer men (37%) than the control group (CG, 49%) and more users of antihypertensive medication (IG = 57%, CG = 43%; $p < 0.05$). No significant baseline differences existed in cardiovascular risk factors and dietary intakes between intervention and control groups (Table 5.1).

After 3 years, the BMI increased by 2% in both IG and CG, and systolic blood pressure increased by 1.4 mmHg (1%) in the IG and by 2.9 mmHg (2%) in the CG. Serum total cholesterol levels decreased by 4% in the IG and by 6% in the CG. During the study period, approximately 12% of the IG and 6% of the CG started to use lipid lowering drugs. The use of lipid lowering medication was self-reported and some misclassification may have occurred. When persons with decreases over 1.5 mmol/l are excluded from the analyses (IG n = 2, CG n = 13), the total cholesterol level dropped by 4% in the IG and by 2% in the CG.

No significant differences between IG and CG were observed regarding total cholesterol and BMI during 3 years of intervention (Table 5.2). The intervention group tended to have lower blood pressure after 1 year (mean net difference = −2.6 mmHg; $p = 0.14$). When the analyses excluded users of antihypertensive drugs at baseline (IG n = 40, CG n = 88), systolic blood pressure decreased by −2.9 mmHg in the IG and increased by +0.8 mmHg in the CG after 1 year of follow-up (p of net difference = 0.10). However, this positive effect did not remain after 2 and 3 years of follow-up (data not shown).

Regarding dietary intake, the IG had consistently lower intakes of total and saturated fat and higher fish intakes during the study period. The initial positive effect of fruit consumption was not statistically significant after 2 and 3 years of follow-up (Table 5.2).

TABLE 5.1
Baseline Characteristics of MARGARIN Population

	Intervention Group		Control Group	
	Men n = 38	Women n = 64	Men n = 78	Women n = 83
Age	52.9 (8.8)	56.1 (10.4)	52.3 (10.3)	54.5 (8.5)
Serum total cholesterol (mmol/l)	6.6 (0.7)	6.9 (0.7)	6.6 (0.7)	6.7 (0.8)
Systolic blood pressure (mmHg)	143 (21)	148 (24)	144 (22)	145 (22)
Present smoking (%)	58%	41%	62%	40%
Body mass index (kg/m²)	29.6 (2.7)	29.9 (4.4)	28.7 (3.4)	30.9 (5.7)
	Dietary intake:			
Total fat (% of energy)	38.0 (6.3)	37.5 (7.2)	39.0 (5.7)	37.4 (7.7)
Saturated fat (% of energy)	14.3 (3.2)	13.8 (2.9)	14.1 (3.1)	14.4 (3.6)
Fruits (g/day)	228 (187)	293 (171)	256 (174)	277 (172)
Median	209	271	271	277
Vegetables (g/day)	140 (60)	139 (53)	155 (86)	134 (51)
Median	136	125	129	125
Fish (g/day)	15 (15)	21 (22)	32 (43)[a]	17 (20)
Median	9	14	19	10

[a] Difference with intervention group $p < 0.05$.

5.5 DISCUSSION: HOW DO RESULTS COMPARE TO OTHER RESEARCH?

The MARGARIN study showed that group nutritional education had no additional positive effects on cardiovascular risk factors when compared to distribution of a printed leaflet. Regarding dietary intake, however, the nutritional education program significantly decreased intake of total and saturated fat and increased fish consumption in the intervention group.

The study had three main limitations. First, the subjects of the control group had free access to a margarine rich in polyunsaturated fat during the first 2 years of the project. This type of intervention alone is expected to decrease serum total cholesterol. As a result, it became more difficult for the education program to establish additional positive effects, especially during the first 2 years. Second, randomization to type of education was not performed on an individual basis and some baseline differences existed. For example, the intervention group contained a higher proportion of users of antihypertensive medication. Third, the study population reported sufficient fruit intake at baseline. This may indicate that the subjects were already eating according to guidelines ("ceiling effect") or that fruit consumption was overestimated and thus not validly assessed.

In general, characteristics of nutritional intervention studies that influence the effect on cardiovascular risk factors include (1) the intensiveness of the education, (2) period of follow-up, (3) baseline levels of risk factors and dietary intake, and

TABLE 5.2
Net Differences (95% Confidence Interval) between Intervention and Control Groups in Effects on Cardiovascular Risk Factors and Dietary Intake after 1, 2, and 3 Years of Follow-Up[a]

	1 Year	2 Years	3 Years
	IG n = 98; CG n = 155	IG n = 94; CG n = 142	IG n = 73; CG n = 108
Serum total cholesterol (mmol/l) [b]	0.1 (–0.1, 0.2)	0.0 (–0.2, 0.2)	0.1 (–0.1, 0.4)
Systolic blood pressure (mmHg) [c]	–2.6 (–6.2, 0.9)	0.2 (–3.6, 3.9)	–2.0 (–7.2, 3.1)
Body mass index (kg/m²)	0.0 (–0.3, 0.3)	0.2 (–0.2, 0.6)	0.1 (–0.4, 0.5)
Dietary intake	IG n = 92; CG n = 148	IG n = 81; CG n = 130	IG n = 67; CG n = 110
Total fat (% of energy)	–2.4 (–3.6, –1.1)[d]	–2.0 (–3.4, –0.6)[d]	–2.0 (–3.7, –0.2)[d]
Saturated fat (% of energy)	–1.4 (–1.9, –0.9)[d]	0.9 (1.4, –0.3)[d]	–1.2 (–2.0, –0.4)[d]
Fruits (g/day)	56 (16, 96)[d]	35 (–8, 78)	6 (–34, 46)
Vegetables (g/day)	3 (–16, 21)	4 (–10, 19)	21 (1, 41)[d]
Fish (g/day)	18 (11, 25)[d]	15 (8, 22)[d]	11 (4, 18)[d]

[a] Negative numbers indicate larger decreases in the intervention group; all analyses have been adjusted for baseline level and gender.
[b] Users of lipid lowering drugs are excluded.
[c] Adjusted for baseline level, gender, and use of antihypertensive drugs at baseline.
[d] $p < 0.05$.

(4) established effects on dietary habits, in particular saturated fat intake. Reviews and meta-analyses of nutritional intervention studies are difficult to interpret because the individual studies have heterogeneous designs. Nevertheless, an indication of the average effects is provided. A review by Yu-Poth et al. concluded that serum total cholesterol can be decreased on average by 10%.[9] Ebrahim et al. found an average net difference between intervention and control groups of –0.14 mmol/l for serum total cholesterol and –2.7 mmHg for systolic blood pressure.[10] Since Ebrahim et al. included studies with a follow-up for only 26 weeks, it is not surprising that the MARGARIN study results (serum total cholesterol decrease of 4% in IG and no difference in CG; mean net difference in systolic blood pressure of –2.6 mmHg after 1 year) are in line with their conclusion.

In general, nutritional education studies with longer periods of follow-up report disappointing effects on established cardiovascular risk factors. However, high quality research in this field of research is scarce[7] and the positive results of individual long-term studies should not be denied. For example, Wing et al. reported a net difference in serum total cholesterol between intervention and control groups of –0.30 mmol/l after 2 years of follow-up. The participants were recruited through a newspaper and may have been highly motivated to change their dietary behaviors.[11] A large beneficial effect on serum total cholesterol when motivated persons are included was noted by Baer et al.[12] In their nonrandomized study, serum total cholesterol decreased by 12% (–0.72 mmol/l) after 1 year of follow-up. The refusals were included as a control group and group serum total cholesterol did not change at all in the control group. It may be concluded that, depending on study characteristics, some moderate positive effects can be achieved on cardiovascular risk factors after longer periods of follow-up.

The MARGARIN study did not succeed in this respect — partly because of limitations of the study design described above. However, regarding dietary intake, the nutritional education program significantly decreased intake of total and saturated fats and increased fish consumption in the intervention group. These results can be considered important regarding prevention of cardiac events. As cited in the introduction, not all positive effects of changed dietary habits are mediated by effects on established cardiovascular risk factors. For example, increased fish intake can be cardioprotective by preventing cardiac arrhythmias.[13] It is noteworthy that we could verify the reported fish intake by changes in the fatty acid composition of the cholesteryl ester (unpublished results). Hence, it can be concluded that group nutrition education actually changed dietary behavior. Eventually, these changes are expected to delay onset of coronary heart disease. However, due to limited power, the MARGARIN study could not examine the effects of the nutritional education program on final cardiac events.

5.6 CONCLUSION

The nutritional education program had no additional positive effects on cardiovascular risk factors as compared to a printed leaflet sent by regular mail. However, long-term beneficial effects were established for intake of fish and saturated fats. These dietary changes may prevent occurrence of coronary heart disease by mechanistic pathways that are partially independent of effects on established cardiovascular risk factors.

REFERENCES

1. Expert Panel on Population Strategies for Blood Cholesterol Reduction, A statement from the National Cholesterol Education Program, National Heart, Lung, and Blood Institute, National Institutes of Health, *Circulation*, 83, 2154, 1991.
2. Kromhout, D., Menotti, A., Kesteloot, H., and Sans, S., Prevention of coronary heart disease and lifestyle: evidence from prospective cross-cultural, cohort, and intervention studies, *Circulation*, 105, 893, 2002.
3. de Lorgeril, M., Renaud, S., Mamelle, N., et al., Mediterranean alpha-linolenic acid-rich diet in secondary prevention of coronary heart disease, *Lancet*, 343, 1454, 1994.
4. Singh, R.B., Dubnov, G., Niaz, M.A., et al., Effect of an Indo-Mediterranean diet on progression of coronary artery disease in high risk patients (Indo-Mediterranean Diet Heart Study): a randomised single-blind trial, *Lancet*, 360, 1455, 2002.
5. Expert Panel on Detection, Evaluation, and Treatment of High Blood Cholesterol in Adults (Adult Treatment Panel III), Executive summary of the Third Report of the National Cholesterol Education Program (NCEP), *JAMA*, 285, 2846, 2001.
6. World Health Organization, 1999 International Society of Hypertension guidelines for the management of hypertension, *J. Hypert.*, 17, 151, 1999.

7. Thompson, R.L., Summerbell, C.D., Hooper, L., Higgins, J.P.T., Little, P.S., Talbot, D., and Ebrahim, S., Dietary advice given by a dietitian versus other health professional or self-help resources to reduce blood cholesterol, Cochrane Library Issue 3, Update Software, Oxford, 2002.

8. Bemelmans, W.J.E., Broer, J., Feskens, E.J.M., Smit, A.J., Muskiet, F.A.J., Lefrandt, J.D., Bom, V.J.J., May, J.F., and Meyboom-de Jong, B., Effect of an increased intake of α-linolenic acid and group nutritional education on cardiovascular risk factors: the Mediterranean Alpha-linolenic Enriched Groningen Dietary Intervention (MARGA-RIN) study, *Am. J. Clin. Nutr.*, 75, 221, 2002.

9. Yu-Poth, S., Zhao, G, Etherton, T., Naglak, M., Jonnalagadda, S., and Kris-Etherton, P.M., Effects of the National Cholesterol Education Program's step I and step II dietary intervention programs on cardiovascular disease risk factors: a meta-analysis, *Am. J. Clin. Nutr.*, 69, 632, 1999.

10. Ebrahim, S. and Davey-Smith, G., Systematic review of randomised controlled trials of multiple risk factor interventions for preventing coronary heart disease, *BMJ*, 314, 1666, 1997.

11. Wing, R.R., Venditti, E., Jakicic, J.M., Polley, B.A., and Lang, W., Lifestyle intervention in overweight individuals with a family history of diabetes, *Diabetes Care*, 21, 350, 1998.

12. Baer, J.T., Improved plasma cholesterol levels in men after a nutrition education program at the worksite, *J. Am. Diet. Assoc.*, 93, 658, 1993.

13. Leaf A., The electrophysiological basis for the antiarrhythmic actions of polyunsaturated fatty acids, *Eur. Heart J.*, 3 (Suppl. D), D98, 2001.

Section II

Nutrients and Heart Disease

6 Micronutrients and Cardiovascular Disease

Klaus K.A. Witte and Andrew L. Clark

CONTENTS

0-8493-1674-X/04/$0.00+$1.50
© 2004 by CRC Press LLC

6.1 INTRODUCTION

Cardiovascular disease is the greatest cause of mortality in developed countries and diet plays an important role in contributing to the development and progression of ischemic heart disease (IHD). The influences of general nutrition and micronutrients such as vitamins and minerals on the progression of IHD are poorly understood and recent studies have done little to clarify the situation.

A micronutrient can be regarded as any essential dietary component present in trace amounts. Micronutrients have multiple roles both as participants in many important metabolic processes throughout the body and to counter the oxidative stress resulting from normal metabolism and daily exposure to environmental agents. They can also serve to facilitate communications, aid muscle contraction, and maintain stable tissue environments.

The most common cause of micronutrient deficiency is a consequence of reduced dietary intake and the role of a particular micronutrient is often uncovered when the consequences of dietary deficiencies such as selenium deficiency (Keshan disease) in China and iodine deficiency (thyroid disease) in the U.K. manifest themselves. (Table 6.1 provides a summary of particular micronutrient deficiencies and their possible contribution to cardiovascular disease.) However, micronutrient deficiency in cardiovascular disease could also be a product of increased losses resulting from the condition, medical therapy, or increased requirements, for example, due to greater levels of oxidative stress. Acute supplementation of individual agents in patients with established coronary disease or at high risk of future events has generally been unsuccessful in randomised trials. This chapter reviews the potential cardiovascular benefits of individual micronutrient supplementation using animal and *in vitro* studies, and examines studies aimed at prevention and treatment of cardiovascular disease in humans.

6.2 MINERALS

6.2.1 Calcium

Ninety-nine percent of the body's calcium is stored as hydroxyapatite $[Ca_{10}(OH)_2(PO_4)_6]$ in the skeleton. Plasma calcium increases under the influence of vitamin D and its metabolites and parathormone. Calcitonin, a thyroid hormone, lowers plasma calcium by inhibiting bone resorption.

Dietary salt, protein, and caffeine all increase urinary calcium loss. Calcium absorption is reduced in individuals over 70 because the gut may become less sensitive to vitamin D and also because of lower renal vitamin D synthesis. Vitamin D_3 or cholecalciferol is derived from the effect of ultraviolet radiation on 7-dehydrocholesterol. Elderly patients in temperate climates who tend to have less exposure to sunlight also have less 7-dehyrocholesterol in their skin and therefore produce less vitamin D after exposure to ultraviolet light.[1]

Postmenopausal women with low intakes of calcium have higher mortality from IHD.[2] Intriguing evidence from an experiment using chick embryos incubated without their shells, i.e., without their usual sources of calcium, suggests that severe calcium deficiency accelerates smooth muscle hypertrophy and cardiomyocyte proliferation

TABLE 6.1
Potential Contribution of Micronutrient Deficiency to Cardiovascular Disease (CVD)

Micronutrient	Deficiency State	Possible Relevance to CVD
Thiamine	Beri beri	Specific cardiomyopathy and frusemide-induced thiamine deficiency worsening heart failure and renal failure
Riboflavin		Increased prevalence in children with chronic heart failure; possible abnormal lipid metabolism
Magnesium	Arrhythmias	Arrythmogenic, particularly with digoxin; can worsen heart failure and increase symptoms of fatigue; may accelerate atherosclerosis
Calcium/Vitamin D	Osteoporosis	Hypertension, smooth muscle hypertrophy, and increased effects of endothelin; arrythmogenesis, long QT, torsades de pointes, and ventricular fibrillation; osteoporosis common in CHF patients; hypocalcemia-induced cardiomyopathy
Zinc		Contractile dysfunction, particularly in combination with ethanol; increased oxidative stress
Copper		Myocyte damage; myofibrillar disarray; copper-deficient cardiomyopathy
Selenium		Decreased antioxidant capacity; reduced smooth muscle relaxation; increased myocyte electrical vulnerability; Keshan disease; peripartum cardiomyopathy
Vitamin A		Impaired cell-mediated immunity; reduced antioxidant capacity
Niacin	Pellagra	Unknown
Vitamin B_6		Can lead to impaired immunity; elevation of homocysteine levels
Pantothenic acid (vitamin B_5)		None
Folate	Macrocytic anemia	Common in the elderly; homocysteine levels raised; increased risk of symptomatic coronary disease; impaired endothelial function
Vitamin B_{12}	Pernicious anemia	Homocysteine levels raised
Vitamin C	Scurvy	Increased risk of stroke; impaired endothelial function; reduced antioxidant capacity
Vitamin E		Increased susceptibility to free radicals; reduced platelet aggregation; inhibition of smooth muscle proliferation
Ubiquinone		Associated with increased mortality and increased oxidative stress in CHF

(accelerated heart weight gain), decelerates sarcomeric protein expression, and induces atherogenic disorders (higher blood pressure) *in vivo.*[3]

Hypocalcemia is potentially proarrhythmogenic. It is associated with QT prolongation[4] and torsades de pointes[5] and hypocalcemic-associated ventricular fibrillation has been reported.[6] Patients with heart failure demonstrated increased bone turnover and a higher incidence of osteoporosis.[7] Hypocalcemia can lead to cardiomyopathy, usually in young children with congenital causes for the hypocalcemia, but the response to calcium supplementation can often be dramatic.[8–10]

6.2.2 MAGNESIUM

Magnesium, the major intercellular divalent cation, is a cofactor in reactions utilizing adenosine triphosphate (ATP) and is essential for deoxyribonucleic acid (DNA) replication and ribonucleic acid (RNA) and protein synthesis. Magnesium is absorbed from the small intestine and excreted in the urine. Loop and thiazide diuretics increase magnesium loss.

Magnesium deficiency is associated with an increase in the rate of ventricular ectopic beats, both in the presence of left ventricular dysfunction[11] and normal cardiac function.[12] In rats, magnesium deficiency can increase the rate of adrenaline-induced ventricular tachycardia.[13] Hypomagnesemia may potentiate the contractile response of smooth muscle to oxidizing agents, thereby accelerating atherosclerosis.[14] In animal studies, hypomagnesemia leads to hypertension, heart failure, and myocardial fibrosis.[15–17] More than 30% of patients with CHF are magnesium-deficient,[19] which is associated with a worse prognosis in CHF.[19–21] The deficiency is a particular problem in patients with heart failure and atrial fibrillation; it can precipitate digoxin toxicity.[22,23] Hypomagnesemic heart failure is described in anorexia nervosa and correction of the electrolyte imbalance leads to improvement in left ventricular function.[24] Muscular magnesium deficiency, which often follows prolonged serum deficiency, may contribute to symptoms of fatigue and also causes positive sodium and negative potassium balances.[25]

Magnesium supplementation is associated with a fall in the rate of ventricular arrhythmias in patients with chronic heart failure,[26,27] atrial fibrillation,[28-30] and digoxin toxicity.[30] It may also be useful in the management of atrial fibrillation in patients with Wolff–Parkinson–White syndrome.[32] Torsades de pointes also often responds to magnesium,[33–35] even if there is no overt biochemical deficiency. Two randomised studies have demonstrated no benefit of intravenous magnesium in acute myocardial infarction in humans.[36,37]

6.2.3 ZINC

Zinc is absorbed mainly through the duodenum, and although absorption is unaffected by age, it is reduced by low protein diets. Elderly patients may show a 5% incidence of frank biochemical deficiency, with 20% displaying symptoms suggestive of moderate deficiency such as loss of taste acuity.[38]

Zinc is a powerful site-specific antioxidant.[39] Deficiency leads to elevated oxidative stress and cholesterol levels in rats.[40,41] A combination of zinc deficiency and ethanol can lead to contractile dysfunction in pre-ischemic conditions in the rat model.[42] Zinc deficiency has been noted in patients using angiotensin-converting enzyme inhibitors (ACEi) for hypertension.[43]

6.2.4 COPPER

Copper is absorbed through active processes from the stomach and duodenum. Excretion occurs mainly via the gastrointestinal tract. Deficiency is rare but has been seen in patients receiving total parenteral nutrition (TPN) and premature infants. Copper is also a powerful antioxidant and is involved in the acute phase reaction. As such it is involved in the regulation of oxidative free radicals and deficiency increases lipoprotein peroxidation.[44] Copper-deficient cardiomyopathy has been described in patients on TPN.[45] This may be due to decreased cytochrome C oxidase activity[46] that causes a reduction in mitochondrial activity. Experimental copper deficiency in rats leads to increased risk of myocyte oxidative damage[47] and long-term copper restriction can lead to myofibrillar disarray and mitochondrial fragmentation.[48] Copper deficiency in humans is associated with elevated cholesterol levels.[49,50]

6.2.5 SELENIUM

Selenium is absorbed principally in the duodenum. Its main function is as an antioxidant in glutathione peroxidase (GSHPx) — an enzyme and major intracellular antioxidant. Selenoprotein P is postulated to serve as a major extracellular antioxidant.[51] Selenium is a powerful antioxidant in its own right and also supports other antioxidant processes.[52] Pure selenium deficiency is rare, but symptoms may occur in cases of additional oxidative stress due to deficiency of other antioxidant systems such as vitamin E. Selenium may preserve the ability of myocardial cells to produce ubiquinone, another powerful antioxidant, and also reduce its breakdown[53,54] (see Section 6.4.2).

Low selenium levels may predispose an individual to ischemic heart disease and peripheral vascular disease.[55] Selenium given to pigs during induced acute myocardial infarction suppressed the electrical vulnerability of myocardial cell membranes.[55] Selenium also causes smooth muscle relaxation and may therefore become useful in the therapy of hypertension.[56]

Selenium deficiency correlates with clinical assessments of severity of chronic heart failure (n = 21).[57] Selenium deficiency impairs the ability of rat sarcoplasmic reticulum to take up calcium[58] and leads to ultrastructural changes such as loss of cristae in the mitochondria.[59] Selenium deficiency is the cause of an endemic cardiomyopathy known as Keshan disease in China; selenium replacement improved the cardiomyopathy.[60] Cardiomyopathies induced by selenium deficiency have also been described in patients on long-term TPN in Western countries.[61] Selenium deficiency is also a risk factor for peripartum cardiomyopathy.[62]

6.3 VITAMINS

6.3.1 VITAMIN A

Vitamin A originates from two classes of compounds: pre-formed vitamin A (retinol and related compounds) and carotenoids. Vitamin A is involved in cellular differentiation, morphogenesis, glycoprotein synthesis, gene expression, immunity, and growth. Its deficiency reduces cell-mediated immunity[63] and leads to increased susceptibility to infection and increased morbidity from respiratory diseases. Vitamin A deficiency mediates its effects on the cardiovascular system through reduced antioxidant activity.[64] Low vitamin A intake is associated with an increase in the risk of acute myocardial infarction.[64] Some studies, but not all,[66] suggest that vitamin A supplementation may reduce overall cardiovascular mortality. Little clear evidence supports its routine supplementation in patients with heart failure,[67] in combination with vitamin E and selenium[68] or alone.[69]

6.3.2 THIAMINE (B$_1$)

Although thiamine is readily absorbed, its turnover is rapid and body stores are small. Thiamine is lost in the urine, and dietary deficiency can lead to low plasma thiamine within 30 days. Thiamine is a coenzyme for several decarboxylation steps in carbohydrate metabolism. Deficiency leads to impaired tissue oxygenation through inhibition of both the citric acid cycle and hexose monophosphate shunt.

The two main forms of thiamine deficiency in humans are beri beri and Wernicke–Korsakoff syndrome. In Western countries, beri beri is occasionally seen in chronic alcoholics. High output cardiac failure is seen with acute beri beri. The features include a bounding pulse with warm extremities. Peripheral edema due to the accumulation of pyruvate and lactate in the tissues leads to intense vasodilation. Skeletal muscle blood flow increases while cerebral and renal blood flows decrease. Response to thiamine is brisk, with diuresis and full recovery. The accumulation of pyruvate and lactate happens with exercise and does not occur in less active patients, where perhaps the first symptom noticed is encephalopathy (Wernicke–Korsakoff syndrome).

Frusemide-induced thiamine deficiency was first described in rats.[70] Moderate thiamine deficiency can occur in hospitalized elderly patients[71,72] and chronic heart failure patients on loop diuretics.[73,74] Thiamine deficiency reduces myocardial contractile performance.[75] Thiamine uptake by cardiac myocytes is impaired by both digoxin and frusemide; the drugs have an additive effect if taken together.[76] Thiamine supplementation in patients with moderate to severe chronic heart failure can increase left ventricular ejection fraction and improve symptoms (Figure 6.1).[77,78] Post-transplant heart failure can also respond to high dose thiamine supplementation.[79]

6.3.3 RIBOFLAVIN (B$_2$)

Riboflavin forms parts of two important coenzymes, flavin mononucleotide (FMN) and flavin adenine dinucleotide (FAD); both are oxidizing agents. Rats fed riboflavin-deficient diets showed abnormal lipid metabolism and a reduction in the beta-oxidation of fatty acids.[80] Children with chronic heart failure due to congenital heart disease have increased risk of riboflavin deficiency.[81] It is, however, not known whether riboflavin deficiency has a detrimental effect on cardiac functioning.

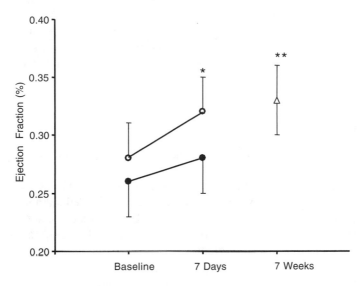

FIGURE 6.1 Left ventricular ejection fraction (mean +/– SEM) at the end of the double-blind study (week 1) and at the end of the open ambulatory phase (week 7). * = $p < 0.05$, thiamine versus placebo, end of week 1. ** = $p < 0.01$, all patients, end of week 7 versus baseline. (From Shimon, I. et al., *Am. J. Med.*, 98, 485, 1995. With permission.)

6.3.4 NIACIN

Niacin is a generic term for nicotinic acid and nicotinamide. Nicotinamide is a component of nicotinamide adenine dinucleotide (NAD), nicotinamide adenine dinucleotide phosphate (NADP), and the pyridine nucleotides. Deficiency causes pellagra. No evidence suggests a consequence of niacin deficiency on the cardiovascular system, although niacin supplementation reduces cellular apoptosis to oxidative stress.[82] Nicotinic acid was used as a lipid lowering agent prior to development of the coenzyme A reductase inhibitors.

6.3.5 PANTOTHENIC ACID (B₅)

Vitamin B_5 is an essential part of coenzyme A and of acyl carrier protein (ACP). Spontaneous pantothenic acid deficiency has never been described because of the ubiquitous nature of the vitamin in foods.

6.3.6 VITAMIN B₆

Vitamin B_6 occurs in three interchangeable forms in the body: pyridoxine, pyridoxal, and pyridoxamine. They all exist as phosphorylated compounds. The principal form is pyridoxal 5′-phosphate (PLP), which is involved in amino acid metabolism. Lack of vitamin B_6 alone is rare; deficiencies most commonly occur in conjunction with other vitamin deficiencies.

The symptoms of PLP deficiency are general weakness, sleepiness, peripheral neuropathy, personality changes, dermatitis, cheilosis, glossitis, anemia, and impaired immunity. Low PLP is an independent risk factor for coronary artery disease even when homocysteine (see below) is taken into account.[83] However, most of its influence is through its effect on homocysteine levels.[84,85] Low B$_6$ levels are also associated with increased risk of extracranial carotid artery disease, although the risk, when corrected for homocysteine, is not as significant as first thought.[87]

6.3.7 FOLATE

Folate is a generic name for compounds related to pteroylglutamic acid (folic acid). Folic acid deficiency is common in hospitalized patients. Many diseases, especially intestinal, neoplastic, and hematological, increase body requirements for folate. Methotrexate, aminopterin, pyrimethamine, and cotrimoxazole inhibit normal folate metabolism. Tissue levels of vitamin B$_{12}$, vitamin B$_6$, and folate are not well-related to blood levels and many more elderly patients may be deficient than are recognized.[88] Folate deficiency leads to reduced ability of cells to double their nuclear DNA in order to divide because of impaired synthesis of thymidylate. Megaloblastic anemia results with similar changes in leukocytes, platelets, and epithelial cells. Folate deficiency also causes infertility and diarrhea.

Folate is required for the conversion of homocysteine to methionine (Figure 6.2) and a strong inverse relationship exists between folate consumption and homocysteine levels among patients with and without hyperhomocysteinemia (see Section

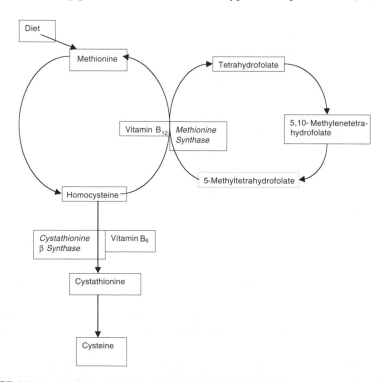

FIGURE 6.2 Interactions of homocysteine, folate, and vitamin B$_{12}$.

6.6).[88,89] Individuals with low folate intake are at higher risk of coronary heart disease.[90–92] Patients with coronary heart disease are more likely to have reduced serum folate and raised homocysteine.[93] Folic acid supplementation improves coronary endothelial function in patients with coronary artery disease by an effect on homocysteine[94] and also by a homocysteine-independent mechanism.[95]

6.3.8 VITAMIN B$_{12}$

Vitamin B$_{12}$ (cobalamin) is a generic term for a group of large complex compounds only synthesized by bacteria. Malabsorption due to gastric atrophy or disease of the terminal ileum is the commonest cause of selective B$_{12}$ deficiency. In the elderly population, the deterioration in gastric production of intrinsic factor due to gastric atrophy leads to pernicious anaemia. This is characterized by megaloblastic anaemia due to the trapping of folate and reduction in DNA synthesis with interruption of normal nuclear division. Vitamin B$_{12}$ deficiency is associated with elevated homocysteine and consequent elevated risk for coronary artery disease,[84,85] but no published work has looked at B$_{12}$ status in patients with heart disease.

6.3.9 VITAMIN C

Vitamin C (ascorbic acid) can be synthesized from glucose or galactose in a wide variety of plants and most animal species. The ability to participate in redox reactions is the basis for most of the functions of this antioxidant vitamin. Cigarette smokers have lower plasma and leukocyte levels of vitamin C;[96] overt deficiency of vitamin C is rare.

Higher levels of intake of vitamin C correlate with a reduced risk of death from stroke as closely as diastolic blood pressure in otherwise normal elderly subjects.[97] Low vitamin C levels increase the risk of stroke, particularly in hypertensive overweight men.[98] However, except for one study,[99] little correlation was shown between vitamin C levels and death from coronary disease.[97,100] High-dose ascorbic acid supplementation might therefore be a useful adjunct in the treatment of hypertension.[101]

Infusions of vitamin C improved peripheral endothelial function in diabetic patients,[102,103] hypercholesterolemic patients,[104] hypertensive patients,[105] patients with chronic heart failure (Figure 6.3),[106] and smokers.[107] Coronary artery endothelial function in patients with hypertension and hypercholesterolemia also improves with vitamin C,[108] and some benefit on acetylcholine-induced vasospasm may be gained by patients with coronary spastic angina.[109]

Vitamin C supplementation can reduce oxidative stress-mediated postprandial endothelial dysfunction.[110] Oral vitamin C improves endothelial-dependent vasodilation of the brachial artery.[111,112] In addition to these acute effects, vitamin C also reduces apoptosis in cardiomyocytes in rats with experimental heart failure, suggesting a potential long-term benefit in CHF patients.[113]

6.3.10 VITAMIN E

Vitamin E (tocopherol) is a powerful antioxidant and is ubiquitous in cell membranes, protecting them from free radical damage. Vitamin E levels predict cardiovascular events and death more accurately in elderly patients (>80 years) than serum cholesterol.[114]

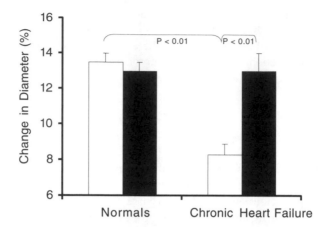

FIGURE 6.3 Change in radial artery diameter (%) during reactive hyperemia (flow-dependent dilation) after wrist occlusion in normal individuals (n = 8) and patients with CHF (n = 10). The filled bars demonstrate the effect of vitamin C infusion prior to occlusion on flow-dependent dilation. (Adapted from Hornig, B. et al., *Circulation,* 97, 363, 1998. With permission.)

High vitamin E intake is associated with a lower incidence of coronary heart disease in middle-aged subjects.[116] Men with high vitamin E intakes have a 40% reduced risk[117] and women a 34% reduction.[118] This effect is, however, not confined to the middle-aged. Additional reductions in risk were noted in subjects over 65 years of age if they took both vitamin E and vitamin C.[118] High-dose vitamin E reduces the oxidation of LDL.[119,120] Oxidized LDL may enhance the generation of foam cells in the arterial walls, proliferation of smooth muscle cells, and platelet adhesion and aggregation, and trigger thrombosis.[121] In healthy volunteers, diabetics, and cardiac transplant patients, vitamin E can lead to a reduction of platelet aggregation.[122–124] This is a direct effect of vitamin E on platelet activity[125] through the inhibition of platelet protein kinase C.[126,127] Alpha-tocopherol can also control the proliferation of smooth muscle cells through a similar mechanism.[128] A transient reduction in endothelial function that occurs after a high-fat meal is inhibited by pretreatment with high doses of vitamin E.[129] Alpha-tocopherol can also improve endothelial function in cholesterol-fed rabbits.[130]

Leukocyte–endothelium cell interactions are reduced by vitamin E due to attenuated surface expression of adhesion molecules on both cell types.[131] In experimental coronary artery occlusion lasting 45 minutes, high-dose vitamin E supplementation prior to ischemia combined with intravenous vitamin C infusion prior to reperfusion led to significantly less myocardial damage in pigs.[132] This suggests further that water-soluble vitamin C aids the antioxidant action of lipid-soluble vitamin E. There is strong evidence that vitamin C is able to regenerate vitamin E radicals at the borders of the lipids and aqueous phases in cell membranes.[133]

Despite these theoretical bases for benefits from vitamin E, few clear data suggest that routine supplementation would benefit patients with ischemic heart disease.[66,134] The CHAOS trial showed a significant reduction in nonfatal myocardial infarction with vitamin E, but a 22% increase in all-cause mortality was found in the vitamin E group.[135] The use of vitamin E in post-acute myocardial infarction also has little supportive evidence.[136,137] The GISSI Prevenzione trial showed no benefit from vitamin E on post-infarct mortality.[138] The HOPE study demonstrated no benefit from vitamin E in primary prevention of coronary events in patients at high risk of coronary disease.[139,140] Vitamin E can reduce oxidative stress in patients with chronic heart failure,[141] but no clinical data support its routine use.

6.3.11 VITAMIN D

Vitamins D_2 and D_3 are derived from the effects of ultraviolet radiation on the skin. Older individuals produce less vitamin D after exposure to ultraviolet light because their skin contains lower amounts of steroid precursors.[1]

Vitamin D can reduce the hypertrophic effects of endothelin on rat myocytes.[142] The requirement for calcium in myocardial contraction is discussed in Section 6.2.1, and vitamin D also seems to be an essential agent. Rats fed vitamin D-deficient diets with calcium levels maintained by high-dose calcium supplements developed deteriorating myocardial contractile function. The myocardial contraction returned to normal only when vitamin D was supplemented.[143]

Patients with chronic heart failure have low serum vitamin D metabolites and increased bone turnover with high levels of osteopenia or osteoporosis.[7,240]

6.4 OTHER COMPOUNDS

6.4.1 UBIQUINONE (COENZYME Q_{10})

Coenzyme Q_{10} (2,3-dimethoxy-5 methyl-6-decaprenyl-1,4-benzoquinone) was first isolated in 1957 in bovine cardiac muscle.[144] It is an endogenous fat-soluble quinone found in high concentrations in the mitochondria of myocardium, liver, and kidney. It functions as an electron carrier during the synthesis of adenosine triphosphate (ATP), but also has membrane stabilizing properties and is a powerful antioxidant.

Myocardial biopsies in patients with heart disease have shown mitochondrial ubiquinone depletion, so ubiquinone deficiency may therefore play a role in the pathogenesis of both heart failure and ischemic heart disease.[145] Patients with heart failure have lower myocardial levels of ubiquinone than normal individuals,[146] and low serum ubiqinone levels are associated with increased mortality in heart failure.[147] The production of ubiquinone is reduced by HMG CoA reductase inhibitors (statins) leading to low serum levels[148,149] although tissue levels remain stable with short-term statin therapy.[150,151]

Non-randomised studies in patients with dilated cardiomyopathy and ischemic heart disease-induced systolic dysfunction have shown positive results for ejection fraction, exercise tolerance, and New York Heart Association (NYHA) status with ubiquinone supplementation.[152–154] Most placebo-controlled trials,[155,156] but not all of them,[157] support these findings and also show reductions in hospitalizations. Ubiquinone may also be of some benefit in left ventricular diastolic dysfunction.[158]

6.4.2 Carnitine

Carnitine supplementation improves the utilization of pyruvate in the Krebs cycle,[227] and thereby improves muscle metabolism. It has been investigated in patients undergoing cardiac surgery,[228] and in those with angina pectoris,[229–232] acute myocardial infarction,[233,234] shock,[235] and peripheral vascular disease.[236,237] Some improvement of exercise tolerance in patients with limiting ischemic symptoms was noted, but a lack of strong evidence for the use of carnitine in these situations remains. Oral propionyl-L-carnitine in some studies[227] but not all[238] has shown improved exercise tolerance (but not hemodynamic variables) in patients with chronic heart failure. The compound may also reduce apoptosis in skeletal muscle cells, suggesting a potential benefit in the myopathy of chronic heart failure.[239]

6.4.3 Creatine Phosphate

Creatine is used to improve athletic performance. Patients with chronic heart failure develop skeletal myopathies.[240] Muscle contraction and relaxation are fueled through the dephosphorylation of ATP, which must be rapidly resynthesized. Creatine serves as a phosphate donor to maintain high levels of intracellular ATP, and creatine supplementation increases the rate of phosphocreatine resynthesis.[241] Skeletal muscle strength and endurance were improved in patients with chronic heart failure after short-term oral creatine supplementation, but no effect on cardiac contractility was noted.[242] Creatine administered intravenously improved ejection fraction.[243,244] The improvements in skeletal muscle function were seen predominantly in patients with low levels of creatine and phosphocreatine in their skeletal muscles.[245] This was not a ubiquitous finding in patients with chronic heart failure.[245,246]

It is possible that creatine is of benefit in some chronic heart failure patients, but long-term safety issues have yet to be addressed, the improvements have not been shown to be sustained, and the patient group most likely to benefit can only be identified by muscle biopsy.

6.5 OXIDATIVE STRESS

Free radicals are highly active by-products of many metabolic processes that have the potential to damage biomolecules. The presence of these molecules represents oxidative stress. Systems for removing free radicals have evolved and include superoxide dismutase and glutathione peroxidases. Once they have been involved in the reactions to remove the free radicals, however, these enzymes are dependent upon continued antioxidant intake for reconstitution to their active state.

Elevated levels of markers of oxidative stress, such as exhaled pentane[159] and plasma or urinary malondialdehyde, have been reported in heart failure patients.[160,161] The presence of these markers in CHF patients correlates with functional class and inversely with exercise tolerance, antioxidant levels, and indices of prognosis.[162–165] Patients with coronary artery disease also show evidence of greater oxidative stress, which correlates with endothelial dysfunction and predicts cardiac events.[166]

Free radicals are linked to the gradual progression of myocardial dysfunction that is a hallmark of chronic heart failure.[167–169] Some stimuli for free radical production such as catecholamines,[170] cardiac sympathetic tone,[171] cytokine activation,[172] and microvascular reperfusion injury[173] are elevated in heart failure. Chronic elevation of angiotensin II in rats can stimulate increases in vascular superoxide production.[174] The cytokine-stimulated cardiomyocyte production of free radicals in CHF can be inhibited by antioxidant vitamins.[175] Oxidative stress also reduces endothelium-mediated vasodilation in CHF patients,[176–178] which leads to an increase in afterload.[179]

In the presence of free radicals, LDL is oxidized. Oxidized LDL is highly atherogenic and encourages arterial mural thrombus formation,[180] perhaps as a consequence of prostacyclin inhibition and nitric oxide synthesis.[181] LDL oxidation leads also to the generation of reactive oxygen species (ROS), in particular superoxide anion. The oxidation of LDL can be inhibited by superoxide dismutase and vitamin C,[182] which may explain some of the antiatherogenic effects of vitamin C. Vitamin C also prevents leukocyte adhesion to the microvascular endothelium and the formation of leukocyte–platelet aggregates in response to the oxidized LDL.[180] This may be due to reduced vascular cell adhesion molecule-1 (VCAM-1) gene transcription and expression, which is regulated through an antioxidant-sensitive mechanism.[183]

Vitamins C and E suppress free radical production in the leukocytes of patients with acute myocardial infarction.[133,184] They also retard the progression of transplant-associated coronary arteriosclerosis.[185]

A study examining the effects of profound lipid lowering and antioxidant vitamin therapy in patients at high risk for cardiovascular events confirmed the results of retrospective studies of reported vitamin intake and the incidence of cardiovascular events.[186] In the Heart Protection Society (HPS), which included over 20,000 patients with coronary artery disease, previous myocardial infarction, peripheral vascular disease, diabetes mellitus, and hypertension, no benefit arose from a combination of antioxidant vitamins (vitamin E, vitamin C, and beta-carotene) despite significant increases in plasma levels of these vitamins.[187] There was also no benefit from an antioxidant combination on angiographically determined coronary artery progression.[188] To date, no data suggest a therapeutic role for specific antioxidant therapy.

6.6 HOMOCYSTEINE AND HEART DISEASE

Several vitamins interact through the metabolism of homocysteine. Most studies[189–191] but not all[192] demonstrate a link between hyperhomocysteinaemia and increased risk of cardiovascular disease. Levels of only 12% above the upper limit of normal are associated with a three-fold increase in risk of acute myocardial infarction.[190] Individuals of Asian Indian origin living in the U.K. who have higher mortality rates from cardiovascular disease also have higher average homocysteine levels.[193] A genetic mutation in the methylenetetrahydrofolate reductase gene that causes hyperhomocysteinemia increased the risk for vascular disease in some[194] but not all studies.[195]

A hyperhomocysteinemic state may promote atherosclerosis by (1) alteration of platelet function and coagulation factors to promote coagulation,[196–198] (2) endothelial

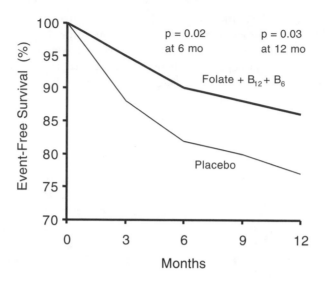

FIGURE 6.4 Kaplan–Meier survival curves for freedom from major adverse events in 553 patients following percutaneous transluminal coronary angioplasty. (From Schnyder, G. et al., *JAMA*, 288, 973, 2000. With permission.)

damage and dysfunction,[199,206] (3) encouraging oxidation of LDL,[207,208] (4) smooth muscle proliferation,[209,210] and (5) endothelium–leukocyte interactions.[211] Although endothelial cells initially respond to homocysteine by increasing nitric oxide synthesis,[212] prolonged exposure[213] and high homocysteine concentrations[214] lead eventually to a fall in nitric oxide production.

Homocysteine may also promote thrombogenesis both by increasing factor V activity,[215] reducing antithrombin III[216] and protein C[217] activity, and impairing fibrinolysis.[218]

Homocysteine levels rise with age, which may be a reflection of particularly poor intake of vitamins B_{12} and B_6 and folate in the elderly population.[219] High folate levels seem to be protective for cardiovascular disease.[192,220] Homocysteine can be lowered with folic acid and vitamin B_6.[221,222] This therapy is associated with a decreased occurrence of abnormal exercise tests[223] and an improvement in endothelial function.[224] Homocysteine-lowering therapy reduced the incidence of events[225] and restenosis[226] in 533 patients randomised to vitamin supplementation (B_{12}, folate, and vitamin B_6) or placebo following percutaneous coronary intervention (Figure 6.4).

6.7 CONCLUSIONS

Micronutrients are involved in numerous essential physiological functions from protection from energy production to muscular contraction and intercellular communication. They are also essential as cofactors for many intracellular metabolic processes and act as antioxidants, for example, in the regulation of a stable environment. Despite this ubiquitous involvement in the processes essential for life, the evidence of benefit of antioxidant or multivitamin supplementation to prevent or treat coronary disease remains unconvincing. Recent data from HPS and other large randomised trials demonstrate that high-dose vitamin supplementation in these patients does no harm but probably produces no benefit either. The data for homocysteine-lowering therapy are more impressive.

Good evidence supports the use of folate and the other B vitamins to lower homocysteine in patients with coronary disease. In addition, it is possible that the inexpensive adjunctive treatment of patients undergoing percutaneous intervention for coronary disease with B vitamins to reduce the rate of restenosis and subsequent acute events might become more common as further evidence appears. There remain few data in patients with chronic heart failure who have potentially the most to gain from both antioxidant and homocysteine-lowering strategies.

REFERENCES

1. Maclaughlin J and Holick MF. Ageing decreases the capacity of human skin to produce vitamin D_3. *J Clin Invest* 1985;**76**:1536-8.
2. Bostick RM, Kushi LH, Wu Y, Meyer KA, Sellars TA, and Folsom AR. Relation of calcium, vitamin D, and dairy food intake to ischaemic heart disease mortality among postmenopausal women. *Am J Epidemiol* 1999;**149**:151-61.
3. Koide M, Harayama H, Iio A, Obata K, Matsuda N, Ono T, Yokota M, and Tuan RS. Major risk factors for atherosclerosis are manifested in experimental Ca-deficiency. *Hypertens Res* 1996 (**Suppl 1**):S35-40.
4. Varma N and Kerrigan GN. Electrocardiographic Q-Tc prolongation associated with infusion of intravenous pamidronate disodium. *Postgrad Med J* 1993;**69**:497-8.
5. Akiyama T, Batchelder J, Worsman J, Moses HW, and Jedlinski M. Hypocalcaemic torsades de pointes. *J Electrocardiol* 1989;**22**:89-92.
6. Gmehlin U, Marx T, and Dirks B. Ventricular fibrillation due to hypocalcaemia after parathyroidectomy with autotransplantation of parathyroid tissue in a dialysis patient. *Nephron* 1995;**70**:110-1.
7. Shane E, Mancini D, Aaronson K, Silverberg SJ, Seibel MJ, Addesso V, and McMahon DJ. Bone mass, vitamin D deficiency, and hypoparathyroidism in congestive heart failure. *Am J Med* 1997;**103**:197-207.
8. Brunvand L, Haga P, Tangsrud SE, and Haug E. Congestive heart failure caused by vitamin D deficiency? *Acta Paediatr* 1995;**84**:106-8.
9. Rimailho A, Bouchard P, Schaison G, Richard C, and Auzepy P. Improvement of hypocalcaemic cardiomyopathy by correction of serum calcium level. *Am Heart J* 1985;**109**:611-3.
10. Palazzuoli V, Martini G, Giovani S, Mondillo S, Giusti R, D'Arpino A, Ricci D. Dilated cardiomyopathy secondary to idiopathic hypoparathyroidism in adults (description of a case). *Recenti Prog Med* 1990;**81**:263-5.
11. Eichorn EJ, Tandon PK, and Di Bianco R. Clinical and prognostic significance of serum magnesium concentration in patients with severe CHF: the PROMISE study. *J Am Coll Cardiol* 1993;**21**:634-40.
12. Tsuji H, Venditti FJ, and Evans JC. The association of serum potassium and magnesium levels with the occurrence of complex or frequent ventricular arrhythmias. *Circulation* 1993;**88**:I-354.

13. Tomiyasu T, Chishaki A, and Nakamura M. Magnesium deficiency in adult rats promotes the induction of ventricular tachycardia by the administration of ephinephrine. *Heart Vessels* 1998;**13:**122-31.

14. Li W, Zheng T, Altura BT, and Altura BM. Magnesium modulates contractile responses of rat aorta to thiocyanate: a possible relationship to smoking-induced atherosclerosis. *Toxicol Appl Pharmacol* 1999;**157:**77-84.

15. Murasato Y, Harada Y, Ikeda M, Nakashima Y, and Hayashida Y. Effect of magnesium deficiency on autonomic circulatory regulation in conscious rats. *Hypertension* 1999;**34:**247-52.

16. Wu F, Zou L, Altura BT, Barbour RL, and Altura BM. Low extracellular magnesium results in cardiac failure in isolated perfused rat hearts. *Magnes Trace Elem* 1991-92;**10:**364-73.

17. Kartha CC, Eapen JT, Radhakumary C, Kutty VR, Ramani K, and Lal AV. Pattern of cardiac fibrosis in rabbits periodically fed a magnesium-restricted diet and administered rare earth chloride through drinking water. *Biol Trace Elem Res* 1998;**63:**19-30.

18. Wester PO and Dyckner T. Intracellular electrolytes in cardiac failure. *Acta Med Scand Suppl* 1986;**707:**33-6.

19. Gottlieb SS, Baruch L, Kukin ML et al. Prognostic importance of the serum magnesium concentration in patients with congestive heart failure. *J Am Coll Cardiol* 1990;**16:**827-31.

20. Eichorn EJ, Tandon PK, and Di Bianco R. Clinical and prognostic significance of serum magnesium concentration in patients with severe CHF: the PROMISE study. *J Am Coll Cardiol* 1993;**21:**634-40.

21. Cohen N, Almoznino-Sarafian D, Zaidenstein R, Alom I, Gorelik O, Shteinshnaider M, Chachahvily S, Averbukh Z, Golik A, Chen-Levy, and Modai D. Serum magnesium aberrations in furosemide (frusemide) treated patients with congestive heart failure: pathophysiological correlates and prognostic evaluation. *Heart* 2003;**89:**411-6.

22. Martin BJ, McAlpine JK, and Devine BL. Hypomagnesaemia in elderly digitalised patients. *Scot Med J* 1988;**33:**273-4.

23. DeCarli C, Sprouse G, LaRosa JC. Serum magnesium levels in symptomatic atrial fibrillation and their relation to rhythm control by intravenous digoxin. *Am J Cardiol* 1986;**57:**956-9.

24. Fonseca V, Havard CW. Electrolyte disturbances and cardiac failure with hypomagnesaemia in anorexia nervosa. *Br Med J (Clin Res Ed)* 1985;**291:**1680-2.

25. Shils ME. Experimental production of magnesium deficiency in man. *Ann NY Acad Sci* 1969;**162:**847-55.

26. Bashir Y, Sneddon JF, and Staunton A. Effects of oral magnesium chloride replacement in CHF secondary to coronary artery disease. *Am J Cardiol* 1993;**72:**1156-62.

27. Gottlieb SS, Baruch L, and Kuklin ML. Prognostic importance of the serum magnesium concentration in patients with congestive heart failure. *J Am Coll Cardiol* 1990;**16:**827-31.

28. Hays JV, Gilman JK, and Rubal BJ. Effect of magnesium sulfate on ventricular rate control in atrial fibrillation. *Ann Emerg Med* 1994;**24:**61-4.

29. Lewis RV, Tregaskis B, McLay J, Service E, and McDevitt DG. Oral magnesium reduces ventricular ectopy in digitalised patients with chronic atrial fibrillation. *Eur J Clin Pharmacol* 1990;**38:**107-10.

30. Lewis R, Durnin C, McLay J, McEwen J, and McDevitt DG. Magnesium deficiency may be an important determinant of ventricular ectopy in digitalised patients with chronic atrial fibrillation. *Br J Clin Pharmacol* 1991;**31**:200-3.

31. Kinlay S and Buckley NA. Magnesium sulfate in the treatment of ventricular arrhythmias due to digoxin toxicity. *J Toxicol Clin Toxicol* 1995;**33**:55-9.

32. Merrill JJ, DeWeese G, and Wharton JM. Magnesium reversal of digoxin-facilitated ventricular rate during atrial fibrillation in the Wolff–Parkinson–White syndrome. *Am J Med* 1994;**97**:25-8.

33. Verduyn SC, Vos MA, van der Zande J, van der Hulst FF, and Wellens HJ. Role of interventricular dispersion of repolarization in acquired torsade-de-pointes arrhythmias: reversal by magnesium. *Cardiovasc Res* 1997;**34**:453-63.

34. Perticone F, Ceravolo R, De Novara G, Torchia L, and Cloro C. New data on the antiarrhythmic value of parenteral magnesium treatment: magnesium and ventricular arrhythmias. *Magnes Res* 1992;**5**:265-72.

35. Hasan RA, Zureikat GY, and Nolan BM. Torsade de pointes associated with Astemizole overdose treated with magnesium sulfate. *Pediatr Emerg Care* 1993;**9**:23-5.

36. Woods KL, Fletcher S, Roffe C, and Haider Y. Intravenous magnesium sulphate in suspected acute myocardial infarction: results of the second Leicester Intravenous Magnesium Intervention Trial (LIMIT-2). *Lancet* 1992;**339**:1499-503.

37. ISIS-4 Collaborative Group. ISIS-4: a randomised factorial trial assessing early oral captopril, oral mononitrate, and intravenous magnesium sulphate in 58,050 patients with suspected acute myocardial infarction. *Lancet* 1995;**345**:669-85.

38. Greger JL. Dietary intake and nutritional status in regard to zinc of institutionalised aged. *J Gerontol* 1977;**32**:549-53.

39. Oteiza PI, Clegg MS, Zago MP, and Keen CL. Zinc deficiency induces oxidative stress and AP-1 activation in 3T3 cells. *Free Radic Biol Med* 2000;**28**:1091-99.

40. Coudray C, Charlon V, de Leiris J, and Favier A. Effect of zinc deficiency on lipid peroxidation status and infarct size in rat hearts. *Int J Cardiol* 1993;**41**:109-13.

41. Faure P, Roussel AM, Richard MJ, Foulon T, Groslambert P, Hadjian A, and Favier A. Effect of an acute zinc depletion on rat lipoprotein distribution and peroxidation. *Biol Trace Elem Res* 1991;**28**:135-46.

42. Coudray C, Boucher F, Richard MJ, Arnaud J, de Leiris J, and Favier A. Zinc deficiency, ethanol, and myocardial ischaemia affect lipoperoxidation in rats. *Biol Trace Elem Res* 1991;**30**:103-18.

43. Golik A, Zaidenstein R, Dishi V, Blatt A, Cohen N, Cotter G, Berman S, and Weissgarten J. Effects of captopril and enalapril on zinc metabolism in hypertensive patients. *J Am Coll Nutr* 1998;**17**:75-8.

44. Rayssiguier Y, Gueux E, Bussiere L, and Mazur A. Copper deficiency increases the susceptibility of lipoproteins and tissues to peroxidation in rats. *J Nutr* 1993;**123**:1343-8.

45. Kopp SJ, Klevay LM, and Feliksik JM. Physiological and metabolic characterisation of a cardiomyopathy induced by chronic copper deficiency. *Am J Physiol* 1983;**245(Part 1)**:H855-66.

46. Rossi L, Lippe G, Marchese E, de Martino A, Mavelli I, Rotilio G, and Ciriolo MR. Decrease of cytochrome C oxidase protein in heart mitochondria of copper-deficient rats. *Biometals* 1998;**11**:207-12.

47. Chen Y, Saari JT, and Kang YJ. Weak antioxidant defenses make the heart a target for damage in copper-deficient rats. *Free Radic Biol Med* 1994;**17**:529-36.

48. Wildman RE, Medeiros DM, and Jenkins J. Comparative aspects of cardiac ultrastructure, morphometry, and electrocardiography of hearts from rats fed restricted dietary copper and selenium. *Biol Trace Elem Res* 1994;**46:**51-66.
49. Klevay LM, Inman L, Johnson LK, Lawler M, Mahalko JR, Milne DB, Lukaski HC, Bolonchuk W, and Sandstead HH. Increased cholesterol in plasma in a young man during experimental copper depletion. *Metabolism* 1984;**33:**1112-8.
50. Klevay LM. Dietary copper: a powerful determination of cholesterolaemia. *Med Hypotheses* 1987;**24:**111-9.
51. Burk RF and Hill KE. Selenoprotein P: a selenium-rich extracellular glycoprotein. *J Nutr* 1994;**124:**1891-7.
52. May JM, Mendiratta S, Hill KE, and Burk RF. Reduction of dehydroacorbate to ascorbate by the selenoenzyme thioredoxin reductase. *J Biol Chem* 1997;**272:**22607-10.
53. Vadhanavikit S and Ganther HE. Decreased ubiquinone levels in tissues of rats deficient in selenium. *Biochem Biophys Res Commun* 1993;**190:**921-6.
54. Vadhanavikit S and Ganther HE. Selenium deficiency and decreased coenzyme Q levels. *Mol Aspects Med* 1994;**15 (Suppl):**103-7.
55. Köhler H, Peters HJ, Pankau H, and Duck HJ. Selenium in cardiology and angiology. *Biol Trace Elem Res* 1988;**15:**157-66.
56. May SW and Pollock SH. Selenium-based antihypertensives. Rationale and potential. *Drugs* 1998;**56:**959-64.
57. de Lorgeril M, Salen P, Accominotti M, Cadau M, Stephens JP, Boucher F, and de Leiris J. Dietary and blood antioxidants in patients with chronic heart failure. *Eur J Heart Failure* 2001;**3:**661-9.
58. Wang YZ, Jia XA, Zhao JY, and Xu GL. Effects of selenium deficiency on Ca transport function of sarcoplasmic reticulum and lipid peroxidation in rat myocardium. *Biol Trace Elem Res* 1993;**36:**159-66.
59. Rani P and Lalitha K. Evidence for altered structure and impaired mitochondrial electron transport function in selenium deficiency. *Biol Trace Elem Res* 1996;**51:**225-34.
60. Yang GQ and Xia YM. Studies on human dietary requirements and safe range of dietary intakes of selenium in China and their application in the prevention of related endemic diseases. *Biomed Environ Sci* 1995;**8:**187-201.
61. Lockitch G, Taylor GP, Wong LT, Davidson AG, Dison PJ, Riddell D, and Massing B. Cardiomyopathy associated with nonendemic selenium deficiency in a Caucasian adolescent. *Am J Clin Nutr* 1990;**52:**572-7.
62. Cenac A, Simonoff M, Moretto P, and Djibo A. Low plasma selenium is a risk factor for peripartum cardiomyopathy. *Int J Cardiol* 1992;**36:**57-9.
63. West CE, Rombout JHWM, Sijtsma SR, and van der Zijpp A. Vitamin A and the immune response. *Proc Nutr Soc* 1991;**50:**249-60.
64. Zobali F, Avci A, Canbolat O, and Karasu C. Effects of vitamin A and insulin on the antioxidative state of diabetic rat heart: a comparison study with combination treatment. *Cell Biochem Funct* 2002;**20:**75-80.
65. Tavani A, Negri E, D'Avanzo B, and La Vecchia C. Beta-carotene intake and risk of nonfatal acute myocardial infarction in women. *Eur J Epidemiol* 1997;**13:**631-7.
66. Alpha-Tocopherol–Beta-Carotene Cancer Prevention Study Group. The effect of vitamin E and beta-carotene on the incidence of lung cancer and other cancers in male smokers. *New Engl J Med* 1994;**330:**1029-35.
67. Palace VP, Khaper N, Qin Q, and Singal PK. Antioxidant potentials of vitamin A and carotenoids and their relevance to heart disease. *Free Radic Biol Med* 1999;**26:**746-61.

68. Blot WJ. Nutrition intervention trials in vitamin/mineral combinations, cancer incidence, and disease-specific mortality in the general population. *J Natl Cancer Inst* 1993;**85:**1483-92.

69. Manson JE et al. Aspirin in the primary prevention of angina pectoris in a randomised trial of United States physicians. *Am J Med* 1990;**89:**772-6.

70. Yui Y, Itokawa Y, and Kawai C. Furosemide-induced thiamine deficiency . *Cardiovasc Res* 1980;**14:**537-40.

71. Pepersack T, Garbusinski J, Robberecht J, Beyer I, Willems D, and Fuss M. Clinical relevance of thiamine status amongst hospitalised elderly patients. *Gerontology* 1999;**45:**96-101.

72. O'Keefe ST, Tormey WP, Glasgow R, and Lavan JN. Thiamine deficiency in hospitalised elderly patients. *Gerontology* 1994;**40:**18-24.

73. Seligmann H, Halkin H, Rauchfleisch S, Kaufmann N, Tal R, Motro M, Vered Z, and Ezra D. Thiamine deficiency in patients with congestive cardiac failure receiving long-term furosemide therapy: a pilot study. *Am J Med* 1991;**91:**151-5.

74. Brady JA, Rock CL, and Horneffer MR. Thiamine status, diuretic medications, and the management of congestive heart failure. *J Am Diet Assoc* 1995;**95:**541-4.

75. Capelli V, Bottinelli R, Polla B, and Reggiani C. Altered contractile properties of rat cardiac muscle during experimental thiamine deficiency and food deprivation. *J Mol Cell Cardiol* 1990;**22:**1095-6.

76. Zangen A, Botzer D, Zangen R, and Shainberg A. Furosemide and digoxin inhibit thiamine uptake in cardiac cells. *Eur J Pharmacol* 1998;**13:**151-5.

77. Shimon I, Shlomo A, Vered Z, Seligmann H, Shefi M, Peleg E, Rosenthal T, Motro M, Halkin H, and Ezra D. Improved left ventricular function after thiamine supplementation in patients with congestive heart failure receiving long-term furosemide therapy. *Am J Med* 1995;**98:**485-90.

78. Nakajima H, Miyagi Y, and Sasayama S. Effects of thiamine (vitamin B_1) on exercise capacity in patients with congestive heart failure. *J Am Coll Cardiol* 1986;**74 (Suppl 2):**153.

79. Gennery AR, Bartlett K, and Hasan A. Thiamine deficiency mimicking acute rejection following cardiac transplantation. *Cardiol Young* 1998;**8:**113-5.

80. Olpin SE and Bates CJ. Lipid metabolism in riboflavin-deficient rats. 1. Effect of dietary lipids on riboflavin status and fatty acid profiles. *Br J Nutr* 1982;**47:**577-96.

81. Steier M, Lopez R, and Cooperman JM. Riboflavin deficiency in infants and children with heart disease. *Am Heart J* 1976;**92:**139-43.

82. Crowley CL, Payne CM, Bernstein H et al. The NAD^+ precursors, nicotinic acid and nicotinamide, protect cells against apoptosis induced by a multiple stress inducer, deoxycholate. *Cell Death Differ* 2000;**7:**314-26.

83. Robinson K, Mayer EL, Miller DP, Green R, van Lente F, Gupta A, Kottke-Marchant K, Savon SR, Selhub J, Nissen SE, Kutner M, Topol EJ, and Jacobsen DW. Hyperhomocysteinaemia and low pyridoxal phosphate: common and independent risk factors for coronary artery disease. *Circulation* 1995;**92:**2825-30.

84. Dalery K, Lussier-Cacan S, Selhub J, Davignon J, Latour Y, and Genest J. Homocysteine and coronary artery disease in French Canadian subjects: relation with vitamins B_{12}, B_6, pyridoxal phosphate, and folate. *Am J Cardiol* 1995;**75:**1107-11.

85. Folsom AR, Nieto FJ, McGovern PG, Tsai MY, Malinow MR, Eckfeldt JH, Hess DL, and Davis CE. Prospective study of coronary heart disease incidence in relation to fasting total homocysteine, related genetic polymorphisms, and B vitamins: the Atherosclerosis Risk in Communities (ARIC) study. *Circulation* 1998;**98:**204-10.

86. Selhub J, Jacques PF, Bostom AG, D'Agostino RB, Wilson PWF, Belanger AJ, O'Leary DH, Wolf PA, and Schaefer EJ. Association between plasma homocysteine concentrations and extracranial carotid artery stenosis. *New Engl J Med* 1995;**332**:286-91.

87. Naurath HJ, Joosten E, Riezler R, Stabler SP, Allen RH, and Lindenbaum J. Effects of vitamin B_{12} folate, and vitamin B_6 supplements in elderly people with normal serum vitamin concentrations. *Lancet* 1995;**346**:85-9.

88. Kang SS, Wong PW, and Norusis M. Homocysteinaemia due to folate deficiency. *Metabolism* 1987;**36**:458-62.

89. Nygord O, Refsum H, Ueland PM, and Vollset SE. Major lifestyle determinants of plasma total homocysteine distribution: the Hordaland Homocysteine Study. *Am J Clin Nutr* 1998;**67**:263-70.

90. Panchurinti N, Lewis CA, and Sauberlich HE. Plasma homocysteine, folate, and vitamin B_{12} concentrations and risk for early onset coronary artery disease. *Am J Clin Nutr* 1994;**59**:940-8.

91. Morrison HI, Schaubel D, Desmeules M, and Wigle DT. Serum folate and risk of fatal coronary heart disease. *JAMA* 1996;**275**:1893-6.

92. Voutilainen S, Rissanen TH, Virtanen J, Lakka TA, and Salonen JT. Low dietary folate intake is associated with an excess incidence of acute coronary events: the Kuopio Ischemic Heart Disease Risk Factor Study. *Circulation* 2001;**103**:2674-80.

93. Piechota W, Jozefczak E, Wadowska E, Bejm J, and Tkaczewski K. Homocysteine, folate and vitamin B_{12} in patients with coronary heart disease. *Eur J Heart Failure* 2000;**2**:P11/10173.

94. Willems FF, Aengevaeren WR, Boers GH, Blom HJ, and Verheugt FW. Coronary endothelial function in hyperhomocysteinemia: improvement after treatment with folic acid and cobalamin in patients with coronary artery disease. *J Am Coll Cardiol* 2002;**40**:766-72.

95. Doshi SN, McDowell IF, Moat SJ, Payne N, Durrant HJ, Lewis MJ, and Goodfellow J. Folic acid improves endothelial function in coronary artery disease via mechanisms largely independent of homocysteine lowering. *Circulation* 2002;**105**:22-6.

96. Schectman G, Byrd JC, and Gruchow HW. The influence of smoking on vitamin C status in adults. *Am J Public Health* 1989;**79**:158-62.

97. Gale CR, Martyn CN, and Winter PD, Cooper C. Vitamin C and risk of death from stroke and coronary heart disease in a cohort of elderly people. *BMJ* 1995;**310**:1563-6.

98. Kurl S, Tuomainen TP, Laukkanen JA, Nyyssonen K, Lakka T, Sivenius J, and Salonen JT. Plasma vitamin C modifies the association between hypertension and risk of stroke. *Stroke* 2002;**33**:1568-73.

99. Nyyssönen K, Parviainen M, Salonen R, Tuomilehto J, and Salonen JT. Vitamin C deficiency and risk of myocardial infarction: prospective study of men from eastern Finland. *BMJ* 1997;**314**:634-8.

100. Kushi LH, Folsom AR, Prineas RJ, Mink PJ, Wu Y, and Bostick RM. Dietary antioxidant vitamins and death from coronary heart disease in post-menopausal women. *New Engl J Med* 1996;**334**:1156-62.

101. Duffy SJ, Gokce N, Holbrook M, Huang A, Frei B, Keaney JF Jr, and Vita JA. Treatment of hypertension with ascorbic acid. *Lancet* 1999;**354**:2048-9.

102. Ting HH, Timimi FK, Boles KS, Creager SJ, Ganz P, and Creager M. Vitamin C improves endothelium-dependant vasodilation in patients with non-insulin-dependant diabetes mellitus. *J Clin Invest* 1996;**97**:22-8.

103. Timimi FK, Ting HH, Haley EA, Roddy M-A, Ganz P, and Creager M. Vitamin C improves endothelium-dependant vasodilation in patients with insulin-dependant diabetes mellitus. *J Am Coll Cardiol* 1998;**31:**552-7.

104. Ting HH, Timimi FK, Haley EA, Roddy M-A, Ganz P, and Creager MA. Vitamin C improves endothelium-dependant vasodilation in forearm resistance vessels of humans with hypercholesterolaemia. *Circulation* 1997;**95:**2617-22.

105. Taddei S, Virdis A, Ghiadoni L, Magagna A, and Salvetti A. Vitamin C improves endothelium-dependant vasodilation by restoring nitric oxide activity in essential hypertension. *Circulation* 1998;**97:**2222-9.

106. Hornig B, Arakawa N, Kohler C, and Drexler H. Vitamin C improves the endothelial function of conduit arteries in patients with chronic heart failure. *Circulation* 1998;**97:**363-8.

107. Heitzer T, Just H, and Münzel T. Antioxidant vitamin C improves endothelial dysfunction in chronic smokers. *Circulation* 1996;**94:**6-9.

108. Jeserich M, Schindler T, and Olschewski M. Vitamin C improves endothelial function of epicardial coronary arteries in patients with hypercholesterolaemia or essential hypertension assessed by cold pressor testing. *Eur Heart J* 1999;**20:**1676-80.

109. Kugiyama K, Motoyama T, Hirashima O, Ohgushi M, Soejima H, Misumi K, Kawano H, Miyao Y, Yoshimura M, Ogawa H, Matsumura T, Sugiyama S, and Yasue H. Vitamin C attenuates abnormal vasomotor reactivity in spasm coronary arteries in patients with coronary spastic angina. *J Am Coll Cardiol* 1998;**32:**103-9.

110. Ling L, Zhao SP, Gao M, Zhou QC, Li YL, and Xia B. Vitamin C preserves endothelial function in patients with coronary heart disease after a high-fat meal. *Clin Cardiol* 2002;**25:**219-24.

111. Gokce N, Keaney JF, Frei B, Holbrook M, Olesiak M, Zachariah BJ, Leeuwenburgh C, Heinecke JW, and Vita JA. Long-term ascorbic acid administration reverses endothelial vasomotor dysfunction in patients with coronary artery disease. *Circulation* 1999;**99:**3234-40.

112. Levine GN, Frei B, Koulouris SN, Gerhard MD, Keaney JF, and Vita JA. Ascorbic acid reverses endothelial vasomotor dysfunction in patients with coronary artery disease. *Circulation* 1996;**93:**1107-1113.

113. Rossig L, Hoffmann J, Hugel B, Mallat Z, Haase A, Freyssinet JM, Tedgui A, Aicher A, Zeiher AM, and Dimmeler S. Vitamin C inhibits endothelial cell apoptosis in congestive heart failure. *Circulation* 2001;**104:**2182-7.

114. Mezzetti A, Zuliani G, Romano F, Costantini F, Pierdomenico SD, Cuccurullo F, and Fellini R. Associazione Medica Sabin: vitamin E and lipid peroxide plasma levels predict the risk of cardiovascular events in a group of healthy very old people. *J Am Geriatr Soc* 2001;**49:**533-7.

115. Riersma RA, Wood DA, Macintyre CCA, Elton RA, Gey KF, and Oliver MF. Risk of angina pectoris and plasma concentrations of vitamins A, C, and E and carotene. *Lancet* 1991;**337:**1-5.

116. Rimm EB, Stampfer MJ, Ascherio A, Giovannucci E, Colditz GA, and Willett WC. Vitamin E consumption and risk of coronary heart disease in men. *New Engl J Med* 1993;**328:**1450-6.

117. Stampfer MJ, Hennekens CH, Manson JE, Colditz GA, Rosner B, and Willett WC. Vitamin E consumption and the risk of coronary disease in women. *New Engl J Med* 1993;**328:**1444-9.

118. Losonszy KG, Harris TB, and Havlick RJ. Vitamin E and vitamin C supplement use and risk of all-cause and coronary heart disease mortality in older persons: the established populations for epidemiologic studies of the elderly. *Am J Clin Nutr* 1996;**64**:190-6.
119. Reaven PD, Khouw A, Beltz WF, Parthasarathy S, and Witzum JL. Effect of dietary antioxidant combinations in humans: protection of LDL by vitamin E but not by beta-carotene. *Arterioscler Thromb* 1993;**13**:590-600.
120. Princen HM, van Duyvenvoorde W, and Buytenhek R. Supplementation with low doses of vitamin E protects LDL from lipid peroxidation in men and women. *Arterioscler Thromb Vasc Biol* 1995;**15**:325-33.
121. Holvoet P and Collen D. Oxidised lipoproteins in atherosclerosis and thrombosis. *FASEB J* 1994;**8**:1279-84.
122. Calzada C, Bruckdorfer KR, and Rice-Evans CA. The influence of antioxidant nutrients on platelet function in healthy volunteers. *Atherosclerosis* 1997;**128**:97-105.
123. Colette C, Pares-Herbute N, Monnier LH, and Cartry E. Platelet function in type I diabetes: effects of supplementation with large doses of vitamin E. *Am J Clin Nutr* 1988;**47**:256-61.0
124. de Lorgeril M, Boissonnat P, and Salen P. The beneficial effects of dietary antioxidant supplementation on platelet aggregation and cyclosporine treatment in heart transplant recipients. *Transplantation* 1994;**58**:193-5.
125. Cox AC, Rao GHR, Gerrard JM, and White JG. The influence of alpha-tocopherol quinone on platelet structure, function and biochemistry. *Blood* 1980;**55**:907-14.
126. Freedman JE, Farhat JH, Loscalzo J, and Keaney JF. Alpha-tocopherol inhibits aggregation of human platelets by a protein kinase C-dependant mechanism. *Circulation* 1996;**94**:2434-40.
127. Keaney JF, Guo Y, Cunningham D, Shwaery GT, Xu A, and Vita JA. Vascular incorporation of alpha-tocopherol prevents endothelial dysfunction due to oxidised LDL by inhibiting protein kinase C stimulation. *J Clin Invest* 1996;**98**:386-94.
128. Azzi A, Aratri E, and Boscoboinick D. Molecular basis of alpha-tocopherol control of smooth muscle cell proliferation. *Biofactors* 1998;**7**:3-14.
129. Plotnick GD, Corretti MC, and Vogel RA. Effect of antioxidant vitamins on the transient impairment of endothelium-dependant brachial artery vasoactivity following a single high-fat meal. *JAMA* 1997;**278**:1682-6.
130. Keaney JF, Gaziano JM, Xu A, Frei B, Curran-Celentano J, Shwaery GT, Loscalzo J, and Vita JA. Low-dose α-tocopherol improves and high-dose α-tocopherol worsens endothelial vasodilator function in cholesterol-fed rabbits. *J Clin Invest* 1994;**93**:844-51.
131. Yoshikawa T, Yoshida N, Manabe H, Terasawa Y, Takemura T, and Kondo M. Alpha-tocopherol protects against expression of adhesion molecules on neutrophils and endothelial cells. *Biofactors* 1998;**7**:15-9.
132. Klein HH, Pich S, Lindert S, Nebendahl K, Niedmann P, and Kreuzer H. Combined treatment with vitamins E and C in experimental myocardial infarction in pigs. *Am Heart J* 1989;**118**:667-73.
133. Leung H-W, Vang MJ, and Mavis RD. The cooperative interaction between vitamin E and vitamin C in suppression of peroxidation of membrane phospholipids. *Biochem Biophys Acta* 1981;**664**:266-72.
134. Rapola JM, Virtamo J, Ripatti S, Huttunen JK, Albanes D, and Taylor PR. Randomised trial of alpha-tocopherol and beta-carotene supplements on incidence of major coronary events in men with previous myocardial infarction. *Lancet* 1997;**349**:1715-20.

135. Stephens NG, Schofield PM, Parsons A, Kelly F, Cheeseman K, and Mitchinson MJ. Randomised controlled trial of vitamin E in patients with coronary disease: Cambridge Heart Antioxidant Study (CHAOS). *Lancet* 1996;**347**:781-6.

136. Singh RB, Niaz MA, Rastogi SS, and Rastogi S. Usefulness of antioxidant vitamins in suspected acute myocardial infarction (the Indian Experiment of Infarct Survival 3). *Am J Cardiol* 1996;**77**:232-6.

137. Elliott TG, Barth JD, and Mancini GBJ. Effects of vitamin E on endothelial function in men after myocardial infarction. *Am J Cardiol* 1995;**76**:1188-91.

138. GISSI Prevenzione Investigators. Dietary supplementation with n-3 polyunsaturated fatty acids and vitamin E after myocardial infarction: results of the GISSI Prevenzione trial. *Lancet* 1999;**354**:447-55.

139. Heart Outcomes Prevention Evaluation Study Investigators. Vitamin E supplementation and cardiovascular events in high-risk patients. *New Engl J Med* 2000;**342**:154-60.

140. Alpha-Tocopherol–Beta-Carotene Cancer Prevention Study Group. The effect of vitamin E and beta-carotene on the incidence of lung cancer and other cancers in male smokers. *New Engl J Med* 1994;**330**:1029-35.

141. Ghatak A, Brar MJ, Agarwal A, Goel N, Rastogi AK, Vaish AK, Sircar AR, and Chandra M. Oxy free radical system in heart failure and therapeutic role of oral vitamin E. *Int J Cardiol* 1996;**57**:119-27.

142. Wu J, Garami M, Cheng T, and Gardner DG. 1,25(OH) vitamin D_3 and retinoic acid antagonise endothelin-stimulated hypertrophy of neonatal rat cardiac myocytes. *J Clin Invest* 1996;**1**:1577-88.

143. Weisshaar RE and Simpson RU. Involvement of vitamin D_3 with cardiovascular function: direct and indirect effects. *Am J Physiol* 1987;**253**:E675-83.

144. Crane FL, Hatefi Y, Lester RL, and Widmer G. Isolation of a quinone from beef heart mitochondria. *Biochem Biophys Acta* 1957;**25**:220-1.

145. Folkers K, Littani G, and Ho L. Evidence for a deficiency of co-enzyme Q_{10} in human heart disease. *Int J Vitam Nutr Res* 1970;**40**:380-90.

146. Kitamura N, Yamaguchi A, and Otaki M. Myocardial tissue level of co-enzyme Q_{10} in patients with cardiac failure. In Folkers K and Yamamura Y, Eds. *Biomedical and Physical Aspects of Coenzyme Q*, Vol 4. Amsterdam, Elsevier, 1984:243-57.

147. Jameson S. Statistical data support prediction of death within 6 months on low levels of coenzyme Q_{10} and other entities. *Clin Invest* 1993;**71**:S137-9.

148. De Pinieux G, Chariot P, Ammi-Said M, Louarn F, Lejonc JL, Astier A, Jacotot B, and Gherardi R. Lipid-lowering drugs and mitochondrial function: effects of HMG-CoA reductase inhibitors on serum ubiquinone and blood lactate/pyruvate ratio. *Br J Clin Pharmacol* 1996;**42**:333-7.

149. Bargossi AM, Battino M, Gaddi A, Fiorella PL, Grossi G, Barozzi G, Di Giulio R, Descovich G, Sassi S, and Genova ML. Exogenous CoQ_{10} preserves plasma ubiquinone levels in patients treated with 3-hydroxy-3-methylglutaryl coenzyme A reductase inhibitors. *Int J Clin Lab Res* 1994;**24**:171-6.

150. Laaksonen R, Jokelainen K, Laakso J, Sahi T, Harkonen M, Tikkanen MJ, and Himberg JJ. The effect of simvastatin treatment on natural antioxidants in low-density lipoproteins and high-energy phosphates and ubiquinone in skeletal muscle. *Am J Cardiol* 1996;**77**:851-4.

151. Laaksonen R, Jokelainen K, Sahi T, Tikkanen MJ, and Himberg JJ. Decreases in serum ubiquinone concentrations do not result in reduced levels in muscle tissue during short-term simvastatin treatment in humans. *Clin Pharmacol Ther* 1995;**57**:62-6.

152. Baggio E, Gandini R, Plancher AC, Passeri M, and Carmosino G. Italian multicentre study on the safety and efficacy of coenzyme Q_{10} as adjunctive therapy in heart failure. *Mol Aspects Med* 1994;**15(Suppl)**:S287-94.

153. Mortensen SA, Vadhanavikit S, Muratsu, K, and Folkers K. Coenzyme Q_{10}: clinical benefits with biochemical correlates suggesting a scientific breakthrough in the management of chronic heart failure. *Int J Tissue React* 1990;**12**:155-62.

154. Morisco C, Nappi A, Argenziano L, Sarno D, Fontana D, Imbriaco M, Nicolai E, Romano M, Rosiello G, and Cuocolo A. Noninvasive evaluation of cardiac haemodynamics during exercise in patients with chronic heart failure: effects of short-term coenzyme Q_{10} treatment. *Mol Aspects Med* 1994;**15**:S155-63.

155. Hofman-Bang C, Rehnqvist N, Swedberg K, Wiklund I, and Astrom H. Coenzyme Q_{10} as an adjunctive treatment of chronic congestive heart failure. *J Card Fail* 1995;**2**:101-7.

156. Morisco C, Trimarco B, and Condorelli M. Effect of coenzyme Q_{10} therapy in patients with congestive heart failure: a long-term multicentre randomised study. *Clin Invest* 1993;**71**:S134-6.

157. Watson PS, Scalia GM, Galbraith A, Burstow DJ, Bett N, Aroney CN. Lack of effect of coenzyme Q_{10} on left ventricular function in patients with congestive cardiac failure. *J Am Coll Cardiol* 1999;**33**:1549-52.

158. Langsjoen PH, Langsjoen PH, and Folkers K. Isolated diastolic dysfunction of the myocardium and its response to CoQ_{10} treatment. *Clin Invest* 1993;**71**:S140-4.

159. Sobotka PA, Brottman MD, Weitz Z et al. Elevated breath pentane in heart failure reduced by free radical scavenger. *Free Radic Biol Med* 1993;**14**:643-7.

160. McMurray J, McLay J, Chopra M et al. Evidence for free radical activity in chronic congestive heart failure secondary to coronary artery disease. *Am J Cardiol* 1990;**65**:1261-2.

161. Díaz-Vélez CR, García-Castiñeiras S, Mendoza-Ramos E, and Hernández-Lopez E. Increased malondialdehyde in peripheral blood of patients with congestive heart failure. *Am Heart J* 1996;**131**:146-52.

162. Keith M, Geranmayegan A, Sole MJ et al. Increased oxidative stress in patients with congestive heart failure. *J Am Coll Cardiol* 1998;**31**:1352-6.

163. Belch JJF, Bridges AB, Scott N, and Chopra M. Oxygen free radicals and congestive heart failure. *Br Heart J* 1991;**65**:245-8.

164. Nishiyama Y, Ikeda H, Haramaki N et al. Oxidative stress is related to exercise intolerance in patients with heart failure. *Am Heart J* 1998;**135**:115-20.

165. Polidori MC, Savino K, Alunni G, Freddio M, Senin U, Sies H, Stahl W, and Mecocci P. Plasma lipophilic antioxidants and malondialdehyde in congestive heart failure patients: relationship to disease severity. *Free Radic Biol Med* 2002;**32**:148-52.

166. Heitzer T, Schlinzig T, Krohn K, Meinertz T, and Munzel T. Endothelial dysfunction, oxidative stress, and risk of cardiovascular events in patients with coronary artery disease. *Circulation* 2001;**104**:2673-8.

167. Gupta M and Singal PK. Time course of structure, function and metabolic changes due to an exogenous source of oxygen metabolites in rat heart. *Can J Physiol Pharmacol* 1989;**67**:1549-59.

168. Prasad K, Gupta JB, Kalra J et al. Oxidative stress as a mechanism of cardiac failure in chronic volume overload in canine model. *J Mol Cell Cardiol* 1996;**28**:375-85.

169. Dhalla AK, Hill MF, and Singal PK. Role of oxidative stress in transition of hypertrophy to heart failure. *J Am Coll Cardiol* 1996;**28**:506-14.

170. Cohn JN, Levine TB, and Olivari MT. Plasma norephinephrine as a guide to prognosis in patients with congestive heart failure. *New Engl J Med* 1984;**311**:819-23.

171. Daly P and Sole MJ. Myocardial catecholamines and the pathophysiology of heart failure. *Circulation* 1990;**82**:35-43.
172. Levine B, Kalman J, Mager L et al. Elevated circulating levels of tumour necrosis factor in severe chronic heart failure. *New Engl J Med* 1990;**323**:236-41.
173. Factor SM, Minase T, Cho S et al. Microvascular spasm in the cardiomyopathic Syrian hamster: a preventable cause of focal myocardial necrosis. *Circulation* 1982;**66**:342-5.
174. Rajagopalan S, Kurz S, Münzel T et al. Angiotensin II-mediated hypertension in the rat increases vascular superoxide production via membrane NADH/NADPH oxidase activation. *J Clin Invest* 1996;**97**:1916-23
175. Nakamura K, Fushimi K, Kouchi H, Mihara K, Miyazaki M, Ohe T, and Namba M. Inhibitory effects of antioxidants on neonatal rat cardiac myocyte hypertrophy induced by tumour necrosis factor-alpha and angiotensin II. *Circulation 1998;***98**:794-99.
176. Bank AJ, Rector TS, Tschumperlin LK, Kraemer MD, Letouneau JG, and Kubo SH. Endothelium-dependant vasodilation of peripheral conduit arteries in patients with heart failure. *J Card Fail* 1994 ;**1**:35-43.
177. Drexler H, Hayoz D, Munzel T, Just H, Zelis H, and Brunner H. Endothelial function in congestive heart failure. *Am Heart J* 1993;**126**:761-4.
178. Katz SD, Biasucci L, Sabba C, Strom JA, Jondeau G, Galvao N, Solomon S, Nikolic SD, Forman R, and LeJemtel T. Impaired endothelium-mediated vasodilatation in the peripheral vasculature of patients with congestive heart failure. *J Am Coll Cardiol* 1992;**19**:918-25.
179. Zelis R and Flaim S. Alterations in vasomotor tone in congestive heart failure. *Prog Cardiovasc Dis* 1982;**24**:437-59
180. Lehr H-A, Frei B, Olofsson AM, Carew TE, and Arfors K-E. Protection from oxidised LDL-induced leukocyte adhesion to microvascular and macrovascular endothelium *in vivo* by vitamin C but not by vitamin E. *Circulation* 1995;**91**:1525-32.
181. Gryglewski RJ, Palmer RMJ, and Moncada S. Superoxide anion is involved in the breakdown of endothelial-derived vascular relaxing factor. *Nature* 1986;**320**:454-6.
182. Gilligan DM, Sack MN, Guetta V, Casino PR, Quyyumi AA, Rader DJ, Panza JA, and Cannon RO. Effect of antioxidant vitamins on low density lipoprotein oxidation and impaired endothelium-dependant vasodilation in patients with hypercholestero-laemia. *J Am Coll Cardiol* 1994;**24**:1611-7.
183. Marui N, Offermann MK, Swerlick R, Kunsch C, Rosen CA, Ahmad M, Alexander RW, and Medford RM. Vascular cell adhesion molecule-1 (VCAM-1) gene transcription and expression are regulated through an antioxidant-sensitive mechanism in human vascular endothelial cells. *J Clin Invest* 1993;**92**:1866-74.
184. Herbaczynska-Cedro K, Kosiewicz-Wasek B, and Cedro K. Supplementation with vitamins C and E suppresses leukocyte oxygen free radical production in patients with myocardial infarction. *Eur Heart J* 1995;**16**:1044-9.
185. Fang JC, Kinlay S, Beltrame J, Hikiti H, Wainstein M, Behrendt D, Suh J, Frei B, Mudge GH, Selwyn AP, and Ganz P. Effect of vitamins C and E on progression of transplant-associated arteriosclerosis: a randomised trial. *Lancet* 2002;**359**:1108-13.
186. Muntwyler J, Hennekens CH, Manson JE, Buring JE, and Gaziano JM. Vitamin supplement use in a low-risk population of U.S. male physicians and subsequent cardiovascular mortality. *Arch Intern Med* 2002;**162**:1472-6.
187. Heart Protection Study Collaborative Group. MRC/BHF Heart Protection Study of antioxidant vitamin supplementation in 20,536 high-risk individuals: a randomised placebo-controlled trial. *Lancet* 2002;**360**:23-33.

188. Brown BG, Zhao XQ, Chait A, Fisher LD, Cheung MC, Morse JS, Dowdy AA, Marino EK, Bolson EL, Alaupovic P, Frohlich J, and Albers JJ. Simvastatin and niacin, antioxidant vitamins, or the combination for the prevention of coronary disease. *New Engl J Med* 2001;**345:**1583-92.

189. Selhub J, Jacques PF, Bostom AG et al. Association between plasma homocysteine concentrations and extracranial carotid artery stenosis. *New Engl J Med* 1995;**332:**286-91.

190. Nygard O, Nordrehaug JE, Refsum H et al. Plasma homocysteine levels and mortality in patients with coronary artery disease. *New Engl J Med* 1997;**337:**230-36.

191. Verhoef P, Kok FJ, Kruyssen DACM et al. Plasma total homocysteine, B vitamins, and risk of coronary atherosclerosis. *Arterioscler Thromb Vasc Biol* 1997;**17:**989-95.

192. de Bree A, Verschuren WM, Blom HJ, Nadeau M, Trijbels FJ, and Kromhout D. Coronary heart disease mortality, plasma homocysteine, and B-vitamins: a prospective study. *Atherosclerosis* 2003;**166:**369-377.

193. Chambers JC, Obeid OA, Refsum H et al. Plasma homocysteine concentrations and risk of coronary heart disease in U.K. Indian Asian and European men. *Lancet* 2000;**355:**523-27.

194. Nair KG, Nair SR, Ashavaid TF, Dalal JJ, and Eghlim FF. Methylenetetrahydrofolate reductase gene mutation and hyperhomocysteinemia as a risk factor for coronary heart disease in the Indian population. *J Assoc Physicians India* 2002;**50(Suppl):**9-15.

195. Kaye JM, Stanton KG, McCann VJ, Vasikaran SD, Burke V, Taylor RR, and van Bockxmeer FM. Homocysteine, folate, methylene tetrahydrofolate reductase genotype and vascular morbidity in diabetic subjects. *Clin Sci (Lond)* 2002;**102:**631-7.

196. Lentz SR and Sadler JE. Inhibition of thrombomodulin surface expression and protein C activation by the thrombogenic agent homocysteine. *J Clin Invest* 1991;**88:**1906-14.

197. Nappo F, De Rosa N, Marfella R et al. Impairment of endothelial functions by acute hyperhomocysteinemia and reversal by antioxidant vitamins. *JAMA* 1999;**281:**2113-8.

198. Rodgers GM and Kane WH. Activation of endogenous factor V by a homocysteine-induced vascular endothelial cell activator. *J Clin Invest* 1996;**77:**1909-16.

199. Wall RT, Harlan JM, Harker LA, and Striker GE. Homocysteine-induced endothelial cell injury *in vitro*: a model for the study of vascular injury. *Thromb Res* 1980;**18:**113-21.

200. Berman RS and Martin W. Arterial endothelial barrier dysfunction: actions of homocysteine and the hypoxanthine-xanthine oxidase free radical generating system. *Br J Pharmacol* 1993;**108:**920-6.

201. Loscalzo J. The oxidant stress of hyperhomocysteinaemia. *J Clin Invest* 1996;**98:**5-7.

202. Blundell G, Jones BG, Rose FA, and Tudball N. Homocysteine mediated endothelial cell toxicity and its amelioration. *Atherosclerosis* 1996;**122:**163-72.

203. Tsai JC, Perella MA, and Yoshizumi M. Promotion of vascular smooth muscle cell growth by homocysteine: a link to atherosclerosis. *Proc Natl Acad Sci USA* 1994;**91:**6369-73.

204. Tawakol A, Omland T, Gerhard M et al. Hyperhomocysteinaemia is associated with impaired endothelium-dependant vasodilation in humans. *Circulation* 1997;**95:**1119-21.

205. Chambers JC, McGregor A, Jean-Marie J et al. Demonstration of rapid onset vascular endothelial dysfunction after hyperhomocysteinaemia: an effect reversible with vitamin C therapy. *Circulation* 1999;**99:**1156-60.

206. Kanani PM, Sinkey CA, Browning RL et al. Role of oxidant stress in endothelial dysfunction produced by experimental hyperhomocysteinaemia in humans. *Circulation* 1999;**100:**1161-8.
207. Blom HJ, Engelen DP, and Boers GH. Lipid peroxidation in homocysteinaemia. *J Inherit Metab Dis* 1992;**15:**419-22.
208. Blom HJ, Kleinveld HA, and Boers GH. Lipid peroxidation and susceptibility of low-density-lipoprotein to *in vitro* oxidation in hyperhomocysteinaemia. *Eur J Clin Invest* 1995;**25:**149-54.
209. Tyagi SC. Homocysteine redox receptor and regulation of extracellular matrix components in vascular cells. *Am J Phsiol* 1998;**274**(Part 1)**:**C396-405.
210. Tsai JC, Perella MA, and Yoshizumi M. Promotion of vascular smooth muscle cell growth by homocysteine: a link to atherosclerosis. *Proc Natl Acad Sci USA* 1994;**91:**6369-73.
211. Dudman NP, Temple SE, Guo XW et al. Homocysteine enhances neutrophil-endothelial interactions in both cultured human cells and rats *in vivo*. *Circ Res* 1999;**84:**409-16.
212. Upchurch GR Jr, Welch GN, Fabian AJ et al. Stimulation of endothelial nitric oxide production by homocysteine. *Atherosclerosis* 1997;**132:**177-85.
213. Stamler JS, Osborne JA, and Jaraki O. Adverse vascular effects of homocysteine are modulated by endothelial derived relaxing factor and related oxides of nitrogen. *J Clin Invest* 1993;**91:**308-18.
214. Upchurch GR Jr., Welch GN, and Loscalzo J. Homocysteine, EDRF, and endothelial function. *J Nutr* 1996;**126**(4Suppl):1290S-4S.
215. Rodgers GM and Kane WH. Activation of endogenous factor V by a homocysteine-induced vascular endothelial cell activator. *J Clin Invest* 1986;**77:**1909-16.
216. Giannini MJ, Coleman M, and Innerfield I. Antithrombin activity in homocysteinuria [letter]. *Lancet* 1977;**1:**1094.
217. Rodgers GM and Conn MT. Homocysteine, an atherogenic stimulus, reduces protein C activation by arterial and venous endothelial cells. *Blood* 1990;**75:**895-901.
218. Hajjar KA. Homocysteine-induced modulation of tissue plasminogen activator binding to its endothelial cell membrane receptor. *J Clin Invest* 1993;**91:**2873-9.
219. Selhub J, Jacques PF, Wilson PWF et al. Vitamin status and intake as primary determinants of homocysteinaemia in an elderly population. *JAMA* 1993;**270:**2693-8.
220. Hernandez-Diaz S, Martinez-Losa E, Fernandez-Jarne E, Serrano-Martinez M, and Martinez-Gonzalez MA. Dietary folate and the risk of nonfatal myocardial infarction. *Epidemiology* 200;**13:**700-6.
221. Naurath HJ, Joosten E, Rizler R et al. Effects of vitamin B12, folate, and vitamin B6 supplementation in elderly people with normal serum vitamin concentrations. *Lancet* 1995;**346:**85-89.
222. Neal B, MacMahon S, Ohkubo T, Tonkin A, and Wilcken D. Dose-dependent effects of folic acid on plasma homocysteine in a randomised trial conducted among 723 individuals with coronary heart disease. *Eur Heart J* 2002;**23:**1509-15.
223. Vermeulen EGJ, Stehouwer CDA, Twisk JWR et al. Effect of homocysteine-lowering treatment with folic acid plus vitamin B_6 on progression of subclinical atherosclerosis: a randomised, placebo-controlled trial. *Lancet* 2000;**355:**517-22.
224. Thambyrajah J, Landray MJ, Jones HJ, McGlynn FJ, Wheeler DC, and Townend JN. A randomised double-blind placebo-controlled trial of the effect of homocysteine-lowering therapy with folic acid on endothelial function in patients with coronary artery disease. *J Am Coll Cardiol* 2001;**37:**1858-63.

225. Schnyder G, Roffi M, Flammer Y, Pin R, and Hess OM. Effect of homocysteine-lowering therapy with folic acid, vitamin $B_{(12)}$, and vitamin $B_{(6)}$ on clinical outcome after percutaneous coronary intervention: the Swiss Heart study: a randomised controlled trial. *JAMA* 2002;**288**:973-9.

226. Schnyder G, Roffi M, Pin R, Flammer Y, Lange H, Eberli FR, Meier B, Turi ZG, and Hess OM. Decreased rate of coronary restenosis after lowering of plasma homocysteine levels. *New Engl J Med* 2001;**345**:1593-600.

227. Anand I, Chandrashekhan Y, De Giuli F et al. Acute and chronic effects of propionyl-L-carnitine on the hemodynamics, exercise capacity, and hormones in patients with congestive heart failure. *Cardiovasc Drugs Ther* 1998;**12**:291-9.

228. Pastoris O, Dossena M, Foppa P et al. Effect of L-carnitine on myocardial metabolism: results of a balanced, placebo-controlled, double-blind study in patients undergoing open heart surgery. *Pharmacol Res* 1998;**37**:115-22.

229. Bartels GL, Remme WJ, Holwerda KJ, and Kruijssen DA. Anti-ischaemic efficacy of L-propionylcarnitine: a promising novel metabolic approach to ischaemia? *Eur Heart J* 1996;**17**:414-20.

230. Bartels GL, Remme WJ, den Hartog FR et al. Additional anti-ischaemic effects of long-term L-propionylcarnitine in anginal patients treated with conventional antianginal therapy. *Cardiovasc Drugs Ther* 1995;**9**:749-53.

231. Bartels GL, Remme WJ, Pillay M et al. Effects of L-propionylcarnitine on ischaemia-induced myocardial dysfunction in men with angina pectoris. *Am J Cardiol* 1994;**74**:125-30.

232. Iyer RN, Khan AA, Gupta A, Vajifdar BU, and Lokhandwala YY. L-carnitine moderately improves the exercise tolerance in chronic stable angina. *J Assoc Physicians India* 2000;**48**:1050-2.

233. Singh RB, Niaz MA, Agarwal P et al. A randomised, double-blind, placebo-controlled trial of L-carnitine in suspected acute myocardial infarction. *Postgrad Med J* 1996;**72**:45-50.

234. Iliceto S, Scrutinio D, Bruzzi P et al. Effects of L-carnitine administration on left ventricular remodelling after acute anterior myocardial infarction: the L-Carnitine Ecocardiografia Digitalizzata Infarto Miocardico (CEDIM) Trial. *J Am Coll Cardiol* 1995;**26**:380-7.

235. Gasparetto A, Corbucci GG, De Blasi RA et al. Influence of acetyl-L-carnitine infusion on haemodynamic parameters and survival of circulatory-shock patients. *Int J Clin Pharmacol Res* 1991;**11**:83-92.

236. Corsi C, Pollastri M, Marrapodi E et al. L-propionylcarnitine effect on postexercise and postischemic hyperaemia in patients affected by peripheral vascular disease. *Angiology* 1995;**46**:705-13.

237. Hiatt WR, Regensteiner JG, Creager MA, Hirsch AT, Cooke JP, Olin JW, Gorbunov GN, Isner J, Lukjanov YV, Tsitsiashvili MS, Zabelskaya TF, and Amato A. Propionyl-L-carnitine improves exercise performance and functional status in patients with claudication. *Am J Med* 2001;**110**:616-22.

238. Investigators of the Study on Propionyl-L-Carnitine in chronic heart failure. Study on propionyl-L-carnitine in chronic heart failure. *Eur Heart J* 1999;**20**:70-6.

239. Vescovo G, Ravara B, Gobbo V, Sandri M, Angelini A, Della Barbera M, Dona M, Peluso G, Calvani M, Mosconi L, and Dalla Libera L. L-Carnitine: a potential treatment for blocking apoptosis and preventing skeletal muscle myopathy in heart failure. *Am J Physiol Cell Physiol* 2002;**283**:C802-10.

240. Clark AL, Poole-Wilson PA, and Coats AJS. Exercise limitation in chronic heart failure: the central role of the periphery. *J Am Coll Cardiol* 1996;**28**:1092-1102.

241. Greenhaff PL, Bodin K, Soderland K, and Hultman E. Effect of oral creatine supplementation on skeletal muscle phosphocreatine resynthesis. *Am J Physiol* 1994;**266**:E725-30.

242. Gordon A, Hultman E, and Kaijser L. Creatine supplementation in chronic heart failure increases skeletal muscle creatine phosphate and muscle performance. *Cardiovasc Res* 1995;**30**:413-8.

243. Ferraro S, Maddalena G, and Fazio S. Acute and short-term efficacy of high doses of creatine phosphate in the treatment of cardiac failure. *Curr Ther Res Clin Exp* 1990;**47**:17-23.

244. Romagnoli GF, Naso A, Carraro G, and Lidestri V. Beneficial effects of L-carnitine in dialysis patients with impaired left ventricular function: an observational study. *Curr Med Res Opin* 2002;**18**:172-5.

245. Gordon A, Hultman E, and Kaijser L. Creatine supplementation in chronic heart failure increases skeletal muscle creatine phosphate and muscle performance. *Cardiovasc Res* 1995;**30**:413-8.

246. Schaufelberger M, Eriksson BO, Held P, and Swedberg K. Skeletal muscle alterations in patients with chronic heart failure. *Eur Heart J* 1997;**18**:971-80.

7 Leptin and Blood Pressure

Steven J. Swoap and J. Michael Overton

CONTENTS

7.1 INTRODUCTORY COMMENTS

The relationship between obesity and cardiovascular disease is well established and has been extensively reviewed.[1-4] The coexistence of obesity and hypertension provides a compelling rationale to examine specific mechanisms that contribute to obesity and evaluate whether these mechanisms explain the relationship between blood pressure (BP) and increased levels of body fat. The discovery of leptin, an adipocyte-derived hormone, in 1994[5] marked the beginning of rapid progress in understanding signals involved in responding to nutritional input, central pathways regulated by these signals, and efferent mechanisms regulated by leptin and these signals. Because human obesity is a disease of elevated leptin levels, the purpose of this review is to examine the evidence testing the hypothesis that increased leptin levels contribute to elevated BP in obesity.

7.2 LEPTIN AND CENTRAL NERVOUS SYSTEM

7.2.1 CIRCULATING LEPTIN GAINS ACCESS TO CNS

Leptin is a 167-amino acid protein produced predominantly by adipocytes, although other organs and tissues including the placenta, stomach, and skeletal muscle also produce leptin.[6,7] Circulating levels are generally low (5 to 10 ng/ml) and are elevated in obese individuals in proportion to body fat, typically two- to four-fold.[8,9] Indeed, the levels of circulating leptin exhibit a close relationship to body fat stores, although time of day, gender, age, sleep apnea, and acute variations in energy balance can all influence leptin levels.[7,10–12]

Leptin appears to enter the central nervous system (CNS) via a saturable transport system. Thus, it is likely that this hormone gains access to hypothalamic receptors and regulates neural pathways that control appetite and energy expenditure through this saturable system and via circumventricular organs such as the median eminence.[13,14] This saturable system appears to be one reason why obesity is associated with reduced responsiveness to leptin, broadly termed leptin resistance (see below).[14,15] In addition, limited access to relevant CNS neurons may explain the minimal weight loss observed in the initial leptin trials for treatment of obesity in humans.[16,17]

7.2.2 LEPTIN REGULATES COMPLEX NEURAL NETWORKS IN MEDIOBASAL HYPOTHALAMUS

Leptin receptors (LRs) are located in cell groups within the hypothalamus and the brain stem in regions known to be important in the regulation of ingestive behavior, pituitary function, and autonomic nervous system activity. LRs are multiple protein products of a single LR gene as a result of alternative splicing of the primary transcript.[18–20] The "long" form of the LR (LRb) contains an intact cytoplasmic domain necessary for intracellular leptin signaling.[18,20,21] Upon ligand binding to LRb, Jak2 tyrosine kinase is activated, and this initiates a number of intracellular signaling events, including activation of the transcription factor STAT3 and activation of SHP-2/GRB-2 pathways.[22]

The short forms of the receptor that lack most of the cytoplasmic domain may serve as transporters at the choroid plexus for leptin entry into cerebrospinal fluid, as circulating binding proteins or performing other as-yet-undetermined functions. Careful studies probing for only LRb demonstrate that while it can be detected in many tissues, LRb is most abundantly expressed within the hypothalamus.[18] Several regions in the hypothalamus express LRb including primarily the arcuate (ARC), dorsomedial (DMH), and ventromedial nuclei, with less expression in the lateral (LHA), posterior, and paraventricular (PVN) nuclei.[23] Many of these regions exhibit leptin-induced c-fos expression, supporting their involvement in mediating the physiologic actions of leptin.[23] Leptin signaling regulates multiple neuronal groups in these areas in complex ways that have not yet been unraveled adequately to explain leptin physiology.

Although much of the current focus on leptin is as an anti-obesity hormone, accumulating evidence indicates that additional (and more important) biologic roles for leptin are preventing the excess deposition of triglyceride in nonadipose tissue[24] and signalling reduced nutrient availability.[25] Many of the hypothalamic neurons expressing LRb are regulated by starvation and are responsive to leptin administration.[26] One key set of neurons in the medial ARC synthesizes both neuropeptide Y (NPY) and agouti-related protein (AgRP) and projects within the hypothalamus to the PVN, DMH, and LHA.[23,26,27] AgRP and NPY are both up-regulated by negative energy balance, and stimulate increased food intake and reduced metabolic rate upon exogenous administration. Leptin infusion inhibits starvation-induced activation of NPY and AgRP gene expression.[28]

Another set of neurons located in the lateral ARC and exhibiting a similar projection pattern expresses pro-opiomelanocortin (POMC) and cocaine- and amphetamine-related transcript (CART).[23,26] These neurons are generally inhibited by starvation and activated by leptin. Multiple lines of evidence support the possibility that second order neurons expressing corticotrophin releasing hormone (CRH), thyrotropin releasing hormone (TRH), melanin-concentrating hormone (MCH), and hypocretin/orexin may ultimately produce many of the physiological effects of leptin. The reader is directed to recent reviews for more information on these pathways.[23,26,29] The putative roles of some of these neurotransmitters in the sympathetic and cardiovascular actions of leptin are discussed later.

7.3 CARDIOVASCULAR AND AUTONOMIC EFFECTS OF LEPTIN

7.3.1 LEPTIN AND HEART RATE

Increasing attention is focused on the cardiovascular disease risk linked to the tachycardia commonly seen in obese patients.[4,30,31] Is increased circulating leptin a primary cause of the tachycardia associated with obesity? Some human studies have observed correlations between circulating leptin levels and resting heart rate (HR), although the results are quite variable.[32–34] In one study where HR was not correlated with leptin per se, spectral analysis suggested a relationship between elevated leptin and increased relative cardiac sympathetic tone.[33]

There have been several difficulties in delineating the effect of leptin on regulation of HR in animal studies. It is a common observation that anesthetized animals have reduced chronotropic responsiveness. Thus, it is not surprising that acute leptin administration to anesthetized animals generally has no effect on HR.[35–37] Acute peripheral leptin administration to conscious rats has also been reported to have no effect on HR.[38] In contrast, acute intracerebral ventricular (ICV) leptin administration to conscious animals produces modest tachycardias in rats and rabbits.[39,40] The issue becomes more complex with chronic leptin administration, as reductions in food intake and body weight (mediated by the potent anorexic and thermogenic effects of leptin in rodents) are normally associated with bradycardia in mice,[41,42] rats,[42–45] and humans.[46,47] Nonetheless, chronic central or peripheral administration of leptin is generally associated with tachycardia.[48–52] The evidence strongly supports the concept that leptin increases HR and thus may participate in obesity-related tachycardia.

7.3.2 LEPTIN AND BLOOD PRESSURE

7.3.2.1 Peripheral Leptin Infusion

Like the effects on HR, several mitigating factors complicate attempts to understand the effect of leptin on BP regulation. In initial studies, it was somewhat surprising that, despite marked increases in sympathetic nerve activation, intravenous leptin infusion did not increase arterial BP.[53] In addition to the issues of anesthesia and weight loss discussed above, it also appears that leptin influences endothelial function and may cause vasodilation.[54–57] Thus, it is not surprising that acute peripheral infusion of leptin into anesthetized animals generally does not increase BP.[38,53] The role of nitric oxide in opposing leptin-mediated BP effects remains unresolved. In conscious rats, nitric oxide synthase inhibition does not uncover a pressor effect of acute peripheral leptin infusion,[38,56,57] and leptin may instead regulate endothelium-derived hyperpolarizing factor.[56]

Chronic infusions of leptin performed in the lab of John Hall provided the first evidence that peripheral leptin administration may increase BP.[52] Leptin infusion raised plasma levels to about 90 ng/ml, reduced food intake and body weight, and increased both HR and BP. The chronic pressor effects of leptin are augmented by NOS inhibition[48] and attenuated by combined treatment with teraozin and propranolol.[49] The findings are consistent with the hypothesis that the pressor effects of leptin are mediated by increased sympathetic outflow.

A second approach toward altering peripheral leptin levels is a genetic one. Mice that overexpress leptin to levels reaching 50 ng/ml have been generated.[58] Consistent with the role of leptin on the sympathetic nervous system, urinary epinephrine and norepinephrine were elevated two- to three-fold. Systolic BP, measured with tail-cuff methodologies, was elevated 15 mmHg in these animals.[58] Thus, it appears that elevation of peripheral leptin levels through infusion or genetic manipulation causes an elevation in BP independent of adiposity and total body weight.

If elevated leptin levels increase BP, do reduced leptin levels have the opposite effect? We will examine this possibility with regard to the effects of weight loss and leptin below; but another strategy to evaluate this possibility is to study mice lacking leptin (ob/ob mice). Experimental observations are conflicting in this area in that two groups have found these animals to be normotensive[42,58] while a third found a mean BP of about 90 mmHg as compared to the mean BP of control littermates of 106 mmHg.[59] Based on the multiple neuroendocrine abnormalities and morbid obesity of ob/ob mice, other approaches including evaluation of cardiovascular responses to leptin receptor antagonists may be needed to determine the direct effects of reduced leptin signaling on blood pressure.

7.3.2.2 Central Leptin Infusion

Central administration of leptin avoids the potential counteracting effects of peripheral vasodilation and generally increases BP.[37,39,40,50] However, the physiological relevance of studies injecting high levels of leptin directly into the brain is uncertain. Recently, a dose–response study of centrally administered leptin carefully addressed this important issue. At a relatively low dose (200 ng/h), leptin decreased food intake and increased HR, but had no effect on BP in rats fed normal diets.[50] In rats fed high salt diets, central infusion of a higher dose of leptin (1000 ng/h) also decreased food intake and increased HR and had a small and transient effect on BP.[50] The finding is consistent with a recent report from Overton et al.,[51] showing infusion of a lower dose of leptin (42 ng/h) decreased food intake yet had no significant effect on BP or HR (although HR increased 20 bpm in spite of weight loss).

Hence, it appears that leptin-mediated anorexic effects are observed at lower doses than cardiovascular effects and that pharmacological doses of leptin may be required to produce physiologically important increases in BP. Careful studies are needed to determine whether chronic, long-term peripheral elevations of leptin in the physiologic range indeed have important effects on HR and BP.

7.3.3 Leptin and Sympathetic Nervous System

Consistent with the cardiovascular effects of leptin, it is not surprising that leptin increases sympathetic nervous system outflow. Allyn Mark and colleagues at the University of Iowa provided the first direct evidence that peripheral leptin infusion increased sympathetic nerve activity (SNA) to multiple targets.[53] It is generally agreed that leptin-mediated increases in SNA proceed via central nervous system action. Central administration of much lower doses of leptin increases plasma catecholamine levels,[60,61] directly measured SNA,[40,62] and UCP1 mRNA levels in brown adipose tissue.[63] Large electrolytic regions of the ventromedial hypothalamus prevent peripherally administered, leptin-mediated sympathoexcitation.[61]

As noted earlier, LRs are widely distributed and account for the complex biological actions of this peptide. LRs are clearly evident in adipocytes, and recent evidence suggests that leptin may activate a reflex pathway originating in adipose tissue and regulating both sympathetic and vagal activity.[64,65] Nonetheless, the observations that leptin administration augments sympathetic activity to multiple targets including the kidneys[35,40,53] are consistent with the hypothesis that leptin may contribute to obesity-induced sympathoexcitation and hypertension.

7.4 LEPTIN-RESPONSIVE NEURAL PATHWAYS AND CARDIOVASCULAR SYSTEM

Although it has been nearly 10 years since the discovery of leptin, the mechanisms by which this hormone produces its biologic actions are only beginning to be understood. As described above, hypothalamic neurons that express either POMC/CART or NPY/AgRP are likely candidates to serve as the initial and primary mediators of leptin, including the sympathetic and cardiovascular responses to altered CNS leptin levels. Downstream mechanisms ultimately regulating preganglionic autonomic neurons controlling HR and vascular tone must be identified to gain a more complete understanding of the cardiovascular and sympathetic effects of leptin.

7.4.1 POMC/CART Neurons and Cardiovascular Effects

One of the primary neurotransmitters in the POMC/CART neuron is alpha melanocyte-stimulating hormone (αMSH). This peptide is cleaved from the POMC precursor and is a ligand for the melanocortin receptor (MC-R). The MC-R family consists of five known receptors. αMSH binds to the MC4-R within the hypothalamus and reduces food intake.[66,67] Several lines of evidence support the hypothesis that the POMC pathway is a critical target for leptin action with respect to both SNA and cardiovascular parameters. Central administration of αMSH or MT-II, an MC4-R agonist, increases BP.[35,68,69] Importantly, central administration of agouti, an antagonist of MC4-R, prevents increases in BP and SNA with either leptin[62] or αMSH administration.[69] Furthermore, leptin-mediated increases in renal SNA, but not brown adipose SNA, were prevented by central administration of the MC4-R antagonist SHU9119.[35] The findings suggest that renal, but not thermogenic, sympathoexcitatory effects of leptin are mediated by POMC pathways.[35]

Leptin has been shown to activate CART-containing neurons that innervate sympathetic preganglionic neurons.[70] However, much less is known about the cardiovascular effects of CART. As with administration of αMSH, central CART administration elevates HR, BP, renal SNA, and plasma catecholamine levels.[71] Collectively, both αMSH and CART are induced by leptin, and central administration of either of these neuropeptides mimics the elevation in cardiovascular parameters elicited by leptin.

7.4.2 NPY/AgRP Neurons and Cardiovascular Effects

Elevated body mass and leptin injections decrease hypothalamic NPY expression in a leptin-receptor dependent fashion.[28,72] Central NPY administration produces a reduction in BP, HR, and sympathetic activity.[73,74] However, little evidence suggests that the reduced arcuate hypothalamic NPYergic activity directly contributes to the physiologic effects of elevated leptin levels. Indeed, studies with NPY knockout mice indicate that the anorexic effects of leptin do not depend on the NPY axis.[75] Further, central infusions of an NPY antagonist had no effect on HR and MAP in ad-lib fed rats.[76] Evidence that hypothalamic NPYergic neurons provide tonic sympathoexcitatory input would provide the basis for more careful examination of the hypothesis that reduced NPY activity contributes to leptin-mediated cardiovascular effects.

AgRP is the endogenous antagonist to MC4-R, blocking binding of αMSH to MC4-R Overexpression of AgRP in the hypothalamus can lead to obesity, indicating the importance of the neuropeptide in leptin-mediated function.[77,78] Central administration of AgRP prevents the increases in BP and RSNA associated with αMSH administration.[68] In sum, both NPY and AgRP are diminished by leptin administration, and when administered centrally, both elicit the opposite effects on body weight maintenance and the cardiovascular system compared to leptin administration. However, we have little compelling evidence that down-regulation of these neuropeptides is required for the cardiovascular and sympathetic effects of leptin.

7.4.3 SECOND ORDER NEURONS AND CARDIOVASCULAR EFFECTS

Some neuron types that appear downstream of POMC/CART and NPY/AgRP neurons have been shown to influence cardiovascular parameters. These neurons include those that express corticotrophin-releasing hormone (CRH), hypocretin/orexin, and thyrotropin-releasing hormone (TRH).

CRH is a 41-amino acid protein that, in addition to regulation of the pituitary–adrenal stress response, is involved with the regulation of energy balance and cardiovascular control. Negative energy balance inhibits expression of CRH, whereas central administration of leptin induces CRH production.[79,80] Central administration of CRH increases plasma epinephrine and norepinephrine and elicits increases in BP, HR, and cardiac output.[81–83] Leptin-induced increases in brown adipose SNA are significantly blunted by pretreatment with a CRH inhibitor, alpha-helical CRF9-41.[84] However, leptin-induced increases in BP were not prevented by pretreatment with alpha-helical CRF9-41, suggesting other downstream pathways are likely to contribute to the cardiovascular actions of leptin.

Orexin-A and orexin-B are 33- and 28-amino acid peptides cleaved from the same protein.[85,86] The cell bodies of orexin neurons are located in the lateral hypothalamus, but these neurons have targets distributed widely in the CNS. Several lines of evidence indicate that the neurons are regulated by leptin and melancortins.[23,87] However, the role of orexin as a downstream mediator of leptin action remains to be determined. Similar to NPY, central administration of orexins induces hunger. However, ICV injection of low doses (10 to 3000 pmol) of either orexin-A or orexin-B elicits the opposite effect of NPY, that is, increased HR and mean arterial BP, although only orexin-A increased renal SNA.[88] The role of orexins in leptin-mediated cardiovascular control remains to be determined.

Another leptin-responsive neuropeptide proposed to mediate the hypertensive effects of leptin is thyrotropin-releasing hormone (TRH). Leptin administration stimulates TRH gene expression, an effect that appears to be mediated by increased αMSH binding to MC4-R receptors on TRH neurons in the paraventricular nucleus of the hypothalamus.[89,90] When administered centrally, TRH has been shown to produce pressor effects.[91,92] ICV administration of antisense TRH, which decreases expression of the endogenous TRH peptide, lowers BP in spontaneously hypertensive rats.[93] Furthermore, antisense TRH blocked leptin-induced increases in both TRH and BP.[94] These findings suggest an important role for TRH neurons in mediating the cardiovascular effects of leptin.

7.5 LEPTIN RESISTANCE, OBESITY, AND CARDIOVASCULAR EFFECTS

The early observations that human obesity is associated with elevated leptin levels (in contrast to the obesity caused by the lack of leptin in the ob/ob mouse) led to the general concept of leptin resistance. Although genetic models of leptin resistance can be well defined, as in db/db mice and Koletsky rats that are missing LRb, acquired leptin resistance is currently a poorly defined and understood condition. In contrast to insulin resistance, no precise definition covers leptin resistance; instead, it is generally defined as reduced responsiveness of some dependent measure (e.g., food intake, body fat, intracellular signaling, gene expression) after exogenous administration of leptin. Experimental animals with diet-induced obesity frequently exhibit attenuated responses to exogenous leptin.[15,95-97] However, the considerable differences in the effects of obesity on leptin responsiveness are dependent on modes of leptin administration, rearing conditions, and strains of mice.[98]

Few studies have addressed whether the cardiovascular and sympathetic effects of leptin administration are reduced by obesity. Mark et al. observed that leptin-induced anorexic effects, but not renal sympathetic effects, are blunted in obese mice.[99] These authors advanced the hypothesis that obesity is associated with selective leptin resistance, so that leptin could potentially contribute to obesity-induced hypertension, while failing to prevent excess adipose accumulation.

7.6 WEIGHT LOSS, LEPTIN, AND BLOOD PRESSURE

The relationship between weight loss and lowered BP has been identified.[43,100-103] Leptin levels fall precipitously during weight loss in humans and rodents. Recently, it was shown that the drop in leptin that accompanies weight loss in humans positively correlates with a drop in BP.[104] Further, reduction of sympathetic nervous system activity occurs during weight loss and is responsible for the drop in BP.[102,103,105,106] However, data obtained from the direct examination of the hypothesis that leptin signaling is requisite to elicit sympathetic nervous system and cardiovascular response to restriction of caloric intake using animal models has been somewhat conflicting. Overton et al.[45] have shown that fasting induced nearly identical cardiovascular changes in the obese Zucker rat, an animal model of reduced leptin-mediated signaling, and in its lean littermate controls. Further, ob/ob mice also exhibited drops in BP during caloric restriction and weight loss,[42] suggesting that the drop in leptin levels that normally occurs in mammals is not requisite for the lowered BP observed during dieting.

Evidence supporting the role of lack of leptin signaling influences of BP during dieting is two-fold. BP of the Koletsky rat, an obese rat with complete leptin resistance due to lack of LRb expression,[107] did not change in response to 7 days of 50% caloric restriction, whereas littermate control BPs dropped significantly.[42] The second line of evidence involves the leptin-sensitive NPY pathway. Although downregulation of NPY with excess leptin may not be responsible for the hypertensive effect of leptin administration as discussed above, some evidence suggests that activation of this neuron type may play an important role in the hypotensive effect of dieting. Decreased caloric intake clearly up-regulates NPY expression and central administration of NPY lowers HR and BP. Thus, increased activation of NPYergic activity in the hypothalamus may contribute to sympathoinhibitory and hypotensive effects observed during dieting. This conclusion is further supported by the finding that central blockade of NPY receptors blunts the hypotensive effect of caloric restriction in hypertensive animals.[76]

The gastrointestinal tract-derived hormone, ghrelin, not only acts as a growth hormone secretagogue, but also participates in regulation of energy balance.[108] Ghrelin levels are increased during weight loss.[108] In addition, ghrelin has orexigenic and cardiovascular effects that may be mediated through NPY/AgRP neurons. Administration of ghrelin centrally or peripherally lowers BP, HR, and renal SNA in rabbits.[109] Peripheral administration of ghrelin also lowers BP in humans.[110] The action of ghrelin appears to be mediated through the NPY pathway, as central ghrelin induces expression of hypothalamic NPY and the orexigenic actions of ghrelin can be prevented using an NPY receptor antagonist.[111] Hence, available evidence suggests that leptin and leptin-regulated neural pathways may be involved with the hypotensive effects of dieting, although leptin-independent pathways may be invoked as well.

7.7 FUTURE DIRECTIONS

Several lines of evidence suggest that chronic elevated leptin levels may contribute to the sympathoexcitation, tachycardia, and hypertension that are common cardiovascular sequelae of obesity. However, the relative importance of elevated leptin in obesity-induced hypertension and the role of reductions in leptin in lowered BP associated with weight loss are not yet known. Carefully controlled studies that monitor and control both peripheral and central leptin levels are required to firmly establish the role of leptin in regulation of cardiovascular function. Certainly, the discovery of leptin has reinvigorated the scientific community's understanding that fat pads are not simply depots for fuel storage; rather, adipose tissue is an important endocrine organ. It may be that other adipocyte-derived hormones present in obese patients, but not yet elucidated in experimental animal studies, are required for the hypertensive effect of leptin when leptin levels are elevated two- to four-fold as seen in obese patients.

Finally, because elevated leptin levels can impact certain physiological characteristics (like HR) and not others (like inhibition of appetite) in obese individuals, "selective" leptin resistance must be explored further to determine the potential mechanisms and neuropeptides involved. Much of the evidence presented in this review has suggested that pharmaceuticals utilizing leptin-regulated pathways to treat obesity may have undesirable cardiovascular side effects. An understanding of selective leptin resistance may result in the generation of a leptin-related antiobesity compound that does not impact the cardiovascular system.

ACKNOWLEDGMENTS

This work was supported by National Science Foundation grant IBN 9984170 to SJS and National Institutes of Health grant HL56732 to JMO.

REFERENCES

1. Montani, J.P. et al., Pathways from obesity to hypertension: from the perspective of a vicious triangle, *Int. J. Obes. Relat. Metab. Disord.*, 26 (Suppl. 2), S28, 2002.
2. Engeli, S. and Sharma, A.M., Emerging concepts in the pathophysiology and treatment of obesity-associated hypertension, *Curr. Opin. Cardiol.*, 17, 355, 2002.

3. Hall, J.E. et al., Role of sympathetic nervous system and neuropeptides in obesity hypertension, *Braz. J. Med. Biol. Res.*, 33, 605, 2000.
4. Julius, S., Valentini, M., and Palatini, P., Overweight and hypertension: A two-way street? *Hypertension*, 35, 807, 2000.
5. Zhang, Y. et al., Positional cloning of the mouse obese gene and its human homologue, *Nature*, 372, 425, 1994.
6. Margetic, S. et al., Leptin: a review of its peripheral actions and interactions, *Int. J. Obes. Relat. Metab. Disord.*, 26, 1407, 2002.
7. Considine, R.V., Regulation of leptin production, *Rev. Endocr. Metab. Disord.*, 2, 357, 2001.
8. Maffei, M. et al., Leptin levels in human and rodent: measurement of plasma leptin and ob RNA in obese and weight-reduced subjects, *Nat. Med.*, 1, 1155, 1995.
9. Considine, R.V. et al., Serum immunoreactive leptin concentrations in normal-weight and obese humans, *New Engl. J. Med.*, 334, 292, 1996.
10. Ostlund, R.E., Jr. et al., Relation between plasma leptin concentration and body fat, gender, diet, age, and metabolic covariates, *J. Clin. Endocrinol. Metab.*, 81, 3909, 1996.
11. Rosenbaum, M. et al., Effects of gender, body composition, and menopause on plasma concentrations of leptin, *J. Clin. Endocrinol. Metab.*, 81, 3424, 1996.
12. Kennedy, A. et al., The metabolic significance of leptin in humans: gender-based differences in relationship to adiposity, insulin sensitivity, and energy expenditure, *J. Clin. Endocrinol. Metab.*, 82, 1293, 1997.
13. Caro, J.F. et al., Decreased cerebrospinal-fluid/serum leptin ratio in obesity: a possible mechanism for leptin resistance, *Lancet,* 348, 159, 1996.
14. Schwartz, M.W. et al., Cerebrospinal fluid leptin levels: relationship to plasma levels and to adiposity in humans, *Nat. Med.*, 2, 589, 1996.
15. El-Haschimi, K. et al., Two defects contribute to hypothalamic leptin resistance in mice with diet-induced obesity, *J. Clin. Invest.*, 105, 1827, 2000.
16. Heymsfield, S.B. et al., Recombinant leptin for weight loss in obese and lean adults: a randomized, controlled, dose-escalation trial, *JAMA*, 282, 1568, 1999.
17. Lee, D.W. et al., Leptin and the treatment of obesity: its current status, *Eur. J. Pharmacol.*, 440, 129, 2002.
18. Tartaglia, L.A., The leptin receptor, *J. Biol. Chem.*, 272, 6093, 1997.
19. Chua, S.C., Jr. et al., Phenotypes of mouse diabetes and rat fatty due to mutations in the ob (leptin) receptor, *Science*, 271, 994, 1996.
20. Ahima, R.S. et al., Leptin regulation of neuroendocrine systems, *Front. Neuroendocrinol.*, 21, 263, 2000.
21. Kloek, C. et al., Regulation of JAK kinases by intracellular leptin receptor sequences, *J. Biol. Chem.*, 277, 41547, 2002.
22. Banks, A.S. et al., Activation of downstream signals by the long form of the leptin receptor, *J. Biol. Chem.*, 275, 14563, 2000.
23. Elmquist, J.K., Hypothalamic pathways underlying the endocrine, autonomic, and behavioral effects of leptin, *Physiol. Behav.*, 74, 703, 2001.
24. Unger, R.H., Leptin physiology: a second look, *Regul. Pept.*, 92, 87, 2000.
25. Ahima, R.S. et al., Role of leptin in the neuroendocrine response to fasting, *Nature*, 382, 250, 1996.
26. Williams, G. et al., The hypothalamus and the control of energy homeostasis: different circuits, different purposes, *Physiol. Behav.*, 74, 683, 2001.
27. Morton, G.J. and Schwartz, M.W., The NPY/AGRP neuron and energy homeostasis, *Int. J. Obes. Relat. Metab. Disord.*, 25 (Suppl. 5), S56, 2001.

28. Ahima, R.S. et al., Distinct physiologic and neuronal responses to decreased leptin and mild hyperleptinemia, *Endocrinology,* 140, 4923, 1999.
29. Berthoud, H., Multiple neural systems controlling food intake and body weight, *Neurosci. Biobehav. Rev.*, 26, 393, 2002.
30. Julius, S., Palatini, P., and Nesbitt, S.D., Tachycardia: an important determinant of coronary risk in hypertension, *J. Hypertens.* 16 (Suppl.), S9, 1998.
31. Palatini, P. and Julius, S., The physiological determinants and risk correlations of elevated heart rate, *Am. J. Hypertens.*, 12, 3S, 1999.
32. Winnicki, M. et al., Independent association between plasma leptin levels and heart rate in heart transplant recipients, *Circulation*, 104, 384, 2001.
33. Paolisso, G. et al., Plasma leptin concentrations and cardiac autonomic nervous system in healthy subjects with different body weights, *J. Clin. Endocrinol. Metab.*, 85, 1810, 2000.
34. Narkiewicz, K. et al., Leptin interacts with heart rate but not sympathetic nerve traffic in healthy male subjects, *J. Hypertens.*, 19, 1089, 2001.
35. Haynes, W.G. et al., Interactions between the melanocortin system and leptin in control of sympathetic nerve traffic, *Hypertension*, 33, 542, 1999.
36. Jalali, A. et al., Does leptin cause functional peripheral sympatholysis? *Am. J. Hypertens.*, 14, 615, 2001.
37. Dunbar, J.C., Hu, Y., and Lu, H., Intracerebroventricular leptin increases lumbar and renal sympathetic nerve activity and blood pressure in normal rats, *Diabetes*, 46, 2040, 1997.
38. Gardiner, S.M. et al., Regional haemodynamic effects of recombinant murine or human leptin in conscious rats, *Br. J. Pharmacol.*, 130, 805, 2000.
39. Casto, R.M., Vanness, J.M., and Overton, J.M., Effects of central leptin administration on blood pressure in normotensive rats, *Neurosci. Lett.*, 246, 29, 1998.
40. Matsumura, K. et al., Central effects of leptin on cardiovascular and neurohormonal responses in conscious rabbits, *Am. J. Physiol. Regul. Integr. Comp. Physiol.*, 278, R1314, 2000.
41. Williams, T.D. et al., Cardiovascular responses to caloric restriction and thermoneutrality in c57bl/6j mice, *Am. J. Physiol. Regul. Integr. Comp. Physiol.*, 282, R1459, 2002.
42. Swoap, S.J., Altered leptin signaling is sufficient, but not required, for hypotension associated with caloric restriction, *Am. J. Physiol. Heart Circ. Physiol.*, 281, H2473, 2001.
43. Swoap, S.J., Boddell, P., and Baldwin, K.M., Interaction of hypertension and caloric restriction on cardiac mass and isomyosin expression, *Am. J. Physiol.*, 268, R33, 1995.
44. Vanness, J.M., Casto, R.M., and Overton, J.M., Antihypertensive effects of food-intake restriction in aortic coarctation hypertension, *J. Hypertens.*, 15, 1253, 1997.
45. Overton, J.M. et al., Cardiovascular and metabolic responsese to fasting and thermoneutrality are conserved in obese Zucker rats, *Am. J. Physiol. Regul. Integr. Comp. Physiol.*, 280, R1007, 2001.
46. Minami, J. et al., Acute and chronic effects of a hypocaloric diet on 24-hour blood pressure, heart rate and heart-rate variability in mildly-to-moderately obese patients with essential hypertension, *Clin. Exp. Hypertens.*, 21, 1413, 1999.
47. Hirsch, J. et al., Heart rate variability as a measure of autonomic function during weight change in humans, *Am. J. Physiol.*, 261, R1418, 1991.
48. Kuo, J.J., Jones, O.B., and Hall, J.E., Inhibition of no synthesis enhances chronic cardiovascular and renal actions of leptin, *Hypertension*, 37, 670, 2001.

49. Carlyle, M. et al., Chronic cardiovascular and renal actions of leptin: role of adrenergic activity, *Hypertension*, 39, 496, 2002.
50. Correia, M.L. et al., Leptin acts in the central nervous system to produce dose-dependent changes in arterial pressure, *Hypertension*, 37, 936, 2001.
51. Overton, J.M. et al., Central leptin infusion attenuates the cardiovascular and metabolic effects of fasting in rats, *Hypertension*, 37, 663, 2001.
52. Shek, E., Brands, M., and Hall, J., Chronic leptin infusion increases arterial pressure, *Hypertension*, 31 (Part 2), 409, 1998.
53. Haynes, W.G. et al., Receptor-mediated regional sympathetic nerve activation by leptin, *J. Clin. Invest.*, 100, 270, 1997.
54. Sierra-Honigmann, M.R. et al., Biological action of leptin as an angiogenic factor, *Science*, 281, 1683, 1998.
55. Fruhbeck, G., Pivotal role of nitric oxide in the control of blood pressure after leptin administration, *Diabetes*, 48, 903, 1999.
56. Lembo, G. et al., Leptin induces direct vasodilation through distinct endothelial mechanisms, *Diabetes*, 49, 293, 2000.
57. Mitchell, J.L. et al., Does leptin stimulate nitric oxide to oppose the effects of sympathetic activation? *Hypertension*, 38, 1081, 2001.
58. Aizawa-Abe, M. et al., Pathophysiological role of leptin in obesity-related hypertension, *J. Clin. Invest.*, 105, 1243, 2000.
59. Mark, A.L. et al., Contrasting blood pressure effects of obesity in leptin-deficient ob/ob mice and agouti yellow obese mice, *J. Hypertens.*, 17, 1949, 1999.
60. Van Dijk, G. et al., Central leptin stimulates corticosterone secretion at the onset of the dark phase, *Diabetes*, 46, 1911, 1997.
61. Satoh, N. et al., Sympathetic activation of leptin via the ventromedial hypothalamus: leptin-induced increase in catecholamine secretion, *Diabetes*, 48, 1787, 1999.
62. Dunbar, J.C. and Lu, H., Leptin-induced increase in sympathetic nervous and cardiovascular tone is mediated by proopiomelanocortin (POMC) products, *Brain Res. Bull.*, 50, 215, 1999.
63. Satoh, N. et al., Satiety effect and sympathetic activation of leptin are mediated by hypothalamic melanocortin system, *Neurosci. Lett.*, 249, 107, 1998.
64. Niijima, A., Reflex effects from leptin sensors in the white adipose tissue of the epididymis to the efferent activity of the sympathetic and vagus nerve in the rat, *Neurosci. Lett.*, 262, 125, 1999.
65. Tanida, M. et al., Leptin injection into white adipose tissue elevates renal sympathetic nerve activity dose-dependently through the afferent nerves pathway in rats, *Neurosci. Lett.*, 293, 107, 2000.
66. Benoit, S. et al., CNS melanocortin system involvement in the regulation of food intake, *Horm. Behav.*, 37, 299, 2000.
67. Cone, R.D., The central melanocortin system and energy homeostasis, *Trends Endocrinol. Metab.*, 10, 211, 1999.
68. Matsumura, K. et al., Central alpha-melanocyte-stimulating hormone acts at melanocortin-4 receptor to activate sympathetic nervous system in conscious rabbits, *Brain Res.*, 948, 145, 2002.
69. Dunbar, J.C. and Lu, H., Chronic intracerebroventricular insulin attenuates the leptin-mediated but not alpha melanocyte stimulating hormone increase in sympathetic and cardiovascular responses, *Brain Res. Bull.*, 52, 123, 2000.
70. Elias, C.F. et al., Leptin activates hypothalamic CART neurons projecting to the spinal cord, *Neuron*, 21, 1375, 1998.

71. Matsumura, K., Tsuchihashi, T., and Abe, I., Central human cocaine- and amphetamine-regulated transcript peptide 55-102 increases arterial pressure in conscious rabbits, *Hypertension*, 38, 1096, 2001.
72. Stephens, T.W. et al., The role of neuropeptide Y in the antiobesity action of the obese gene product, *Nature*, 377, 530, 1995.
73. Matsumura, K., Tsuchihashi, T., and Abe, I., Central cardiovascular action of neuropeptide Y in conscious rabbits, *Hypertension*, 36, 1040, 2000.
74. Van Dijk, G. et al., Hormonal and metabolic effects of paraventricular hypothalamic administration of neuropeptide Y during rest and feeding, *Brain Res.*, 660, 96, 1994.
75. Palmiter, R.D. et al., Life without neuropeptide Y, *Recent Prog. Horm. Res.*, 53, 163, 1998.
76. Vanness, J.M., Demaria, J.E., and Overton, J.M., Increased NPY activity in the PVN contributes to food-restriction induced reductions in blood pressure in aortic coarctation hypertensive rats, *Brain Res.*, 821, 263, 1999.
77. Ollmann, M.M. et al., Antagonism of central melanocortin receptors *in vitro* and *in vivo* by agouti-related protein, *Science*, 278, 135, 1997.
78. Graham, M. et al., Overexpression of AGRT leads to obesity in transgenic mice, *Nat. Genet.*, 17, 273, 1997.
79. Raber, J. et al., Corticotropin-releasing factor and adrenocorticotrophic hormone as potential central mediators of ob effects, *J. Biol. Chem.*, 272, 15057, 1997.
80. Van Dijk, G. et al., Metabolic, gastrointestinal, and CNS neuropeptide effects of brain leptin administration in the rat, *Am. J. Physiol.*, 276, R1425, 1999.
81. Overton, J.M., Davis-Gorman, G., and Fisher, L.A., Central nervous effects of CRF and angiotensin II on cardiac output in conscious rats, *J. Appl. Physiol.*, 69, 788, 1990.
82. Overton, J.M. and Fisher, L.A., Differentiated hemodynamic responses to central versus peripheral administration of corticotropin-releasing factor in conscious rats, *J. Auton. Nerv. Syst.*, 35, 43, 1991.
83. Fisher, L.A., Corticotropin-releasing factor: endocrine and autonomic integration of responses to stress, *Trends Pharmacol. Sci.*, 10, 189, 1989.
84. Correia, M.L.G. et al., Role of corticotrophin-releasing factor in effects of leptin on sympathetic nerve activity and arterial pressure, *Hypertension*, 38, 384, 2001.
85. Sakurai, T. et al., Orexins and orexin receptors: a family of hypothalamic neuropeptides and g protein-coupled receptors that regulate feeding behavior, *Cell*, 92, 573, 1998.
86. Kukkonen, J.P. et al., Functions of the orexinergic/hypocretinergic system, *Am. J. Physiol. Cell Physiol.*, 283, C1567, 2002.
87. Rauch, M. et al., Orexin a activates leptin-responsive neurons in the arcuate nucleus, *Pflügers Arch.*, 440, 699, 2000.
88. Shirasaka, T. et al., Sympathetic and cardiovascular actions of orexins in conscious rats, *Am. J. Physiol.*, 277, R1780, 1999.
89. Legradi, G. and Lechan, R.M., Agouti-related protein containing nerve terminals innervate thyrotropin-releasing hormone neurons in the hypothalamic paraventricular nucleus, *Endocrinology*, 140, 3643, 1999.
90. Harris, M. et al., Transcriptional regulation of the thyrotropin-releasing hormone gene by leptin and melanocortin signaling, *J. Clin. Invest.*, 107, 111, 2001.
91. Siren, A.L., Lake, C.R., and Feuerstein, G., Hemodynamic and neural mechanisms of action of thyrotropin-releasing hormone in the rat, *Circ. Res.*, 62, 139, 1988.
92. Koivusalo, F. et al., The effect of centrally administered TRH on blood pressure, heart rate and ventilation in rat, *Acta Physiol. Scand.*, 106, 83, 1979.

93. Garcia, S.I. et al., Antisense inhibition of thyrotropin-releasing hormone reduces arterial blood pressure in spontaneously hypertensive rats, *Hypertension,* 37, 365, 2001.

94. Garcia, S.I. et al., Thyrotropin-releasing hormone decreases leptin and mediates the leptin-induced pressor effect, *Hypertension,* 39, 491, 2002.

95. Lin, L. et al., Acute changes in the response to peripheral leptin with alteration in the diet composition, *Am. J. Physiol. Regul. Integr. Comp. Physiol.,* 280, R504, 2001.

96. Correia, M.L. et al., The concept of selective leptin resistance: evidence from agouti yellow obese mice, *Diabetes,* 51, 439, 2002.

97. Jequier, E., Leptin signaling, adiposity, and energy balance, *Ann. N.Y. Acad. Sci.,* 967, 379, 2002.

98. Bowen, H., Mitchell, T.D., and Harris, R.B., Method of leptin dosing, strain, and group housing influence leptin sensitivity in high fat-fed weanling mice, *Am. J. Physiol. Regul. Integr. Comp. Physiol.,* 284, R87, 2003.

99. Mark, A.L. et al., Selective leptin resistance: a new concept in leptin physiology with cardiovascular implications, *J. Hypertens.,* 20, 1245, 2002.

100. Young, J.B., Mullin, D., and Landsberg, L., Caloric restriction lowers blood pressure in the spontaneously hypertensive rat, *Metabolism,* 27, 1711, 1978.

101. Reisin, E. et al., Effect of weight loss without salt restriction on the reduction of blood pressure in overweight hypertensive patients, *New Eng. J. Med.,* 298, 1, 1978.

102. Einhorn, D., Young, J.B., and Landsberg, L., Hypotensive effect of fasting: possible involvement of the sympathetic nervous system and endogenous opiates, *Science,* 217, 727, 1982.

103. Kushiro, T. et al., Role of sympathetic activity in blood pressure reduction with low calorie regimen, *Hypertension,* 17, 965, 1991.

104. Itoh, K. et al., Relationship between changes in serum leptin levels and blood pressure after weight loss, *Hypertens. Res.,* 25, 881, 2002.

105. Daly, P.A., Young, J.B., and Landsberg, L., Effect of cold exposure and nutrient intake on sympathetic nervous system activity in rat kidney, *Am. J. Physiol.,* 263, F586, 1992.

106. Jung, R.T. et al., Role of catecholamines in hypotensive response to dieting, *Br. Med. J.,* 1, 12, 1979.

107. Takaya, K. et al., Nonsense mutation of leptin receptor in the obese spontaneously hypertensive Koletsky rat, *Nat. Genet.,* 14, 130, 1996.

108. Wang, G. et al., Ghrelin: not just another stomach hormone, *Regul. Pept.,* 105, 75, 2002.

109. Matsumura, K. et al., Central ghrelin modulates sympathetic activity in conscious rabbits, *Hypertension,* 40, 694, 2002.

110. Nagaya, N. et al., Hemodynamic and hormonal effects of human ghrelin in healthy volunteers, *Am. J. Physiol. Regul. Integr. Comp. Physiol.,* 280, R1483, 2001.

111. Shintani, M. et al., Ghrelin, an endogenous growth hormone secretagogue, is a novel orexigenic peptide that antagonizes leptin action through the activation of hypothalamic neuropeptide y/y1 receptor pathway, *Diabetes,* 50, 227, 2001.

8 Retinol, Beta-Carotene, and Alpha-Tocopherol in Heart Disease

Carla Lopes, Susana Casal, Beatriz Oliveira, and Henrique Barros

CONTENTS

8.1 INTRODUCTION

In 1984, Burton and Ingold published a paper in *Science*[1] that noted as a departure observation a weak epidemiological association between cancer incidence and intake of beta-carotene and other carotenoids. Their paper opened a new era for epidemiology and put forward a new biochemical hypothesis centered on the role of antioxidants.

A large body of laboratorial, epidemiological, and clinical research followed these earlier findings without obvious gains in understanding cancer causation. However, these findings stimulated interest in antioxidant and anti-inflammatory mechanisms of vitamins and trace elements in health and disease. The apparent limits of the lipid and mechanical paradigms for understanding atherosclerosis and acute coronary events stimulated searches for other contributing factors for cardio-vascular diseases. This chapter reviews the biochemical features and epidemiological findings relating retinol, beta-carotene, and alpha-tocopherol to coronary disease incidence and mortality.

8.2 CHEMISTRY AND NOMENCLATURE

Retinol is the parent compound of the lipid-soluble vitamin A group. *Vitamin A is a nutritional descriptor* for a group of essential fat-soluble dietary compounds that are structurally related to the lipid alcohol all-*trans*-retinol and share its biological activity.[2] These compounds are also called retinoids. Vitamin A-active retinoids occur in nature in three forms: the alcohol (retinol; see Figure 8.1), the aldehyde (retinal or retinaldehyde), and the acid (retinoic acid). Certain plant pigments called caro-tenoids can yield retinoids via metabolism. Those that yield retinol are designated provitamin A. Common provitamin A carotenoids in foods are beta-carotene, alpha-carotene, gamma-carotene, and beta-cryptoxanthin. Beta-carotene, a retinol dimer (Figure 8.1), is the most active.

Alpha-tocopherol is the major and most potent natural form of vitamin E activity, another fat-soluble vitamin. *Vitamin E is a generic descriptor* for all tocol and tocotrienol derivatives that qualitatively exhibit the biological activities of alpha-tocopherol.[2] The class has four natural forms (alpha, beta, gamma, and delta) that differ in the numbers and positions of methyl groups attached to the chromanol rings or the saturated carbon side chains (Figure 8.1). The multiple forms differ in vitamin E potency. The most active is the *RRR*-alpha-tocopherol natural isomer that accounts for about 90% of the vitamin E present in humans. The tocotrienols are less potent biologically and provide only a little vitamin E activity from diet. Unlike most other vitamins, synthetic alpha-tocopherol, designated all-*rac*-alpha-tocopherol

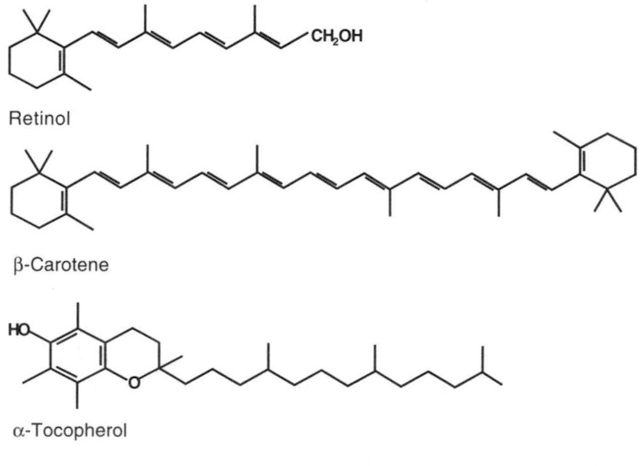

Retinol

β-Carotene

α-Tocopherol

FIGURE 8.1 Structures of retinol, beta-carotene, and alpha-tocopherol.

or dl-alpha-tocopherol, is not identical to the naturally occurring form; it is a mixture of eight stereoisomers.

8.3 BIOLOGIC FUNCTIONS

Vision effects were the first recognized and are the best defined effects of vitamin A, a constituent of the rhodopsin retinal pigment that is essential for normal eyesight. The second major function is cell differentiation; vitamin A is required for the integrity of epithelial tissues. Other documented effects include modulating immune function, affecting gap junction communications, influencing cell and growth factor interactions, and protection against atherosclerosis, lipid oxidation[2], and cancer.[3,4]

Beta-carotene, a provitamin A, performs the same vitamin A functions after hydrolysis. It is also a particularly effective antioxidant capable of physically quenching reactive oxygen species (ROS) at a diffusion-controlled rate and inhibiting free radical chain reactions and lipoxygenase activity.[4,5]

Vitamin E's physiological role is not completely understood. The main *in vivo* function of vitamin E seems to be as a chain-breaking antioxidant that prevents propagation of free radical damage in biological membranes. Because it is a potent peroxyl radical scavenger, it protects polyunsaturated fatty acids in biologic membranes and in plasma lipoproteins and stabilizes other active agents (vitamin A, hormones, and enzymes) against oxidation.[6]

Antioxidant synergism between alpha-tocopherol and vitamin C is well established. The chain-breaking reaction converts alpha-tocopherol into its radical, and the radical is converted back to alpha-tocopherol by reaction with vitamin C (or other reductants serving as hydrogen donors, namely glutathione). In addition to preventing oxidative degradation of cellular constituents and contributing to membrane repair, alpha-tocopherol also blocks the formation of nitrosamines, protects human low density lipoproteins (LDLs), is involved in the conversion of arachidonic acid to prostaglandins, and reduces exercise-induced oxidative damage. The physiological effects of alpha-tocopherol include altering membrane fluidity, enhancing certain immune functions while decreasing human neutrophil chemotaxis, and reducing ischemic heart disease mortality, platelet aggregation, and clot formation.[7]

8.4 METABOLISM

After release from digested food and emulsified with bile salts and lipids, dietary vitamins A and E are first processed in the lumen of the small intestine. Esterases are required for the hydrolytic cleavage of retinyl and tocopheryl esters, and the retinol and tocopherol formed are taken up by enterocytes by means of passive diffusion. In contrast, carotenoids are taken up as such and partially converted to retinol in the enterocytes by enzymatic cleavage.

Within the intestinal epithelia, retinol is bound to a cellular retinoid-binding protein (RBP) and re-esterified by two specific enzymes. The resulting retinyl esters are incorporated in the chylomicrons, followed by secretion in the lymph and transport to the liver. The liver is the essential organ for vitamin A storage (50 to 85%), is a major site for retinoid oxidation and catabolism, and is responsible for regulated secretion of retinol bound to RBP. Other target tissues for retinol include adipose tissue, lung, bone marrow, eye, and kidney.

The main retinoid form present in most tissues is esterified retinol, mainly palmitate and stearate, and it serves as a concentrated storage pool that can be readily hydrolyzed. The carotenoids are transported in the blood by lipoproteins and distributed to human tissues, mainly adipose tissue (80 to 85%) followed by liver and muscle. Their conversion to vitamin A may occur in the intestinal mucosa, liver, and other organs, mainly by central cleavage (see References 3 through 5 for details).

After incorporation in chylomicra and secretion into the lymph, some vitamin E is transported nonspecifically in plasma lipoproteins and then distributed to cells and tissues. Plasma vitamin E concentration depends upon secretion of vitamin E in very low density lipoproteins (VLDLs) from the liver. A specific protein, alpha-tocopherol transfer protein, present in the hepatocytes transfers alpha-tocopherol between liposomes and microsomes. The mechanisms for vitamin E release from tissues are unknown and no specific organ is known to function as a storage organ, releasing the vitamin on demand. Most vitamin E is located in the adipose tissue (>90%; see Reference 6 for details).

Overall absorptive efficiency for physiologic amounts of preformed vitamin A is high (70 to 90%), but relatively low for beta-carotene (10 to 50%) and vitamin E (<45%) even in healthy individuals.

8.5 SOURCES

Plants and some lower organisms synthesize carotenoids that serve as vitamin A precursors, but they do not synthesize retinoids directly. Humans and other animals convert carotenoids to retinol and its metabolites, but may obtain preformed vitamin A in foods of animal origin or through nutritional supplements. Common dietary vitamin A sources are liver, dairy products such as milk, cheese, and butter, and fish oil. Common dietary sources of preformed provitamin A carotenoids include carrots, dark green leafy vegetables, corn, tomatoes, papayas, mangoes, oranges, and artificially colored foods.

It is possible to obtain adequate intakes of vitamin A from diets of diverse types, ranging from strictly vegetarian to strictly carnivorous. Preformed vitamin A comprises two-thirds of dietary vitamin A in the U.S. and Europe, whereas provitamin A predominates in many other parts of the world.

The primary dietary sources of vitamin E are vegetable oils and derivatives such as margarine; secondary sources include liver, eggs, cheese, olives, unprocessed cereals, fruits, and vegetables. Vitamin E is also extensively used as a food additive due to its antioxidant activity.

Food processing and storage can lead to 5 to 40% losses of vitamin A and carotenoids and up to 80% for vitamin E.[7]

8.6 UNITS

The common nutritional unit of vitamin A is the microgram retinol equivalent (μg RE) equal to 1 μg of all-*trans*-retinol. The U.S. Pharmacopeia (USP) unit and international unit (IU) are sometimes used to quantify vitamin A activity. One USP unit or IU equals 0.30 μg of retinol, 0.344 μg of retinyl acetate, and 0.55 μg of retinyl palmitate, all as their all-*trans*-isomers. Because preformed and provitamin A differ in biologic activities, it has been necessary to develop factors to equate the biologic activities of carotenoids and retinol in foods. Generally, it is assumed that 6 μg of all-*trans*-beta-carotene or 12 μg of other all-*trans*-provitamin A carotenoids are equivalent nutritionally to one RE (μg) of all-*trans*-retinol due to the limited extent of carotenoid cleavage.

Système International d'unités (SI units) are preferred for expressing vitamin A concentrations in tissues. Conversion factors are (a) 1 μmol retinol/L equals 286.46 μg retinol/L of fluid or 286.46 μg retinol/g of tissue and (b) 1 μmol/L retinyl palmitate equals 524.86 μg/L of retinyl palmitate or 286.46 μg/L of retinol.

For vitamin E, 1 IU equals 1 mg all-*rac*-alpha-tocopheryl acetate (the synthesized form of vitamin E commonly used in food enrichment), 0.67 mg *RRR*-alpha-tocopherol, or 0.74 mg *RRR*-alpha-tocopheryl acetate, based on their relative biological activities.

8.7 RECOMMENDED DIETARY ALLOWANCES

The recommended dietary allowance (RDA) for vitamin A expressed in RE/day ranges from 375 μg RE/day for infants to 1000 μg RE/day for male adults. No consensus exists for an RDA for vitamin E. The requirement increases when the diet is rich in unsaturated fatty acid and in the presence of environmental factors that increase oxidative stress (smoking, exercise, drugs, etc.). Generally it is assumed as about 8 to 10 mg/day of *RRR*-alpha-tocopherol,[8] although ideally the requirement for vitamin E should be defined in terms of polyunsaturated fatty acid intake.[9]

Commercial supplements of vitamin A and/or vitamin E as pills are available in most countries in doses that generally equal and sometimes exceed the recommended dietary allowances.

8.8 STATUS ASSESSMENT

The most commonly used biochemical measure of vitamin A status in the past has been serum and/or plasma retinol concentration. Although instructive, the concentration of holo-RBP is homeostatically controlled over a wide range of total body reserves (0.5% of total body reserves are catabolized each day). Also during fever and infections or inadequate intakes of other nutrients such as zinc and proteins, circulating retinol is depressed and decreases extensively only when liver vitamin A stores are nearly exhausted. Thus, serum/plasma retinol concentrations are not very sensitive indicators of vitamin A status, which can best be defined in terms of total body reserves of the vitamin, especially in liver and adipose tissue.

Provitamin A concentration in the body is also an important factor for vitamin A status assessment.

Speed of vitamin E turnover in body tissues ranges from very fast in the liver, small bowel, and spleen, to slow in the heart, muscles, and particularly the brain.[6] As with vitamin A, the analysis of the adipose tissue yields a useful estimate of long vitamin E status, rather than serum/plasma levels that vary greatly.

8.8.1 METHODS OF ANALYSIS

The most general method for assessing vitamin A and E status is the isotope dilution technique, in which a dose of deuterated vitamin is allowed to equilibrate with endogenous reserves. This procedure, although currently being simplified and improved, is still too technically demanding for general survey use.[4]

The most common fat-soluble vitamin analysis procedures are based on solvent extraction, usually after saponification of samples followed by separation, usually by high-performance liquid chromatography and detection by ultraviolet absorption at a single or multiple wavelengths (see References 10 and 11 for review). The analysis must be conducted in the presence of antioxidants in order to reduce vitamin losses, particularly those due to oxidation. Accurate determinations of vitamin A and E activities are possible only if the distributions of isomers are known due to their different biological potencies.[7]

8.9 DEFICIENCIES

Nutritionally, vitamin A deficiency still exists in parts of the developing world, especially in young children. It is the most important cause of blindness and also leads to dedifferentiation (metaplasia), epithelial keratinization, appetite changes that contribute to poor growth, and xerophthalmia. Animal and human studies have shown that the liver vitamin A content is low at birth and after liver vitamin A reserves are established, they can supply retinol to other tissues for several months or even longer.[3]

Vitamin E deficiency rarely occurs because of the nearly ubiquitous distribution of tocopherols in foods. The deficiency is usually associated with genetic abnormalities or fat malabsorption syndromes. The primary manifestations include spinocerebellar ataxia, skeletal myopathy, fetal death, and pigmented retinopathy. Vitamin E deficiency also makes red blood cells sensitive to peroxide which causes their destruction and leads to anemia.[6]

8.10 TOXICOLOGICAL EFFECTS

Hypervitaminosis A may result from acute or chronic excessive intake of preformed vitamin A (acute oral LD_{50} in mice is 1510 to 2570 mg/kg), but not from excess carotenoids.[3,5] After the intake of excessive amounts, most processes such as uptake, sterification, hydrolysis, and binding to proteins may become saturated and an increase in free retinol concentration and induction of toxic effects ensue. Generally, signs of toxicity are associated with chronic consumption of doses in excess of 10 times the RDA. Dose-dependent manifestations of retinoid toxicity include headache, vomiting, diplopia, alopecia, dryness of the mucous membranes, desquamation, bone and joint pain, liver damage, hemorrhage, and coma.[3,12]

The most important toxicological effect is probably the teratogenic effect. A high prevalence (>20%) of spontaneous abortions and birth defects in fetuses was observed in women ingesting therapeutic doses of 13-*cis*-retinoic acid (as prescribed for dermatological diseases) during the first trimester of pregnancy, and similar retinoid-induced birth defects are well documented in several animal studies. A generally recognized safe upper limit of intake for vitamin A is 8,000 to 10,000 IU (~3,000 mg RE/day).[3,12]

Beta-carotene has been used extensively as a colorant in the food and cosmetic industries and also as a drug and a dietary supplement. Although associated with very low toxicity when judged by conventional toxicological methodology, apparent deleterious effects noted in subjects at high risk for cancer must be taken seriously. However, we can assume that beta-carotene supplementation at levels up to 10 to 12 mg/day is entirely safe. Daily intakes of as much as 30 mg are without side effects other than the reversible yellowing of the skin.[5,12,13.]

Compared to other lipophilic vitamins, vitamin E is relatively nontoxic when taken orally (LD_{50} unknown). Dosages up to 1000 mg/day are considered entirely safe and without side effects. There is no evidence of detrimental effects attributable to vitamin E, and similar conclusions are possible with respect to its teratogenicity and reproductive toxicity in animals even at large levels of intake. Oral intake of vitamin E may result in liver damage and symptoms associated with its pro-oxidant action and exacerbate the blood coagulation defect of vitamin K deficiency.[12,13]

8.11 MECHANISMS OF ACTION

Laboratorial, animal, and human data suggest that oxidation of lipids in low density lipoproteins (LDLs) is an important step in the pathogenesis of atherosclerotic lesions.[14-16] An unbalanced excess of reactive oxygen species (ROS) caused by a deficiency of antioxidants may result in the development of atheroma and the formation of the fibrous plaque, partly dependent on incorporation of oxidized cholesterol into monocytes and macrophages within the arterial walls.[15, 17-18]

LDLs initially cross the endothelium in a concentration- and size-dependent manner and become trapped in the subendothelial space where they can be oxidized by resident vascular structures such as smooth muscle cells, endothelial cells, and macrophages. Monocytes differentiate into macrophages that internalize oxidized LDL, leading to foam cell formation. Further oxidation leads to endothelial dysfunction and injury as well as foam-cell necrosis.[15] The presence of antioxidants inhibits LDL oxidation and limits cellular responses to oxidized LDL, resulting in less monocyte adhesion, less foam-cell formation, less cytotoxicity to vascular cells, and improved vascular function.[17-19] The role of antioxidants in preventing the clinical manifestations of coronary heart disease (CHD) may additionally comprise mechanisms such as plaque stability, modification of vasomotor function, and reduction of thrombosis.[17,20]

Antioxidants may also be useful to counterbalance the harmful reactive oxygen species formed during the reperfusion process after the occurrence of an event.[16]

The oxidant–antioxidant balance is an important determinant of immune cell function,[21-23] including maintenance of the integrity and functionality of membrane lipids, cellular proteins, and nucleic acids and controlling signal transduction and gene expression in immune cells. Recent research suggests that focal inflammation in the coronary arteries is an important step in the genesis of unstable coronary syndromes,[24-26] indicating that optimal amounts of antioxidants are needed for maintenance of immune responses across all age groups.[27]

8.12 EPIDEMIOLOGIC EVIDENCE

Observational studies of dietary intake and serum levels of antioxidants including descriptive, case–control, and cohort studies point toward preventive effects of antioxidants on coronary heart disease. However the protective effects were consensually described only for high consumption of antioxidant-rich foods, particularly for vitamin E from dietary sources. This inverse relation has been consensually described only for the upper levels of consumption of fruits, vegetables, and other foods containing vitamins, particularly vitamin E.[28-32]

A review[33] reporting measures of association between fruit and vegetable intakes and coronary heart disease found nine of ten ecological studies, two of three case-control studies, and six of sixteen cohort studies that reported significant protective associations of consumption of fruit and vegetables or their antioxidant constituents with the disease.

Additional observations among large North American cohorts of the effects of consuming more than 100 IU of vitamin E daily on decreasing coronary event rates[34,35] and effects of lower doses on the rates of progression of coronary artery lesions[36] led to several studies with experimental designs. However, the results of intervention studies using supplements were deceptive. The apparent benefit from high intakes of antioxidant vitamins reported in observational studies was not confirmed in large randomized trials. All of eight randomized trials[37-44] of antioxidant vitamins as dietary supplements for primary prevention in healthy subjects failed to show beneficial effects of antioxidant supplementation on cardiovascular events.

Large secondary prevention studies of antioxidant vitamins in people who already had clinical manifestations of cardiovascular disease were conducted.[45-53] The initial enthusiasm for using antioxidants for secondary prevention, in part due to positive results of the Cambridge Heart Antioxidant Study (CHAOS)[46] faded after analysis of results of later studies.

8.12.1 CASE–CONTROL STUDIES

A systematic review of published case–control studies[54] showed significantly lower plasma, serum, or tissue levels of carotene/carotenoids in cases in five[55-59] of eleven studies.[55-65] Four of sixteen case–control studies[55-70] assessing tocopherol effects showed significantly lower risks at high levels of alpha-tocopherol[58,61] or reported significant lower levels in cases.[56,69] In the European Multicenter Case–Control Study on Antioxidants, Myocardial Infarction, and Breast Cancer (EURAMIC), one of the largest case–control studies,[67] tissue adipose content of carotene and tocopherol were similar in cases and controls. Only one study[71] evaluated the effect of beta-carotene intake using food frequency questionnaires and described a lower nonfatal myocardial infarction (MI) risk for high versus low intake (OR = 0.4). No case–control studies showed any effect of high antioxidant vitamin levels in increasing risk of acute coronary events.

8.12.2 Cohort Studies

Several prospective cohort studies were conducted to evaluate the effects of antioxidant vitamins on the occurrence of heart disease. Results of some of the largest studies are presented in Table 8.1.

The two emblematic cohort studies are the Nurses' Health Study (NHS)[72,73] and the Health Professionals' Follow-Up Study (HPS)[74] designed in the U.S. and published in 1993. The nurses' study showed a 34% reduction in the risk of any cardiac events in nurses taking vitamin E over 8 years. The follow-up study found a statistically significant 40% reduction in heart attack risk. In both groups, the association concerned mainly vitamin E supplements. Daily use of 100 IU (74 mg alpha-tocopherol) of the vitamin for 2 or more years was associated with a 41% decrease in heart disease risk among women and a 37% decrease in men. Supplement doses greater than 100 to 250 IU/day (74 to 185 mg alpha-tocopherol) were associated with further reductions in risk.

The same study of male health professionals also described an association between high dietary beta-carotene intakes and reduced coronary risk in smokers. Current smokers in the highest quintile of intake showed a 70% reduction in heart disease risk and former smokers showed a 40% reduction. Neither study found an association between vitamin C supplementation and heart disease.

The Established Populations for Epidemiologic Studies on the Elderly (EPESE),[75] the Iowa Women's Health Study (IWHS),[76] and a study conducted in Finland by Knekt et al.,[77] also found declines in cardiac mortality with high vitamin E intake. EPESE showed that long-term use of vitamin E supplements was associated with a 63% (95% confidence interval [CI], 10 to 85%) decrease in risk of death from coronary heart disease. The study also suggested the possibility of a short-term effect of the vitamin because the use of vitamin E at any time was associated with a 47% reduction (CI of 95%, 16 to 64%) in mortality. In the IWHS, an inverse association between vitamin E intake from food (but not from supplements) and cardiac events (RR = 0.38 for women in the highest quintile of vitamin E intake) was found. In the Finnish study,[77] the association found for disease occurrence and higher intakes of alpha-tocopherol was 0.58 (CI of 95%, 0.42 to 0.81) and beta-carotene was 0.97 (CI of 95%, 0.71 to 1.34).

The Rotterdam Study[78] conducted with elderly Dutch people supported the hypothesis that high dietary beta-carotene intakes may protect against cardiovascular disease. No association was observed between vitamin C or vitamin E and MI. The EPIC–Norfolk 2001 study[79] of a British population described beneficial effects of high levels of plasma ascorbic acid on death from cardiovascular disease.

According to the systematic review[54] of the set of cohort studies, high intakes of antioxidant vitamins as regular food or supplements seem to produce modest

TABLE 8.1
Effects of Antioxidant Vitamins on Heart Disease: Results of Large Prospective Observational Studies

Study	Population	Follow-Up (years)	Exposure	Outcome	Conclusions
NHS 1993[72,83]	87,245 U.S. female nurses	8	α-tocopherol (diet + supplement)	Nonfatal and fatal AMI	Risk reduction = 41%
HPS 1993[74]	39,910 U.S. male health professionals	4	Carotene, ascorbic acid, α-tocopherol (diet + supplement)	Nonfatal and fatal AMI	Risk reduction = 37%; reduction highest in those receiving supplements (>100 IU/day for at least 2 years)
Knekt 1994[77]	5133 men and women	14	Carotene, ascorbic acid, α-tocopherol	Coronary mortality	Vitamin E risk reduction = 32% and 65% for men and women, respectively; Vitamin C risk reduction = 51% in women
EPESE 1996[75]	11,178 men and women >65 years old	10	α-tocopherol and ascorbic acid (supplement)	Coronary mortality	Risk reduction = 53%
IWHS 1996[76]	34,387 U.S. postmenopausal women	6	Carotenoids, ascorbic acid, α-tocopherol (diet + supplement)	Coronary mortality	Risk reduction = 62%; benefit only from diet
Rotterdam Study 1999[78]	4,802 men and women	4	β-carotene, ascorbic acid, α-tocopherol (diet)	AMI	Risk reduction = 45% for β-carotene; no effect of ascorbic acid or α-tocopherol
EPIC–Norfolk 2001[79]	19,496 men and women	4	Plasma levels of ascorbic acid	Cardiovascular mortality	Risk reduction = 30% for 20 μmol/L rise

NHS = Nurses' Health Study; HPS = Health Professionals' Follow-Up Study; EPESE = Established Populations for Epidemiologic Studies on the Elderly; IWHS = Iowa Women's Health Study; EPIC = European Prospective Investigation into Cancer and Nutrition; AMI = acute myocardial infarction.

reductions of the risk of cardiovascular events. The risk reductions appear to be of similar magnitude for carotene, tocopherol, and ascorbic acid.

8.12.3 RANDOMIZED CONTROLLED TRIALS

Table 8.2 lists the results of the largest randomized controlled trials on primary or secondary prevention of heart disease.

The Alpha-Tocopherol–Beta-Carotene Cancer Prevention Study (ATBC),[37] the first randomized primary prevention study involving 29,133 male smokers followed for 5 to 8 years, showed no effect on the risk of death from coronary heart disease of a daily dose of 50 mg of alpha-tocopherol, 20 mg of beta-carotene, both, or placebo. A significantly increased risk of fatal and nonfatal intracerebral and sub-arachnoid haemorrhage was found in subjects taking alpha-tocopherol. The other studies on primary prevention[33,39,43] also failed to show beneficial effects of antioxidant supplementation on heart disease.

The Cambridge Heart Antioxidant Study[46] that randomly assigned 2002 patients with coronary atherosclerosis to receive vitamin E for a median of 1.4 years showed benefits from the use of the vitamin for nonfatal MI risk but failed to demonstrate any mortality benefit. A reduction in the number of patients with nonfatal MI was observed when comparing the vitamin E group to the placebo group (n = 14 vs. n = 41, RR = 0.53, 95% CI, 0.11 to 0.47), but no difference in number of deaths due to cardiovascular causes (n = 27 vs. n = 23, RR = 1.18, 95% CI, 0.62 to 2.27) was noted. The largest studies on secondary prevention (the GISSI,[48] the HOPE,[51] the SECURE,[52] and the MRC/BHF Heart Protection Study[53]) did not show any benefits of antioxidant vitamins.

Only one study tested with an experimental design the effects of diet antioxidants. In the Lyon Diet Heart Study,[45] patients with MI were randomized to advice focused on Mediterranean diet or to regular diet advice. After a follow-up of 2 years, the risk of severe cardiovascular complications was reduced by half in those exposed to the Mediterranean diet.

The evidence from epidemiologic research on the relationship of antioxidant vitamins and coronary heart disease risk is not conclusive and results from observational and experimental studies are contradictory. For exposures postulated to confer small to moderate protection, as with antioxidant vitamins, the amount of uncontrolled and uncontrollable confounding inherent in case–control and cohort studies is about as large as the most plausible benefits of risk.[80] Large dietary intakes of antioxidant vitamins may act as surrogates for truly protective dietary choices, or it is possible that benefits from antioxidant-rich food intakes result from the inclusion of other compounds with or without antioxidant properties and not from any special effects of vitamins.[81] Also, intakes of antioxidant vitamins from food or supplements may simply be correlated with unmeasured or unknown nondietary lifestyle activities that protect against coronary disease.[82]

Randomized trials are of primary importance because they provide reliable evidence. However, certain aspects of these types of studies deserve special attention.[54,83–84] The inconsistent results of the CHAOS study may be due to the small number of events, the differences seen in several baseline characteristics

TABLE 8.2
Effects of Antioxidant Vitamins on Heart Disease: Results from Randomized Trials

Study	Population	Intervention	Follow-Up (years)	Outcome	Conclusions
ATBC, 1994[37]	29,133 Finnish male smokers	A = α-tocopherol (50 mg/d) B = β-carotene (20 mg/d) C = A + B D = placebo	5 to 8	MI	No effect of either β-carotene or α-tocopherol
CARET, 1996[38]	18,314 U.S. men and women with history of smoking or occupational exposure to asbestos	β-carotene (30 mg/d) in combination with retinol	4	Cardiovascular mortality	No benefit of β-carotene (RR = 1.26; CI 95%, 0.99 to 1.61)
CHAOS, 1996[46]	2,002 British men and women with CAD	α-tocopherol (400 or 800 IU/d versus placebo	1 to 3	MI	77% reduction in nonfatal MI (p = 0.05); no difference in fatal MI
PHS, 1996[40]	22,071 U.S. male physicians	β-carotene (50 mg/d)	12	Incidence and mortality of cardiovascular disease	No effect of β-carotene (RR = 0.99, CI 95%, 0.91 to 1.09)
ATBC (substudy), 1997[47]	1,862 Finnish male smokers with previous AMI	A = β-carotene (200 mg/d) B = α-tocopherol (50 mg/d) C = A + B D = placebo	5.3	First major coronary event	No effect of vitamin supplements on coronary occurrence; increased risk of fatal coronary disease
ATBC (substudy), 1998[50]	1,795 Finnish male smokers with angina at baseline	A = β-carotene (20 mg/d) B = α-tocopherol (50 mg/d) C = A + B D = placebo	4 to 5.5	Recurrence of angina pectoris; incidence of major coronary events	No benefit of β-carotene or α-tocopherol

Study	Population	Intervention	Years	Endpoints	Results
GISSI, 1999[48]	11,324 Italian men and women with MI	A = α-tocopherol (300 mg/d) B = polyunsaturated fat C = A + B D = no supplementation	3.5	Cardiovascular death; nonfatal MI; stroke	No effect of α-tocopherol (RR = 0.98, CI 95%, 0.87 to 1.10)
Lyon Diet Heart Study, 1999[45]	314 French men and women with MI	Mediterranean diet	3.8	Cardiac death; nonfatal myocardial infarction	Protective effect
HOPE, 2000[51]	9,541 U.S. patients with vascular disease or diabetes	A = ramipril B = tocopherol (400 IU/d) C = A + B D = placebo	4.5	MI; stroke; death from cardiovascular causes	No effect of α-tocopherol
SECURE, 2001[52]	4,495 U.S. patients with vascular disease or diabetes	A = aspirin B = α-tocopherol C = A + B D = placebo	3.6	Cardiovascular death; nonfatal MI; nonfatal stroke	α-tocopherol OR = 0.94 (0.75 to 1.18)
MRC/BHF Heart Protection Study, 2001[53]	20,536 British men and women at elevated risk of death from coronary disease	A = antioxidant vitamins (β-carotene + ascorbic acid + α-tocopherol) B = simvastatin C = A + B D = placebo	5.5	CHD; stroke, revascularization or total mortality	No effect of antioxidant vitamins on any vascular endpoint
PPP, 2001[39]	4,495 Italians >65 years old with at least one cardiovascular risk factor	A = aspirin B = α-tocopherol C = A + B D = placebo	3.6	Cardiovascular death; nonfatal MI; nonfatal stroke	α-tocopherol OR = 0.94 (0.75 to 1.18)

ATBC = Alpha-Tocopherol–Beta-Carotene Cancer Prevention Study; CARET = Beta-Carotene and Retinol Efficacy Trial; CHAOS = Cambridge Heart Antioxidant Study; PHS = Physicians' Health Study; GISSI = Grupo Italiano per lo Studio della Sopravivenza nell'Infarto Miocardico; HOPE = Heart Outcomes Prevention Evaluation Study; SECURE = Study to Evaluate Carotid Ultrasound changes in patients treated with Ramipril and vitamin E; PPP = Primary Prevention Project; MI = myocardial infarction; CAD = coronary artery disease; CHD = coronary heart disease.

of participants, and the relatively short time of follow-up (median = 1.4 years). Other general limitations arose because studies were designed for other purposes (e.g., to assess cancer risk) and not specifically to test the effects of antioxidant vitamins on cardiovascular disease risk. Few studies focus on cardiovascular disease risk and antioxidant vitamins. Some of the largest trials included only smokers and the relationship between smoking and oxidation is complex. Another common limitation is not considering the effects of other modifiers such as exercise and ingestion of polyunsaturated fatty acids on the association between antioxidants and cardiovascular disease.[54,85]

Low vitamin doses, particularly of tocopherol, may also influence the lack of effect. Another reason that may justify the lack of effect of vitamin supplementation is the isolated use of vitamins without other antioxidants.[86] In fact, antioxidants interact in synergistic ways. For example, vitamin C reinforces the antioxidant effect of vitamin E by regenerating the active form of the vitamin after it has reacted with a reactive oxygen species. It is possible that vitamin combinations rather than isolated use may produce a beneficial effect. Large-scale clinical trials are in development[53] or are ongoing[87] in attempts to clarify the role of vitamins in association with other antioxidants in the prevention of atherosclerotic coronary disease. However, recent studies showed no effects of an antioxidant vitamin combination (beta-carotene + ascorbic acid + alpha-tocopherol) on any vascular endpoint.[53]

The American Heart Association[88] considers that only the total diet influences disease risk and recommends for the general population a balanced diet with emphasis on antioxidant-rich fruits, vegetables, and whole grains. Better definition of diet influences and disease processes in which antioxidants may intervene will allow the optimization of conditions for better understanding of the impacts of these compounds on disease prevention.

REFERENCES

1. Burton, G.W. and Ingold, K.U., Beta-carotene: an unusual type of lipid antioxidant, *Science*, 224, 569, 1984.
2. IUPAC–IUB Joint Commission on Biochemical Nomenclature, *Biochemical Nomenclature and Related Documents*, 2nd ed., Portland Press, London, 1992, 239 and 247.
3. Ross, A.C., Vitamin A and carotenoids, in *Modern Nutrition in Health and Disease*, 9th ed., Shils, M.E., Ed., Williams & Wilkins, Baltimore, 1999, chap. 17.
4. Olson, J.A., Loveridge, N., Duthie, G.G., and Shearer, M.J., Fat soluble vitamins, in *Human Nutrition and Dietetics*, 10th ed., Garrow, J.S. et al., Eds., Churchill Livingstone, London, 2000, chap. 13.
5. Olson, J.A., Carotenoids, in *Modern Nutrition in Health and Disease*, 9th ed., Shils, M.E., Ed., Williams & Wilkins, Baltimore, 1999, chap. 33.
6. Traber, M.G., Vitamin E, in *Modern Nutrition in Health and Disease*, 9th ed., Shils, M.E., Ed., Williams & Wilkins, Baltimore, 1999, chap. 19.
7. Belitz, H.D. and Grosch, W., Vitamins, in *Food Chemistry*, 2nd ed., Belitz, H.D. et al., Eds., Springer, Berlin, 1999, chap. 6.
8. NRC Food and Nutrition Board, *Recommended Dietary Allowances*, 10th ed., National Academy of Sciences Press, Washington, D.C., 1989.

9. Vitamin E, in *Reports of the Scientific Comittee for Food*, 31st series, European Commision, Luxembourg, 1993, chap. 17.

10. Su, Q., Rowley, K.G., and Balazs, N.D.H., Carotenoids: separation methods applicable to biological samples, *J. Chromatogr. B*, 781, 393, 2002.

11. Rupérez, F.J., Martín, D., Herrera, E., and Barbas, C., Chromatographic analysis of α-tocopherol and related compounds in various matrices, *J. Chromatogr. A*, 935, 45, 2001.

12. Madhavi, D.L. and Salunkhe, D.K., Toxicological aspects of food antioxidants, in *Food Antioxidants: Technological, Toxicological, and Health Perspectives*, Madhavi, D.L. et al., Eds., Marcel Dekker, New York, 1995, chap. 5.

13. Diplock, A.T., Safety of β-carotene and the antioxidant vitamins C and E, in *Antioxidants and Disease Prevention*, Garewal, H.S., Ed., CRC Press, Boca Raton, FL, 1997, chap. 2.

14. Selwyn, A.P., Kinlay, S., and Ganz, P. Atherogenesis and ischemic heart disease, *Am. J. Cardiol.*, 80, 3, 1997.

15. Witztum, J.L., The oxidation hypothesis of atherosclerosis, *Lancet*, 344, 793, 1994.

16. Jacob, R.A. and Burri, B.J., Oxidative damage and defense, *Am. J. Clin. Nut.*, 63, 985S, 1996.

17. Diaz, M.N., Frei, B., Vita, J.A., and Keaney, J.F., Antioxidants and atherosclerotic heart disease, *New. Eng. J. Med.*, 337, 408, 1997.

18. Oliver, M.F., Antioxidant nutrients, atherosclerosis, and coronary heart disease (editorial), *Br. Heart J.*, 73, 299, 1995.

19. Halliwell, B., Antioxidants and human disease: a general introduction, *Nutr. Rev.*, 55 44S, 1997.

20. Miller, G.J., Effects of diet composition on coagulation pathways, *Am. J. Clin. Nutr.*, 67, 542S, 1998.

21. Schmidt, K., Antioxidants, vitamins and β-carotene: effects on immunocompetence, *Am. J. Clin. Nutr.*, 53, 383S, 1991.

22. Semba, R.D., The role of vitamin A and related retinoids in immune function, *Nutr. Rev.*, 56, 38S, 1998.

23. Meydani, S.N. and Beharka, A.A., Recent developments in vitamin E and immune response, *Nutr. Rev.*, 56, 49S, 1996.

24. Ross, R., Atherosclerosis: an inflammatory disease, *New Engl. J. Med.*, 340, 115, 1999.

25. Alexander, R.W., Inflammation and coronary artery disease, *New Engl. J. Med.*, 331, 468, 1994.

26. Watanabe, T., Haraoka, S., and Shimokama, T., Inflamatory and immunological nature of atherosclerosis, *Int. J. Cardiol.*, 54 (Suppl.), 51S, 1996.

27. Meydani, M., Nutrition, immune cells and atherosclerosis, *Nutr. Rev.*, 1, S177, 1998.

28. Prabhat, J., Flater, M., Lonn, E. et al., The antioxidant vitamins and cardiovascular disease: a critical review of epidemiologic and clinical trial data, *Ann. Intern. Med.*, 123, 860, 1995.

29. Knekt, P., Reunanen, A., Järvinen, R. et al., Antioxidant vitamin intake and coronary mortality in a longitudinal population study, *Am. J. Epidemiol.*, 1390, 1180, 1994.

30. Gaziano, J.M., Branch, L.G., Manson, J.E. et al., A prospective study of beta-carotene in fruits and vegetables and the decreased cardiovascular mortality in the elderly, *Ann. Epidemiol.*, 5, 255, 1995.

31. Kushi, L.H., Folsom, A.R., Prineas, R. et al., Dietary antioxidants and death from coronary heart disease in postmenopausal women, *New Engl. J. Med.*, 334, 1156, 1996.

32. Klipstein-Grobusch, K., Geleijnse, J.M., Breeijen, den J.H. et al., Dietary antioxidants and risk of myocardial infarction in the elderly: the Rotterdam study, *Am. J. Clin. Nutr.*, 69, 261, 1999.

33. Ness, A.R. and Powles, J.W., Fruits and vegetables and cardiovascular disease: a review, *Int. J. Epidemiol.*, 26, 1, 1997.

34. Stampfer, M.J., Hennekens, C.H., Manson, J.A.E. et al., Vitamin E consumption and the risk of coronary disease in women. *New Engl. J. Med.*, 328, 1444, 1993.

35. Rimm, E.B., Stampfer, M.J., Ascherio, A. et al., Vitamin E consumption and the risk of coronary disease in men, *New Engl. J. Med.*, 328, 1450, 1993.

36. Hodis, H.N., Mack, W.J., LaBree, L. et al., Serial coronary angiographic evidence that antioxidant vitamin intake reduces progression of coronary artery atherosclerosis, *JAMA*, 23, 1849, 1995.

37. Alpha-Tocopherol–Beta-Carotene Cancer Prevention Study Group, The effect of vitamin E and beta-carotene on the incidence of lung cancer and other cancers in male smokers, *New Engl. J. Med.*, 330, 1029, 1994.

38. Omenn, G.S., Goodman, E., Thornquist, M.D. et al., Effects of a combination of beta-carotene and vitamin A on lung cancer and cardiovascular disease, *New Engl. J. Med.*, 334, 1150, 1996.

39. Collaborative Group of the Primary Prevention Project (PPP), Low-dose aspirin and vitamin E in people at cardiovascular risk: a randomised trial in general practice, *Lancet*, 357, 89, 2001.

40. Hennekens, C.H., Buring, J.E., Manson, J.E. et al., Lack of effect on long-term supplementation with beta-carotene on the incidence of malignant neoplasms and cardiovascular disease, *New Engl. J. Med.*, 334, 1145, 1996.

41. Blot, W.J., Li, J.Y., Taylor, P.R. et al., Nutrition intervention trials in Linxian, China: supplementation with specific vitamin/mineral combinations, cancer incidence, and disease-specific mortality in the general population, *J. Natl. Cancer Inst.*, 84, 1483, 1993.

42. Greenberg, E.R., Baron, J.A., Karagas, M.R. et al., Mortality associated with low plasma concentration of beta-carotene and the effect of oral supplementation, *JAMA*, 275, 699, 1996.

43. de Klerk, N.H., Musk, A.W., Ambrosini, G.L. et al., Vitamin A and cancer prevention II: comparison of the effects of retinol and β-carotene, *Int. J. Cancer*, 75, 362, 1998.

44. Salonen, J.T., Nyysönen, K., Salonen, R. et al., Antioxidant supplementation in atherosclerosis prevention (ASAP) study: a randomized trial of the effect of vitamins E and C on 3-year progression of carotid atherosclerosis, *J. Intern. Med.*, 248, 377, 2000.

45. de Lorgeril, M., Salen, P., Martin, J.L. et al., Mediterranean diet, traditional risk factors, and the rate of cardiovascular complications after myocardial infarction: final report of the Lyon Diet Heart Study, *Circulation*, 16, 779, 1999.

46. Stephens, N.G., Parson, A., Schofield, P.M. et al., Randomised controlled trial of vitamin E in patients with coronary disease: Cambridge Heart Antioxidant Study (CHAOS), *Lancet*, 347, 781, 1996.

47. Rapola, J.M., Virtamo, J., Ripatti, S. et al., Randomised trial of alfa-tocopherol and beta-carotene supplements on incidence of major coronary events in men with previous myocardial infarction, *Lancet*, 349, 1715, 1997.

48. GISSI Prevenzione Investigators, Dietary supplementation with n-3 polyunsaturated fatty acids and vitamin E after myocardial infarction: results of the GISSI Prevenzione trial, *Lancet*, 354, 447, 1999.

49. Hennekens, C.H. and Gaziano, J.M., Antioxidants and heart disease: epidemiology and clinical evidence, *Clin. Cardiol.*, 16, 10, 1993.

50. Rapola, J.M., Virtamo, J., Ripatti, S. et al., Effects of alpha-tocopherol and beta-carotene supplements on symptoms, progression, and prognosis of angina pectoris, *Heart*, 79, 454, 1998.

51. Heart Outcomes Prevention Evaluation Study Investigators, Vitamin E supplementation and cardiovascular events in high-risk patients, *New Engl. J. Med.*, 342, 154, 2000.

52. Lonn, E.M., Yusuf, S., Dzavik, V. et al., Effects of ramipril and vitamin E on atherosclerosis, *Circulation*, 103, 919, 2001.

53. MRC/BHF Heart Protection Study of cholesterol-lowering therapy and of antioxidant vitamin supplementation in a wide range of patients at increased risk of coronary heart disease death: early safety and efficacy experience, *Eur. Heart J.* 20, 725, 1999.

54. Asplund, K., Antioxidant vitamins in the prevention of cardiovascular disease: a systematic review, *J. Intern. Med.*, 251, 372, 2002.

55. Bobak, M., Brunner, E., Miller, N.J. et al., Could antioxidants play a role in high rates of coronary heart disease in the Czech Republic? *Eur. J. Clin. Nutr.*, 52, 632, 1998.

56. Levy, Y., Bartha, P., Ben-Amotz, A. et al., Plasma antioxidants and lipid peroxidation in acute myocardial infarction and thrombosis, *J. Am. Coll. Nutr.*, 17, 337, 1998.

57. Kim, S.Y., Lee-Kim, Y.C., Kim, M.K. et al., Serum levels of antioxidant vitamins in relation to coronary artery disease: a case–control study of Koreans, *Biomed. Environ. Sci.*, 9, 229, 1996.

58. Rejon, F.R., Pena, G.M., Manglano, L. et al., Niveles plasmaticos de vitaminas A y E y riesgo de infarto agudo de miocardio, *Rev. Clin. Esp.*, 197, 411, 1997.

59. Kontush, A., Spranger, T., Reich, A. et al., Lipophilic antioxidants in blood plasma as markers of atherosclerosis: the role of α-carotene and β-tocopherol, *Atherosclerosis*, 144, 117, 1999.

60. Kardinaal, A.F.M., Kok, F.J., Ringstad, J. et al., Antioxidants in adipose tissue and risk of myocardial infarction: the EURAMIC Study, *Lancet*, 342, 1379, 1993.

61. Riemersma, R.A., Wood, D.A., Macintyre, C.C.A. et al., Risk of angina pectoris and plasma concentrations of vitamins A, C and E and carotene, *Lancet*, 337, 1, 1991.

62. Duthie, G.G., Beattie, J.A., Arthur, J.R. et al., Blood antioxidants and indices of lipid peroxidation in subjects with angina pectoris, *Nutrition*, 10, 313, 1994.

63. Street, D.A., Comstock, G.W., Salkeld, R.M. et al., Serum antioxidants and myocardial infarction: are low levels of carotenoids and alpha-tocopherol risk factors for myocardial infarction? *Circulation*, 90, 1154, 1994.

64. Marzatico, F., Gaetani, P., and Tartara, F., Antioxidant status and alpha-1-antiproteinase activity in subarachnoid hemorrhage patients, *Life Sci.*, 63, 821, 1998.

65. Evans, R.W., Shaten, B.J., Day, B.W., and Kuller, L.H., Prospective association between lipid soluble antioxidants and coronary heart disease in men, *Am. J. Epidemiol.*, 147, 180, 1998.

66. Kohlmeier, L., Kark, J.D., Gomez-Garcia, E. et al., Lycopene and myocardial infarction risk in the EURAMIC study, *Am. J. Epidemiol.*, 146, 618, 1997.

67. Eichholzer, M., Staehelin, H.B., and Gey, K.F., Inverse correlation between essential antioxidants in plasma and subsequent risk to develop cancer, ischemic heart disease and stroke respectively: 12 year follow-up of the Prospective Basel Study, in *Free Radicals and Aging*, Emerit, I. and Chance, B., Eds., Birkhäuser, Basel, 1992.

68. Öhrvall, M., Sundlö, F.G., and Vessby, B., Gamma, but not alpha, tocopherol levels in serum are reduced in coronary heart disease patients, *J. Intern. Med.*, 239, 111, 1996.

69. Kostner, K., Hornykewycz, S., Yang, P. et al., Is oxidative stress causally linked to unstable angina pectoris? A study in 100 CAD patients and matched controls, *Cardiovasc. Res.*, 36, 330, 1997.

70. Kardinaal, A.F., Aro, A., Kark, J.D. et al., Association between beta-carotene and acute myocardial infarction depends on polyunsaturated fatty acid status, *Arterioscler. Thromb. Vasc. Biol.* 15, 726, 1995.

71. Tavani, A., Negri, E., D'Avanzo, B., and La Vecchia, C., Beta-carotene intake and risk of nonfatal acute myocardial infarction in women, *Eur. J. Epidemiol.,* 13, 631, 1997.

72. Manson, J.A., Stampfer, M.J., Willett, W.C. et al., A prospective study of antioxidant vitamins and incidence of coronary heart disease in women, *Circulation,* 84, SII, 1991.

73. Stampfer, M.J., Hennekens, C.H., Manson, J.A.E. et al., Vitamin E consumption and the risk of coronary disease in women, *New Engl. J. Med.,* 328, 1444, 1993.

74. Rimm, E.B., Stampfer, M.J., Ascherio, A. et al., Vitamin E consumption and the risk of coronary disease in men, *New Engl. J. Med.,* 328, 1450, 1993.

75. Losonczy, K.G., Harris, T.B., and Havlik, R.J., Vitamin E and vitamin C supplement use and risk of all cause and coronary heart disease mortality in older persons: the Established Populations for Epidemiologic Studies of the Elderly, *Am. J. Clin. Nutr.,* 64, 190, 1996.

76. Kushi, L.H., Folsom, A.R., Prineas, R. et al., Dietary antioxidants and death from coronary heart disease in postmenopausal women, *New Engl. J. Med.,* 334, 1156, 1996.

77. Knekt, P., Reunanen, A., Järvinen, R. et al., Antioxidant vitamin intake and coronary mortality in a longitudinal population study, *Am. J. Epidemiol.,* 1390, 1180, 1994.

78. Klipstein-Grobusch, K., Geleijnse, J.M., and Breeijen, J.H., Dietary antioxidants and risk of myocardial infarction in the elderly: the Rotterdam study, *Am. J. Clin. Nutr.,* 69, 261, 1999.

79. Khaw, K.-T., Bingham, S., Welch, A. et al., Relation between plasma ascorbic acid and mortality in men and women in EPIC-Norfolk prospective study: a prospective population study, *Lancet,* 357, 657, 2001.

80. Hennekens, C.H. and Buring, J.E., *Epidemiology in Medicine*, Little, Brown, Boston, 1987.

81. Hertog, M.G.L., Feskens, E.J.M., Hollman, P.C.H. et al., Dietary antioxidant flavonoids and risk of coronary heart disease: the Zutphen Elderly Study, *Lancet,* 342, 1007, 1993.

82. Buring, J.E. and Hennekens, C.H., Antioxidant vitamins and cardiovascular disease, *Nutr. Rev.,* 55, S53, 1997.

83. Jha, P., Flather, M., and Lonn, E., The antioxidant vitamins and cardiovascular disease, *Ann. Intern. Med.,* 123, 860, 1995.

84. Parthasarathy, S., Khan-Merchant, N., Penumetcha, M. et al., Did the antioxidant trials fail to validate the oxidation hypothesis? *Curr. Atheroscler Rep.,* 3, 392, 2001.

85. Kok, F.J., van Poppel, G., Melse, J. et al., Do antioxidants and polyunsaturated fatty acids have a combined association with coronary atherosclerosis? *Atherosclerosis,* 31, 85, 1991.

86. Upston, J.M., Terentis, A.C., and Stocker, R., Tocopherol-mediated peroxidation of lipoproteins: implications for vitamin E as a potential antiatherogenic supplement, *FASEB J.,* 13, 977, 1999.

87. Hercberg, S., Galan, P., Preziosi, P. et al., Background and rationale behind the SUVIMAX study, a prevention trial using nutritional doses of a combination of antioxidant vitamins and minerals to reduce cardiovascular diseases and cancers, *Int. J. Vit. Nutr. Res.,* 68, 3, 1998.

88. Krauss, R.M., Eckel, R.H., Howard, B. et al., AHA dietary guidelines revision 2000: a statement for healthcare professionals from the nutrition committee of the American Heart Association, *Circulation,* 102, 2296, 2000.

9 Folate, Homocysteine, and Heart Disease

Pauline Ashfield-Watt, Michael Burr,
and Ian McDowell

CONTENTS

0-8493-1674-X/04/$0.00+$1.50
© 2004 by CRC Press LLC

9.1 INTRODUCTION

With the growing understanding of the parts played by nutritional factors in relation to cardiovascular diseases, many versions of dietary guidelines have been devised in order to prevent these diseases. The underlying principle in the formulation of the guidelines is the need to determine optimal nutrient intakes for different groups in the population. Compliance with traditional dietary guidelines that usually emphasize restrictions in fat intake has been poor. There is now a growing awareness that a wide range of nutrients should be considered. As more risk factors are identified, their dietary determinants need to be investigated so that they can be included when recommendations are issued to the public. This chapter will present evidence connecting folate intake with homocysteine, one of the newly identified risk factors for cardiovascular disease.

Where a nutrient such as folate appears to be protective, the effective dose needs to be established. Other aspects to be considered include method of administration, public attitudes to dietary change, bioavailability, genetics, and environmental influences.

9.2 HOMOCYSTEINE

9.2.1 ASSOCIATIONS WITH CARDIOVASCULAR DISEASE

Homocysteine is a sulfur-containing amino acid produced during the metabolism of methionine that occurs abundantly in animal protein. The association of homocysteine and vascular disease was first observed in patients with certain inborn errors of metabolism that caused homocysteine to accumulate in the blood and be excreted in the urine (homocystinuria). Rare genetic defects of three key enzymes involved in homocysteine metabolism can produce homocystinuria; in the commonest of these, homocysteine concentrations may be in excess of 200 μmol/l compared to the normal range of 5 to 15 μmol/l.[1] Homocystinuria is associated with developmental delay, thromboembolism, and premature arteriosclerosis.

In 1969, McCully linked the vascular outcomes associated with these enzyme defects to the common underlying homocystinuria and speculated that homocysteine may be toxic to the vascular endothelium.[2] Soon after this, Wilcken and Wilcken demonstrated an association between modest elevations in homocysteine and premature vascular disease.[3] Since then, several studies have demonstrated a concurrent association between homocysteine and cardiovascular disease, while an ecological analysis showed a strong correlation between mean plasma homocysteine and cardiovascular mortality among 13 countries participating in the WHO/MONICA Project.[4]

9.2.2 PROSPECTIVE STUDIES

Stampfer et al. reported the first prospective nested case–control study of the association between homocysteine and vascular disease in 1992.[5] Of an original cohort of 14,916 healthy male physicians aged 40 to 84 years who provided plasma samples at baseline, 271 subsequently suffered myocardial infarctions (MIs). Each case was age- and sex-matched to a single control who was free from MI at the time of the case diagnosis. Overall, cases had slightly higher mean homocysteine concentrations than controls, but there was a clear excess of cases with high homocysteine values. The authors concluded that homocysteine was an independent risk factor for MI, but that the excess risk was limited to individuals with markedly high levels.

In 1995, Arnesen et al. reported the results of a Norwegian nested case–control study that challenged the idea of a threshold for homocysteine risk.[6] One hundred twenty-three subjects who developed coronary heart disease among an initial cohort of 21,826 healthy subjects were identified as cases and each matched to four controls. Homocysteine concentrations were 12.4% greater in cases than in controls, but the whole distribution curve for homocysteine was shifted to the right for cases compared to controls, indicating that across the normal range of homocysteine concentrations, there was no threshold level below which homocysteine was not associated with risk of MI.

9.2.3 META-ANALYSIS OF STUDIES OF HOMOCYSTEINE AND CARDIOVASCULAR DISEASE

The meta-analysis of Boushey et al. incorporated data from 27 studies relating homocysteine to arteriosclerotic vascular disease at various sites and included 3 prospective studies, 6 population-based case–control studies, 5 cross-sectional studies, and 13 other case–control studies.[7] The results suggest that homocysteine is an independent graded risk factor for arteriosclerotic diseases, an increment of 5μmol/l having an effect on the risk of heart disease comparable to the effect of 0.5 mmol/l serum cholesterol. They estimated that 10% of coronary disease risk in the U.S. population was attributable to homocysteine and that homocysteine was also strongly associated with cerebrovascular disease and peripheral vascular disease.

During subsequent years, several retrospective and prospective studies were reported. Some failed to show these associations.[8,9] Further meta-analyses have been published,[10–13] and although the component studies were not uniformly positive, overall associations can be inferred between elevated homocysteine concentrations and the risk of ischemic heart disease and stroke. Wald et al. concluded that the relationship is likely to be causal, and they noted that lowering homocysteine concentrations by 3 μmol/l from current levels would reduce the risk of ischemic heart disease by 16% (95% confidence interval [CI], 11 to 20%), deep-vein thrombosis by 25% (8 to 38%), and stroke by 24% (15 to 33%).[13]

9.2.4 MECHANISMS OF HOMOCYSTEINE DAMAGE

The adverse effects of homocysteine associated with vascular disease probably include endothelial damage, smooth muscle proliferation, and thrombogenesis. Homocysteine is considered toxic to the vascular endothelium, which maintains the health of vessels by producing a range of regulatory factors. Impaired endothelial function is an early feature of atherosclerosis.[14] Hence, homocysteine is implicated as a putative agent in the genesis of vascular disease. Noninvasive techniques developed to assess endothelial function include measurement of endothelium-dependent vasodilatation of peripheral arteries in response to increased blood flow.[15] This response is impaired in patients with homocystinuria.[16]

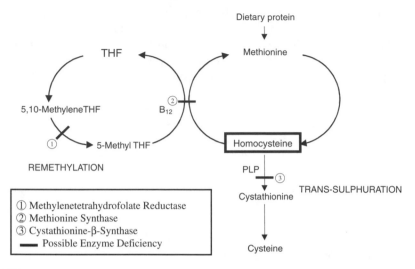

FIGURE 9.1 Metabolism of homocysteine; possible enzyme deficiencies. PLP = pyridoxal phosphate; THF = tetrahydrofolate.

9.3 HOMOCYSTEINE AND FOLATE

9.3.1 BIOCHEMICAL MECHANISMS

Homocysteine is formed by the demethylation of methionine and is removed by remethylation (reconstituting methionine) or by trans-sulfuration (Figure 9.1). In most tissues, remethylation involves a derivative of dietary folate (5-methyltetrahydrofolate, also known as 5-meTHF) as the methyl donor; the process is catalyzed by methionine synthase with vitamin B_{12} (cobalamin) as an essential cofactor. Methionine synthase and another enzyme (methylenetetrahydrofolate reductase, also known as MTHFR) also participate in successive stages of the conversion of dietary folate into the methyl donor. Trans-sulfuration involves conversion of homocysteine into cystathione. Vitamin B_6 (pyridoxine) is an essential cofactor.

9.3.2 OBSERVATIONAL STUDIES

As a consequence of these metabolic pathways, the plasma concentration of homocysteine is inversely related to blood levels of folate, vitamin B_{12}, and vitamin B_6. A survey of a healthy elderly U.S. population led Selhub et al. to conclude that about two-thirds of hyperhomocysteinemia is due to suboptimal blood levels of one or more of these nutrients.[17] Another study among adults with a wide age range showed fasting plasma homocysteine to be negatively associated with the same three nutrients and positively associated with alcohol intake, caffeine intake, smoking, and hypertension.[18]

9.3.3 INTERVENTION STUDIES

The frequency of elevated plasma homocysteine concentrations in subjects with marginal vitamin B_{12} or folate deficiency suggests that hyperhomocysteinemia is due to impaired homocysteine methylation secondary to low B_{12} or folate status. The inverse association between homocysteine and vitamin status has therefore stimulated research into treatment of hyperhomocysteinemia by single and combined vitamin supplementation.

In a study of subjects with very early onset vascular disease, Brattstrom et al. observed that blood vitamin B_{12} and folic acid concentrations were significantly and inversely related to fasting homocysteine concentrations.[19] Folate and B_{12} concentrations explained 23% and 5%, respectively, of the variation in basal homocysteine in cardiovascular disease patients. Pyridoxal phosphate (B_6) was not significantly related to basal homocysteine. A subset of these patients was treated with 240 mg pyridoxine hydrochloride for 2 weeks. The treatment produced no change in basal homocysteine and a 26% reduction in post-methionine load homocysteine elevations. A further 2 weeks of pyridoxine treatment combined with 10 mg folic acid produced a mean 53% reduction in basal homocysteine and a 39% reduction in post-load homocysteine increases. This study highlights the separate effects of folic acid and pyridoxal phosphate on homocysteine metabolism. The effect of pyridoxal phosphate was confined to reduction of post-methionine load homocysteine concentrations.

Another study by the same group reported significant homocysteine reductions in healthy subjects supplemented with 5 mg folic acid, but not in those administered either 1 mg B_{12} or 40 mg pyridoxine hydrochloride. The authors suggest that the greater effect of folic acid compared to vitamins B_6 and B_{12} was explained by the role of the former as a cosubstrate rather than by the B_6 and B_{12}, which act as enzyme cofactors.[20] These studies employed high dose vitamin interventions similar to those used to treat patients with homocystinuria. Progressively lower doses were almost as effective in reducing homocysteine concentrations in subjects with and without hyperhomocysteinemia.

A meta-analysis of randomized controlled trials showed that the proportionate and absolute reductions in blood homocysteine produced by folic acid supplements were greater at higher pretreatment homocysteine concentrations and at lower pretreatment blood folate levels, with similar effects in the range of 0.5 to 5 mg folic acid daily. A small additional effect was produced by vitamin B_{12} (16.5 mg daily), but not by vitamin B_6. It was concluded that in typical Western populations, daily supplementation by these amounts of folic acid and vitamin B_{12} would reduce blood homocysteine by a quarter to a third (for example, from about 12 µmol/l to 8 or 9 µmol/l).[21] Even at lower levels of folic acid, the effects are not entirely proportional to the dose; the reduction in homocysteine concentrations achieved by 2 mg/day is only about one-third more than that produced by a tenth of that dose.[22] Boushey considered that an extra 200 µg/day folic acid reduces homocysteine by about 4 µmmol/l; the full effect is achieved by about 400 µg/day.[7]

9.3.4 FOLATE AND CARDIOVASCULAR DISEASE

The inverse relationships between cardiovascular disease and homocysteine and between homocysteine and folate suggest a cardioprotective role for folate. Only a few studies have directly investigated the link between cardiovascular disease and blood folate concentrations. In a case–control study in white males, Pancharuniti et al. reported that plasma folate and vitamin B_{12} levels were inversely related to homocysteine concentrations in patients with coronary artery disease.[23] Folate and B_{12} accounted for 28% of the variation in homocysteine concentrations in patients and 19% in controls. Plasma folate, but not B_{12}, was significantly lower in cases than in controls.

Coronary disease risk decreased with increasing quartiles of plasma folate and the relationship was unchanged after adjustment for standard risk factors. Adjusting for homocysteine attenuated the relationship slightly, suggesting that the effect of folate on risk may have been mediated, at least in part, through modifying homocysteine concentrations. The authors suggest that the lack of beneficial effect of B_{12} in this cohort may have been due to the lower frequency of poor B_{12} status compared to marginal folate status. They identified threshold plasma vitamin concentrations below which homocysteine appears to increase: for folate about 12.5 nmol/l and for B_{12} about 225 pmol/l. Sixty-five percent of patients had folate and 13% had B_{12} concentrations below these thresholds. These data agree with the World Health Organization (WHO), which recommended a lower limit for folate of 13.6 nmol/l.

Associations between folate status and risk of coronary heart disease have also been investigated in prospective studies. In a large Canadian cohort, Morrison et al. reported that the relative risk of fatal coronary disease increased with decreasing quartiles of serum folate.[24] The relationship was graded throughout the folate distribution, indicating that folate status even within the currently defined normal range is associated with risk of heart disease and that current reference ranges are probably too low. In the Physicians' Health Study, the risk of MI was higher among subjects in the bottom fifth than among those in the top fifth of the plasma folate distribution.[25] Although this difference was not statistically significant, it suggests that low plasma folate may contribute to cardiovascular risk. A Finnish study showed a significant relationship between low dietary folate intake and incidence of acute coronary events.[26] On the other hand, no association was found between folate status and cardiovascular mortality in an Australian cohort followed up for 29 years.[27]

The relationship between folate and cardiovascular disease is probably confounded by other dietary and lifestyle factors. People whose habitual folate intake is high are likely to differ from those with a low intake in various ways, some of which may have important effects on cardiovascular risk. The apparent effect of serum folate may be merely a marker of other factors.

Direct evidence that folate protects against heart disease was obtained from a randomized controlled trial among healthy siblings of patients with premature atherothrombotic disease. A 2-year course of 5 mg folic acid and 250 mg vitamin B_6 reduced the incidence of abnormal exercise electrocardiography tests and plasma homocysteine concentrations.[28] Several large randomized controlled trials are currently in progress to investigate the effect of folate supplementation on clinical outcomes.[29] The results of these studies will show the degree of benefit that can arise from an increased intake of folate and the extent to which this benefit is associated with reduction in homocysteine concentration.

Even if these trials demonstrate a beneficial effect of folic acid associated with a reduction in homocysteine, it will not necessarily follow that homocysteine reduction is the mechanism by which benefit occurs. The benefit may be an epiphenomenon or a side effect of folic acid.[30] It is difficult to distinguish between folate and homocysteine effects within the range of folate intakes where homocysteine lowering occurs (up to 400 to 500 μg/day). An independent effect of folate would be more easily identified at intakes above which no further reduction in homocysteine occurs.

Pharmacological doses (5 mg) of folate (folic acid or 5-meTHF) improve vascular endothelial function as determined by changes in flow-mediated arterial dilatation in the peripheral vasculature in both hypercholesterolemic and coronary artery disease patients.[31,32] In one study, intravenous infusion of 5-meTHF to achieve a plasma concentration of 1 μmol/l significantly improved flow-mediated dilatation without altering plasma homocysteine.[32] This provides some evidence of a direct effect of folic acid not attributable to homocysteine reduction. It does not necessarily imply that homocysteine is irrelevant; it is possible that pharmacological doses have direct effects quite distinct from those of physiological intakes mediated by a reduction in homocysteine.

9.3.5 EFFECT OF GENOTYPE

In 1988, Kang et al. described a common variant of the MTHFR enzyme that exhibited reduced catalytic activity and was heat-sensitive *in vitro*. This thermolabile variant was associated with elevated homocysteine concentrations and also with coronary artery disease.[33,34] It is caused by a C-to-T substitution at nucleotide 677 that converts an alanine to a valine residue. The variant enzyme has 50% normal activity in subjects with two mutant alleles (TT homozygotes) compared to the wild types (CC). Heterozygotes (CT) exhibit MTHFR activity intermediate to those of the other genotypes.[35]

The MTHFR enzyme maintains the supply of 5-meTHF required for the conversion of homocysteine to methionine. Reduced MTHFR activity leads to elevated homocysteine concentrations in TT homozygotes. Population frequencies for the homozygous TT genotype vary with ethnicity and have been reported to range from approximately 1% in African blacks living in the U.S. to 12% in Caucasians in the U.K. and North America to 20% in Italians and Hispanics.[36] The reason for the difference in TT homozygote frequencies is unclear. However, this genetic variation among ethnic groups may explain some of the geographical variations in homocysteine concentrations.

Although the TT genotype is a major cause of hyperhomocysteinemia, a few studies suggest that it is associated with raised plasma homocysteine only when folate status is poor.[37,38] The MTHFR C677T polymorphism is considered a candidate genetic risk factor for vascular disease on the basis of its relationship with elevated homocysteine concentrations. It could also be construed that elevated homocysteine in such individuals is a marker of poor folate intake and reduced 5-meTHF availability for adequate one-carbon metabolism.

A possible mechanism for the relationship between folate status and MTHFR activity was suggested by Frosst et al., who proposed that the C677T substitution occurs in the region of the folate-binding site of the enzyme and that MTHFR may be stabilized by the presence of folate.[35] Deloughery expanded this hypothesis by suggesting that the mutant enzyme may have a reduced folate affinity [K_m], thus requiring significantly higher folate concentrations for efficient functioning.[39] In situations of low folate intake, folate concentrations may fall below the K_m of the mutant enzyme. The consequent reduction in available 5-meTHF would result in elevated homocysteine concentrations.

The greater sensitivity of MTHFR TT homozygotes to folate status implies that these individuals may have greater dietary folate requirements than their CT and CC counterparts, particularly as they also tend to have lower plasma folate levels.[40] Furthermore, the slope of the inverse relationship between plasma homocysteine and folate is steeper in TT homozygotes compared to the other genotypes. This suggests that folate intervention would provoke a greater homocysteine lowering response in TT homozygotes than in the other genotypes,[39] which has in fact been demonstrated in a randomized controlled trial.[40]

Several studies examined the relationship between MTHFR 677 C → T genotype and risk of CHD. People with the TT genotype are at higher risk than those with the CC genotype; this association appeared in European but not in North American populations, possibly because the latter have been more exposed to food fortified with folate.[41]

9.4 DIETARY FOLATE

9.4.1 FOLIC ACID

The nutritional benefit of folate was first reported by Wills who, in 1931, demonstrated that a constituent of yeast cured the macrocytic anaemia of pregnancy.[42] In the early 1940s, the beneficial factor was isolated from spinach and named folic acid, from the Latin *folium* (meaning "leaf"). It was subsequently found that derivatives of folic acid occur widely in nature in both plant and animal sources. Collectively they comprise a family of compounds generically known as folates that exert similar vitamin activities.

The simplest structural form of the vitamin is pteroylglutamic acid monoglutamate (folic acid), composed of an aromatic pteridine ring joined to *p*-amino benzoate and a single glutamic acid residue. This form of the vitamin does not occur naturally, but may be formed from other folate species during the isolation process. Folic acid is chemically stable during food processing and storage and is efficiently absorbed and converted to active forms of folate *in vivo* (80 to 100% bioavailability). It can be synthesized commercially and is the form of folate commonly added to foods or manufactured in supplement form.

9.4.2 NATURALLY OCCURRING FOLATES

Natural food folates are structurally diverse. They differ from the basic folic acid structure in three ways: they exist in the reduced state as dihydrofolate (DHF) or tetrahydrofolate (THF); methyl or other carbon groups are inserted into the pteridine ring at the N-5 or N-10 position; and a polyglutamate side chain is attached to the benzene ring. The different combinations of these variations allow for numerous forms in which the molecule can occur.

TABLE 9.1
Folate Contents of Foods Commonly Eaten in the U.K.

Cooked or Raw Food (As Eaten)	Folate Content (µg/100g)	Folate (µg per portion)
White bread	29	10/slice
Brown bread	40	14/slice
Whole meal bread	39	14/slice
Whole milk	5	28/pt
Semi-skimmed milk	6	34/pt
Eggs	50	25 each
Beef	15	22
Liver	320	320
Chicken	8	14
Green vegetables		
Sprouts	110	99
Broccoli	64	50
Green beans	57	50
Spinach	90	81
Other vegetables		
Cauliflower	51	46
Peas	27	20
Baked beans	22	3
Fruits		
Oranges	31	50 each
Bananas	14	14 each
Orange juice	20	31 (average glass)
Bovril	1040	94 (level tsp)

Rich sources of natural folates include green leafy vegetables (particularly sprouts and spinach), citrus fruits, bananas, liver, and kidney (Table 9.1). Dairy products and potatoes are poorer sources of folates, but contribute substantially to British dietary intakes because of the amounts of these foods eaten in the British diet. In 1999, the mean daily intake of folate from all sources was estimated to be 235 µg per capita in the British population (Table 9.2).[43]

9.4.3 STABILITY AND BIOAVAILABILITY

Most natural food folates exist as reduced tetrahydrofolates that are generally unstable and therefore easily oxidized under aerobic conditions, especially when heat, light, and certain metal ions are present (typical food processing conditions). It has been reported that 50 to 95% of folates originally present in foods can be lost during food processing. The acid environment of the stomach also increases folate instability.[44] Tetrahydrofolates may be partially oxidized to dihydrofolates or fully oxidized to folic acid. Oxidation of reduced folates results in the production of cleavage products that lack vitamin activity. Only a small proportion of these may be converted

TABLE 9.2
Contributions of Food Groups to Total Folate Intake (Natural Folate and Folic Acid) per Capita in the U.K., 1999

Food Group	Total Folate (μg/d)	% Total Intake
Milk and milk products	25	10.6
Whole milk	7	3.0
Skimmed milks	9	2.8
Cheese	5	2.1
Eggs	6	2.6
Meat and meat products	16	6.8
Potatoes	24	10.2
Fresh green vegetables	18	7.7
Other fresh vegetables	15	6.4
Processed vegetables	20	8.5
Fruit	16	6.8
Cereals	75	31.9
Bread	18	7.7
Breakfast cereals	33	11.0
Other foods	20	8.5
Tea	9	3.8
Total	235	100

to biologically active forms.[45] However, some protection is afforded by the presence of antioxidants such as vitamin C.

The bioavailability of folates varies widely among foods, from 96% in lima beans to 25% in romaine lettuce. Overall, natural folates have approximately 50% bioavailability compared to synthetic folic acid.[46] Folates from plant sources are less well utilized than those from animal sources. Factors that affect bioavailability include:

- *Other dietary components.* Folates can bind to food matrices and many foods contain compounds that inhibit folate absorption or transport. For example, oranges, beans, and lentils contain conjugase inhibitors that reduce folate absorption. This may explain the low bioavailability of the plentiful folates found in orange juice.[47,48]
- *Chemical structures of folates.* The various folates differ in biopotency, stability, percentage absorbed, and the amount of processing required *in vivo*.
- *Nutritional status of the host.* Deficiencies of iron, vitamin C, and zinc are associated with impaired utilization of dietary folate.
- *Other host factors.* Marginally acid conditions can increase folate utilization; strongly acid conditions inhibit the enzyme.

9.4.4 FOOD FORTIFICATION

The practice of fortifying foods with folic acid arose from the discovery that low folate status very early in pregnancy increases the risk of neural tube defects. The effect occurs soon after conception, so any intervention should be directed to women intending to become pregnant. Provision of folic acid supplements before pregnancy will inevitably fail to reach many women who may become pregnant; the only feasible method of improving the folate status of most women periconceptually is by adding folic acid to foods they are likely to eat.

Folic acid is converted to a bioactive folate form *in vivo*, and even when incorporated into food, it is much more bioavailable than natural folate polyglutamates. Folic acid fortification is inexpensive and in cereal production does not require any "overage" to guarantee vitamin activity following storage. In contrast, folic acid added to flour must contain an overage, i.e., extra folic acid above the amount specified on the product label in order to counteract losses due to heat of baking and storage.

9.4.5 DIETARY FOLATE AND HOMOCYSTEINE

Plasma folate levels can be raised and homocysteine levels reduced by foods that have been fortified with folic acid so as to supply an extra 200 to 300 µg/day,[40,49–51] and the effect on homocysteine is greatest in the MTHFR TT genotype.[40] Increasing the intake of foods with naturally high folate contents will also elevate plasma folate levels, but the effects on homocysteine are less clear. In some studies, homocysteine was shown to be reduced,[52–54] but in others little or no effect was seen.[50,55] The difference between the effects of natural folate and folate fortification may reflect differences in bioavailability, although it is possible that poor compliance with dietary advice may be a contributory factor.

9.4.6 OPTIMAL FOLATE INTAKES

The folate intake required to produce or maintain maximum homocysteine reduction may not be the same for everyone; 200 µg/day will suffice for many individuals; 400 to 500 µg/day is needed for some[56,57] and people with the TT genotype may require up to 600 µg/day.[40] Some uncertainty surrounds the intake needed to prevent neural tube defects. The protective effect was demonstrated in a placebo-controlled randomized trial using 4 mg folic acid daily among women who had already borne affected children,[58] but the pharmacological dose probably exceeded the amounts required by most women. British and American authorities recommend consumption of at least 400 µg folic acid per day for women who might become pregnant.

9.5 PUBLIC HEALTH ISSUES

9.5.1 FOLATE INTAKE IN POPULATION

The estimated average requirement (EAR) of a nutrient is the level of intake required for the maintenance of normal physiological function. The reference guideline for nutrient intake in the U.K. is known as the reference nutrient intake (RNI). To satisfy the nutrient requirements of the majority of a given population, the RNI is set at two standard deviations above the EAR. Therefore, the RNI should be adequate for 97.5% of the population, assuming that intakes are normally distributed. The lower reference nutrient intake (LRNI) is set at two standard deviations below the EAR and represents a level of intake adequate for only a minority of the population.

The current RNI for dietary folate intakes in the U.K. is 200 µg/day — similar to folate intake recommendations of other countries including France and Germany. The RNI represents the official recommendation of the European Union Scientific Committee for Food. Data from the National Food Survey (NFS) indicates mean intakes in the U.K. exceed the RNI, but these data are based on household food purchases and do not consider wastage or household composition.[43] The National Diet and Nutrition Survey in 1990 reported that 1% of men and 4% of women had folate intakes below the LRNI. Folate intakes in the U.K., Sweden, and Ireland are among the lowest in Europe.[59,60]

Pressure to increase RNIs globally, particularly for certain vitamins, has arisen from the increasing awareness of beneficial actions (e.g., prevention of chronic disease) of nutrients at levels of intake above those required for normal physiological function. The main stimulus for an increase in the RNI for folate has been the risk of neural tube defects associated with suboptimal folate intake and status. In the U.S., this has resulted in a higher RNI for dietary folate of 400 µg/day since 1998.[61] The new recommendation endeavours to overcome some of the difficulties associated with bioavailability of different folate forms by using dietary folate equivalents (DFEs) as the units of measurement. DFEs are calculated on the assumption that the bioavailability of folic acid is 1.7 times greater than that of natural food folates. The DFE is a somewhat crude measurement, given the wide variation in reported bioavailability of natural folates, synthetic folic acid incorporated into a food matrix (fortified food), and synthetic folic acid in tablet form. Nevertheless, these dietary recommendations are the first to acknowledge the difficulty of assessing folate intakes from different sources and the problems of communicating folate recommendations to the general public.

9.5.2 FOLIC ACID FORTIFICATION IN THE U.S.

Mandatory folic acid fortification of flour products at 140 µg/100 g cereal product was introduced in the U.S. on January 1, 1998, in an effort to increase folate status in the general population and specifically reduce the incidence of neural tube defects.[62] Low level fortification was chosen to prevent overexposure to the vitamin by high consumers of flour products, particularly elderly subjects with undiagnosed vitamin B_{12} deficiencies, who are subject to serious neurological damage. It was anticipated that this level of fortification would increase folic acid intake by approximately 100 µg/day for the majority of consumers.

The mandatory enrichment level represents a minimum requirement for fortification in the U.S. To comply with this directive, flour product manufacturers may add variable overages to flour to counteract any losses in vitamin activity during the baking process. Furthermore, the 1996 FDA directive allows for the fortification of ready-to-eat cereals with up to 400 µg folate per serving (i.e., 100% of the daily recommended value).

It is possible that fortification at or above the upper recommended level may have occurred, producing changes in folate intakes in excess of the original calculated average amounts. Lewis et al. updated two U.S. food consumption surveys to include additional folate intakes arising from mandatory fortification policy and reported that 67 to 95% of the population met or surpassed the new estimated average requirement (400 µg/day).[63] It has recently been reported that the mandatory policy has caused folate intakes in the U.S. to increase by about 200 µg/day (twice the predicted rise), probably because of widespread overfortification.[64,65]

9.5.3 FOLIC ACID FORTIFICATION IN THE U.K.

In 1992, the U.K. Department of Health advised all women planning pregnancies to take a daily supplement of 400 µg folic acid before conception and during the first 12 weeks of pregnancy. The advice has had only limited success. Supplementation with folic acid effectively increases folate status, but benefit is restricted to planned pregnancies.[66] Furthermore, supplements are generally taken by those least in need of them.

The use of natural dietary folates to achieve 400 µg/day is virtually impossible, given the difficulties associated with dietary change and the variations in bioavailability of natural folate forms. The simplest way to increase the folate intake throughout the population is by food fortification. If folic acid is added to common foods such as bread and breakfast cereals, the amount obtained will rise without a change in eating habits. Some foods have been fortified since 1987, and the public health policy relating to neural tube defects in 1992 produced an increase in the range and variety of fortified cereal products available in the U.K. Folic acid can be added in large doses, and many cereals now provide up to 70% of the U.K. RNI in a single serving.

Although the government encouraged folic acid fortification of foods, recommended fortification levels were not specified and fortification levels vary widely both within and among brands, particularly in ready-to-eat breakfast cereals. Mandatory fortification of the food supply is likely to be the most effective method of increasing dietary folate intakes at the population level, but levels should be closely monitored to prevent overfortification. This issue is under consideration in the U.K. The Committee on Medical Aspects of Food and Nutrition (COMA) produced a report on folic acid and the prevention of disease that puts forward a strong case for fortifying flour products with folic acid at a level of 240 µg/day.[67] The estimated effect of this dose would be an increase of 201 µg/day in women aged 16 to 45 years, producing a total folate intake of 405 µg/day. To date, however, concerns about long-term exposure to synthetic folic acid and possible masking of B_{12} deficiency have prevented the introduction of mandatory folic acid fortification.

9.6 SUMMARY

Homocysteine is a risk factor for coronary heart disease. Plasma concentrations are inversely related to folate intake, at least up to a dose of about 400 µg/day, above which no further reduction in homocysteine levels occurs in most people. Some interaction of folate intake and genotype exists. Individuals with the homozygous MTHFR 677 C → T genotype tend to have higher homocysteine levels, lower plasma folate levels, and greater folate requirements (about 600 µg/day in terms of homocysteine reduction) than others. Evidence that folate supplementation reduces cardiovascular morbidity and mortality is at present indirect, but the results of trials currently in progress should clarify this issue.

The optimal intake of folate seems to be 400 to 600 µg/day, both with relation to cardiovascular health and to prevent congenital neural tube defects. This intake is not attained by a substantial section of the population, and the simplest method for achieving it is by fortifying foods that are commonly eaten. Increasing the intake of foods with naturally high folate content is less feasible and also less efficient, owing to the lower stability and bioavailability of folates naturally present in foods.

REFERENCES

1. Still, R.A. and McDowell, I.F., ACP Broadsheet 52: clinical implications of plasma homocysteine measurement in cardiovascular disease, *J. Clin. Pathol.,* 51, 183, 1998.
2. McCully, K.S., Vascular pathology of homocysteinemia: implications for the pathogenesis of arteriosclerosis, *Am. J. Pathol.,* 56, 111, 1969.
3. Wilcken, D.E. and Wilcken, B., The pathogenesis of coronary artery disease: a possible role for methionine metabolism, *J. Clin. Invest.,* 57, 1079, 1976.
4. Alfthan, G., Aro, A., and Gey, K.F., Plasma homocysteine and cardiovascular disease mortality, *Lancet,* 349, 397, 2000.
5. Stampfer, M.J. et al., A prospective study of plasma homocyst(e)ine and risk of myocardial infarction in U.S. physicians, *JAMA,* 268, 877, 1992.
6. Arnesen, E. et al., Serum total homocysteine and coronary heart disease, *Int. J. Epidemiol.,* 24, 704, 1995.
7. Boushey, C.J. et al., A quantitative assessment of plasma homocysteine as a risk factor for vascular disease: probable benefits of increasing folic acid intakes, *JAMA,* 274, 1049, 1995.
8. Alfthan, G. et al., Relation of serum homocysteine and lipoprotein (a) concentrations to atherosclerotic disease in a prospective Finnish population-based study, *Atherosclerosis,* 106, 9, 1994.
9. Evans, R.W. et al., Homocyst(e)ine and risk of cardiovascular disease in the Multiple Risk Factor Intervention Trial, *Atheroscler. Thromb. Vasc. Biol.,* 17, 1947, 1997.
10. Ford, E.S. et al., Homocyst(e)ine and cardiovascular disease: a systematic review of the evidence with special emphasis on case-control studies and nested case-control studies, *Int. J. Epidemiol.,* 31, 59, 2002.
11. Bautista, L.E. et al., Total plasma homocysteine level and risk of cardiovascular disease: a meta-analysis of prospective cohort studies, *J. Clin. Epidemiol.,* 55, 882, 2002.
12. Homocysteine Studies Collaboration, Homocysteine and risk of ischemic heart disease and stroke: a meta-analysis, *JAMA,* 288, 2015, 2002.
13. Wald, D.S., Law, M., and Morris, J.K., Homocysteine and cardiovascular disease: evidence on causality from a meta-analysis, *Br. Med. J.,* 325, 1202, 2002.
14. Ross, R., The pathogenesis of atherosclerosis: a perspective for the 1990s, *Nature,* 362, 801, 1993.
15. Ramsey, M. et al., Non-invasive detection of endothelial dysfunction, *Lancet,* 348, 128, 1996.

16. Celermajer, D.S. et al., Impaired endothelial function occurs in the systemic arteries of children with homozygous homocystinuria but not in their heterozygous parents, *J. Am. Coll. Cardiol.*, 22, 854, 1993.

17. Selhub, J. et al., Vitamin status and intake as primary determinants of homocycteinemia in an elderly population, *JAMA*, 270, 2693, 1993.

18. Jacques, P.F. et al., Determinants of plasma total homocysteine concentration in the Framingham Offspring cohort, *Am. J. Clin. Nutr.*, 73, 613, 2001.

19. Brattstrom, L. et al., Impaired homocysteine metabolism in early-onset cerebral and peripheral occlusive arterial disease: effects of pyridoxine and folic acid treatment, *Atherosclerosis*, 81, 51, 1990.

20. Brattstrom, L.E. et al., Folic acid: an innocuous means to reduce plasma homocysteine, *Scand. J. Clin. Lab. Invest.*, 48, 215, 1988.

21. Homocysteine Lowering Trialists' Collaboration, Lowering blood homocysteine with folic acid based supplements: meta-analysis of randomised trials, *Br. Med. J.*, 316, 894, 1998.

22. PACIFIC Study Group, Dose-dependent effects of folic acid on plasma homocysteine in a randomized trial conducted among 723 individuals with coronary heart disease, *Eur. Heart J.*, 23, 1509, 2002.

23. Pancharuniti, N. et al., Plasma homocyst(e)ine, folate, and vitamin B-12 concentrations and risk for early-onset coronary artery disease, *Am. J. Clin. Nutr.*, 59, 940, 1994.

24. Morrison, H.I. et al., Serum folate and risk of fatal coronary heart disease, *JAMA*, 275, 1893, 1996.

25. Chasan-Taber, L. et al., A prospective study of folate and vitamin B6 and risk of myocardial infarction in U.S. physicians, *J. Am. Coll. Nutr.*, 15, 136, 1996.

26. Voutilainen, S. et al., Low dietary folate intake is associated with an excess incidence of acute coronary events: the Kuopio Ischemic Heart Disease Risk Factor Study, *Circulation*, 103, 2674, 2001.

27. Hung, J. et al., Folate and vitamin B_{12} and risk of fatal cardiovascular disease: cohort study from Busselton, Western Australia, *Brit. Med. J.*, 326, 131, 2003.

28. Vermeulen, E.G.J. et al., Effect of homocysteine-lowering treatment with folic acid plus vitamin B_6 on progression of subclinical atherosclerosis: a randomised, placebo-controlled trial, *Lancet*, 355, 517, 2000.

29. Clarke, R. and Collins, R., Can dietary supplements with folic acid or vitamin B_6 reduce cardiovascular risk? Design of clinical trials to test the homocysteine hypothesis of vascular disease, *J. Cardiovasc. Risk*, 5, 249, 1998.

30. Doshi, S.N. et al., Lowering plasma homocysteine with folic acid in cardiovascular disease: what will the trials tell us? *Atherosclerosis*, 165, 1, 2002.

31. Verhaar, M.C. et al., Effects of oral folic acid supplementation on endothelial function in familial hypercholesterolemia: a randomised placebo-controlled trial, *Circulation*, 100, 335, 1999.

32. Doshi, S.M. et al., Folate improves endothelial function in coronary artery disease: an effect mediated by reduction of intracellular superoxide? *Arterioscler. Thromb. Vasc. Biol.*, 21, 1196, 2001.

33. Kang, S.S. et al., Intermediate homocysteinemia: a thermolabile variant of methylenetetrahydrofolate reductase, *Am. J. Hum. Genet.*, 43, 414, 1988.

34. Kang, S.S. et al., Thermolabile methylenetetrahydrofolate reductase in patients with coronary artery disease, *Metabolism*, 37, 611, 1988.

35. Frosst, P. et al., A candidate genetic risk factor for vascular disease: a common mutation in methylenetetrahydrofolate reductase, *Nat. Genet.*, 10, 111, 1995.

36. Botto, L.D. and Yang, Q., 5,10-Methylenetetrahydrofolate reductase gene variants and congenital anomalies: a HuGE review, *Am. J. Epidemiol.,*151, 862, 2000.

37. Harmon, D.L. et al., The common 'thermolabile' variant of methylenetetrahydrofolate reductase in a major determinant of mild hyperhomocysteinaemia, *Q. J. Med.,* 89, 571, 1996.

38. Jacques, P.F. et al., Relation between folate status, a common mutation in methyle-netetrahydrofolate reductase, and plasma homocysteine concentrations, *Circulation,* 93, 7, 1996.

39. Deloughery, T.G. et al., Common mutation in methylenetetrahydrofolate reductase: correlation with homocysteine metabolism and late-onset vascular disease, *Circulation,* 94, 3074, 1996.

40. Ashfield-Watt, P.A.L. et al., Methylenetetrahydrofolate reductase 677 C → T geno-type modulates homocysteine responses to a folate-rich diet or a low-dose folic acid supplement: a randomized controlled trial, *Am. J. Clin. Nutr.,* 76, 180, 2002.

41. Klerk, M. et al., MTHFR 677 C → T polymorphism and risk of coronary heart disease: a meta-analysis, *JAMA,* 288, 2023, 2002.

42. Wills, L., Treatment of "pernicious anaemia of pregnancy and tropical anemia" with special reference to yeast extract as a curative agent, *BMJ,* 1, 1059, 1931.

43. Ministry of Agriculture, Fisheries and Food, National Food Survey, 1999 Annual Report on Food Expenditure, Consumption and Nutrient Intakes, The Stationery Office, London, 2000.

44. Seyoum, E. and Selhub, J., Properties of food folates determined by stability and susceptibility to intestinal pteroylpolyglutamate hydrolase action, *J. Nutr.,*128, 1956, 1998.

45. Gregory, J.F., Chemical and nutritional aspects of folate research: analytical proce-dures, methods of folate synthesis, stability, and bioavailability of dietary folates, *Adv. Food Nutr. Res.,* 33, 1, 1989.

46. Gregory, J.F., The bioavailability of folate, in Bailey, L.B, Ed., *Folate in Health and Disease,* Marcel Dekker, New York, 1995, p. 218.

47. Tamura, T. et al., The availability of folates in man: effect of orange juice supplement on intestinal conjugase, *Br. J. Haematol.,* 32, 123, 1976.

48. Bhandari, S.D. and Gregory, J.F., Inhibition by selected food components of human and porcine intestinal pteroylpolyglutamate hydrolase activity, *Am. J. Clin. Nutr.,* 51, 87, 1990.

49. Schorah, C.J. et al., The responsiveness of plasma homocysteine to small increases in dietary folic acid: a primary care study, *Eur. J. Clin. Nutr.,* 52, 407, 1998.

50. Riddell, L.J. et al., Dietary strategies for lowering homocysteine concentrations, *Am. J. Clin. Nutr.,* 71, 1448, 2000.

51. Ashfield-Watt, P.A.L. et al., Folate-enriched diet lowers plasma homocysteine in patients with hyperlipidaemia: a randomised controlled trial, *Br. J. Cardiol.,* 8, 28, 2001.

52. Brouwer, I.A. et al., Dietary folate from vegetables and citrus fruit decreases plasma homocysteine concentrations in humans in a dietary controlled trial, *J. Nutr.,* 129, 1135, 1999.

53. Appel, L.J. et al., Effect of dietary patterns on serum homocysteine: results of a randomised, controlled feeding study, *Circulation,* 102, 852, 2000.

54. Venn, B.J. et al. Dietary counseling to increase natural folate intake: a randomized, placebo-controlled trial in free-living subjects to assess effects on serum folate and plasma total homocysteine, *Am. J. Clin. Nutr.,* 76, 758, 2002.

55. Ashfield-Watt, P.A.L. et al., A comparison of the effect of advice to eat either five-a-day fruit and vegetables or folic acid fortified foods on plasma folate and homocysteine, *Eur. J. Clin. Nutr.*, 57, 316, 2003.
56. Jacob, R.A. et al., Homocysteine increases as folate decreases in plasma of healthy men during short-term dietary folate and methyl group restriction, *J. Nutr.*, 124, 1072, 1994.
57. Ward, M. et al., Plasma homocysteine, a risk factor for cardiovascular disease, is lowered by physiological doses of folic acid, *Q. J. Med.*, 90, 519, 1997.
58. MRC Vitamin Research Study Group, Prevention of neural tube defects: results of the Medical Research Council Vitamin Study, *Lancet,* 338, 131, 1991.
59. Gregory, J. et al., The Dietary and Nutritional Survey of British Adults, Her Majesty's Stationery Office, London, 1990.
60. de Bree, A. et al., Folate intake in Europe: recommended, actual and desired intake, *Eur. J. Clin. Nutr.*, 51, 643, 1997.
61. Institute of Medicine, Subcommittee on Folate, etc., Dietary reference intakes: thiamin, riboflavin, niacin, vitamin B_6, vitamin B_{12}, National Academy of Sciences, Washington, D.C., 1998.
62. Food standards: amendment of standards of identity for enriched grain products to require addition of folic acid, *Fed. Reg.*, 61, 8781, 1996.
63. Lewis, C.J. et al., Estimated folate intakes: data updated to reflect food fortification, increased bioavailability, and dietary supplement use, *Am. J.Clin. Nutr.*, 70, 198, 1999.
64. Choumenkovitch, S.F. et al., Folic acid intake from fortification in United States exceeds predictions, *J. Nutr.*, 132, 2792, 2002.
65. Quinlivan, E.P. and Gregory, J.F., Effect of food fortification on folic acid intake in the United States, *Am. J. Clin. Nutr.*, 77, 221, 2003.
66. Sillender, M., Continuing low uptake of periconceptual folate warrants increased food fortification, *J. Hum. Nutr. Dietet.*, 13, 425, 2000.
67. Department of Health, Folic Acid and the Prevention of Disease, Report on Health and Social Subjects 50, The Stationery Office, London, 2000.

Section III

*Foods and Macronutrients
in Heart Disease*

10 Flavonoids Extracted and in Foods: Role in Hypertension Prevention and Treatment

Cynthia Mlakar, Katrina Simpson, and Ronald R. Watson*

CONTENTS

10.1 INTRODUCTION

This chapter addresses the possible role of flavonoids in the prevention and treatment of hypertension. It begins with a concise description and the probable causes of hypertension. Comorbidity rates, as well as the resultant widespread financial impacts on the health system associated with hypertension, are mentioned. Current medical antihypertensive treatments are briefly summarized, along with the side effects considered partially responsible for patient noncompliance with therapies. Dietary suggestions and alternative herbal remedies are reviewed, leading into a discussion of flavonoids — plant substances gaining popularity for their prevention and remedial effects on a variety of diseases and ailments. Studies of the blood pressure lowering effects of flavonoid ingestion are cited.

---

* This work was written during the Summer Institute on Medical Ignorance (SIMI) under the guidance of Dr. Watson at the University Medical Center of the University of Arizona in Tucson.

Hypertension, also known as high blood pressure, is the most common reason for patient visits to primary care offices.[1] One study showed that up to 70% of all doctor visits in 1995 were concerned with hypertension.[2] In 1998, 50 million people in the U.S. were diagnosed with hypertension.[3] Hypertension is at the top of the lists of many health care systems[1] and is one of the costliest and most complex diseases to treat. In 1995, $18.7 billion was spent in the U.S. to treat hypertension.[2,4] Approximately 20% of that amount was spent on drug treatment.[2] The costs of treating high blood pressure represent large and increasing proportions of health care costs in many countries.[4] The higher rates of hypertension noted in formerly communist countries were originally presumed to result from the increased consumption of cereals and more obesity.[5] However, the incidence of hypertension is probably influenced more by the lack of fresh fruits and vegetables in winter and spring and the high levels of alcoholism, smoking, and pollution that enhance production of free radicals.[5]

The high cost of treating hypertension is a result of the complexity of the disease. Often referred to as a "silent killer," hypertension has a high degree of comorbidity. In other words, hypertension causes or is connected with many other diseases. This fact makes hypertension more complex to manage because several providers of different types of care may be involved in various treatments, and multiple mechanisms may be required to manage high blood pressure.[4] The inflammatory reaction of chronic venous insufficiency (CVI) may be triggered by venous hypertension.[6] Additionally, hypertension is chronically present over a long period of time in a patient's life.[1]

Hypertension is a significant cause of major organ damage, usually as a result of inadequate treatment.[7] Because it is asymptomatic and produces few or no tangible effects, patients often ignore advice and fail to comply with treatments prescribed for this chronic disease. Hypertension is the most prevalent risk factor for atherosclerosis, which affects approximately 43 million persons in the U.S.[8] Strokes, heart attacks, and other cardiovascular diseases can also be caused by hypertension.[9] Studies indicate hypertension predisposes those who have it to all major atherosclerotic diseases,[4] and researchers cite hypertension as one of the three most preventable causes of cardiovascular mortality.[5] Other sources argue that the risk of heart disease in hypertensive populations is the same as the risk for nonhypertensive populations.[10]

Some studies indicate that only 47% of patients with hypertension achieve optimal blood pressure control (measurements below 140/90 mmHg).[8] Tight blood pressure control is considered more effective than glycemic control in preventing macrovascular events.[11] A strong association exists between high blood pressure and intermittent claudication and other symptoms of peripheral arterial disease (PAD). Type I diabetes mellitus is associated with peripheral macrovascular and microvascular disease.[8]

High blood pressure is defined as an excessive amount of energy generated by the force of blood flowing against the walls of arteries.[12] Over 80% of patients with high blood pressure fall within the borderline to moderate range;[13] that is, they have systolic blood pressures of 120 to 180 mmHg and diastolic blood pressures of 90 to 114 mmHg. High blood pressure is often considered a systolic pressure above 140 and a diastolic pressure above 90 mmHg.[13]

10.2 TYPES AND CAUSES OF HYPERTENSION

Essential or primary hypertension is defined as a medical condition denoted by consecutive high (above 140/90 mmHg) blood pressure readings in the absence of a known causal disease.[14] It is the result of elevated arterial pressure associated with increased cardiac output, total peripheral resistance, or both.[15] Unfortunately, mystery exists about the causes and treatment of this form, even though 95% of all hypertensive patients have essential hypertension.[9] Primary hypertension affects approximately one-third of the world's adult population.[4]

Secondary hypertension is the sudden onset of high blood pressure in children or people over the age of 50.[9] A mere 5% of those with hypertension have the secondary type.[9] Systemic arterial hypertension is one of the most common cardiovascular diseases of industrialized populations. It affects approximately 20% of adults in these societies, and the percentage is higher among the elderly and blacks.[15] Males were at higher risk to develop hypertension, but greater risks for women have been noted in the past decade.[16] Malignant hypertension is the most severe form. It progresses rapidly and proves fatal within 5 years for 90% of its patients.[9]

Essential hypertension can result from narrowed arteries, from circulation of a greater-than-normal volume of blood through the body, or a combination of both factors.[12] Arteriosclerosis is a narrowing of the smaller arteries recognized as a major pathophysiological change in essential hypertension.[17] In order to function well, arteries must have elasticity. Serotonin occurs naturally in the body and is believed responsible for causing constriction of the large arteries while causing arterioles and large veins to vasodilate.[18]

The sympathetic nervous system or insulin resistance can also cause hypertension.[19] Abnormal renin that triggers angiotensin[21] and oxidation that produces aldosterone[21] are further risk factors.[19] Other causes of clinical variable hypertension are physiologic variables.[22] The first is vascular tone, which establishes the elastic properties of veins and arteries, vessel diameter, and vascular resistance.[22] Additional variables causing high blood pressure are inotropic state and heart rate.[22] Hypertension can result also from the use of drugs, medications, and other substances such as oral contraceptives, nonsteroidal anti-inflammatory drugs, licorice, cocaine, and amphetamines.[23]

Obesity and diet factors are other issues considered as causes for hypertension because 50% of obese people have hypertension.[9] Possible dietary causes for hypertension include high intake of salt and fats.[24] Processed foods and many snack foods are high in sodium content. Although modern society embraces the fast food concept, fast foods may not be as healthy as we want or need. Actions to promote awareness of the risks associated with this type of daily dietary intake have met with resistance. "The possible loss of income to the salt and soft-drink industries that might follow moderate sodium reduction has led to the formation of lobbying operations in several countries that work against efforts to reduce sodium intake." [25]

An elevated level of dietary salt (NaCl) is thought to be a cause of hypertension. By the late 1940s, the role of dietary salt as a cause of hypertension had been studied and debated for over 100 years.[26] "The prevalence of hypertension and its consequences is [sic] linearly linked to dietary salt intake in societies throughout the world."[27]

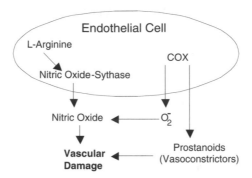

FIGURE 10.1 Vascular damage caused by functions within the endothelial cell.

Endothelial cells are important mediators of vasoconstriction and vasodilatation. This mediation is brought about by the production of nitric oxide (a vasodilator) by the endothelium.[28,29] Inhibition of platelet aggregation relaxation are some ways nitric oxide can affect the body.[30] Alterations in L-arginine, a compound that forms nitric oxide, can lead to a decrease in nitric oxide production and high blood pressure. While not directly related to nitric oxide, cyclooxygenase (COX) can cause vascular damage by producing superoxide anions and prostanions[31] (see Figure 10.1).

10.3 CURRENT MEDICAL TREATMENTS FOR HYPERTENSION

Hypertensive drugs are normally taken on a continuous basis.[9] In diseases such as hypertension, diabetes, and asthma, a relapse following cessation of treatment is considered evidence of the effectiveness of the treatment and the need to continue monitoring the patient.[32] The six main drug treatments for hypertension are diuretics, beta-blockers, calcium antagonists, angiotensin-converting enzyme (ACE) inhibitors, angiotensin II antagonists, and alpha-adrenergic blockers, although no reliable data support the last two regimens.[23]

Beta-blockers interfere with the absorption of epinephrine, leading to decreases of heart rate and blood pressure, although caffeine, alcohol, and salt can reverse the effects.[8] Furthermore, an increase of triglycerides may result from the use of beta-blockers.[33,34] Diuretics may impair lipid profile, cause glucose intolerance, and result in elevation of uric acid.[33] Reserpine and methyldopa are also used in some parts of the world. Aspirin is used as an antiplatelet therapy.[23]

Possible new drugs are constantly on trial, for instance, vasopeptidase inhibitors.[9] Sildenafil specializes in pulmonary vasodilation; while it increases blood flow out of the heart, it has no effect on wedge pressure.[35] One group of researchers attempted to determine whether benazepril or nitrendipine produced a "greater reduction in left ventricular mass." The results were close: benazepril had greater effect on diastolic pressure and nitrendipine decreased systolic pressure more.[32]

Keeping in mind the terrible risks the disease involves, some people with high blood pressure do not feel any warning signs and thus fail to realize they have a major illness.[9] They feel fine and the treatments are expensive and cause uncomfortable side effects. Thus, only 24% of patients with hypertension in the U.S. are adequately treated.[7] Discontinuation of treatments and switching therapies increase the costs of patient care.[4] In the U.S., nearly 75% of patients with hypertension are poorly controlled, and the number is higher in other countries.[4] Tolerability of drug treatment is an important influence; some patients may consider their hypertensive medications more troublesome than the seemingly symptomless disease and stop taking their medications.[16]

Attention is now paid to health-related quality of life (HR-QOL) issues in health services. The most common areas of inquiry on patient-completed questionnaires are cognitive function, symptomatic well-being, adverse effects, sexual function, psychological well-being, sleep dysfunction, social participation, and general health perception.[16] A recent goal of treatment for hypertension, in addition to lowering blood pressure, is to reduce the adverse side effects of medications in order to increase patient compliance.[33] Side effects include nausea, vomiting, muscle twitching, headaches, flushing, hypotension, tachycardia, aggravation of angina pectoris, hyperglycemia, renal failure, bowel and bladder paresis, blurred vision, dry mouth, bronchoconstriction, heartblock, drowsiness, and increased risk of glaucoma.[15]

The comorbidity rate of hypertension with other diseases, the effects of hypertension medications on symptoms, and the effects of the medications for the other diseases on hypertension further increase the adverse side effects and the probability of noncompliance with drug therapy. No single class of hypertensive medication meets the requirements of an ideal drug therapy.[33] Patients clearly have a need to be educated about hypertension therapy in order to increase compliance with prescribed treatments.[1] Greater numbers of television and magazine advertisements urging people with high blood pressure to continue to take their medications and to stay in contact with their doctors, even if they feel fine, are attempts to meet this need.

10.4 OTHER TREATMENTS FOR HYPERTENSION

The disappointing results of some hypertensive therapies have caused doubts about traditional approaches to management of hypertension.[36] Rates of successful blood pressure control remain low among treated patients.[4] Only 47% of patients with hypertension achieve optimal blood pressures below 140/90 mmHg.[37] Hypertension treatments that will help patients establish healthy lifestyle changes and have fewer and less severe side effects would probably lead to more optimum results and higher rates of patient compliance with treatment programs. In fact, the most common reason patients seek complementary alternative medicine (CAM) is dissatisfaction with the ability of conventional medicine to treat chronic diseases. Interestingly, those most likely to utilize CAM have higher educational levels, poorer health, and holistic philosophies.[38]

Herbs are used worldwide to treat a number of ailments alternatively. "Herbs have been used as medical treatments since the beginning of time."[35] *Gingko biloba* is used to treat cerebral insufficiency and intermittent claudication, and St. John's wort (*Hypericum perforatum*) is an herbal remedy for depression. Hawthorne (*Crataegus* spp.) is a treatment for congestive heart failure, and horse chestnut (*Aesculus hippocastanum*) is used for chronic venous insufficiency. Saw palmetto (*Serenoa repens*) fruit is used as a remedy for benign prostatic hyperplasia.[39]

A number of herbs are recommended for the treatment of hypertension. Some have dangerous side effects and can be toxic. The list includes aconite (wolfsbane), American hellebore, bee pollen, cinnamon, coenzyme Q_{10}, cucumber, dandelion, dong quai, garlic, gotu kola, hawthorne, kelp, mistletoe, nettle, parsley, peach, rauwolfia, and yerba maté.[13]

Resperpine is an alkaloid derivative of *Rauwolfia serpentina*. It is also known as snakeroot and has been used since ancient times as a Hindu Ayurvedic remedy for hypertension and psychoses.[40] Resperpine was one of the first drugs used widely to treat systolic high blood pressure. It lowers blood pressure by decreasing cardiac output, heart rate, peripheral vascular resistance, and rennin secretion. It has the ability to block the uptake of biogenic amines,[40] but adversely affects the nervous system and has uncomfortable side effects including nasal congestion, increased gastric secretion, and mild diarrhea.[40]

Tetradrine, an alkaloid extract of *Stephania tetrandra*, a Chinese herb, is a calcium ion channel antagonist. It blocks both T and L calcium channels and therefore stops the smooth muscle cells of the arteries from contracting. It also causes swelling of liver cells and has been deemed responsible for deaths caused by rapidly progressing renal failure (Chinese herb nephropathy) when used as part of a dieting regimen.[35,40] Tetramethylpyrazine inhibits platelet aggregation and non-selectively antagonizes adrenergic receptors. *Veratrum* (hellebore) enhances nerve and muscle excitability, causing reflex hypotension, but also causes nausea and vomiting.[35] *Viscum album L* is a semiparasitic plant that grows on various shrubs and trees, including apple trees, and has been used as an herbal remedy for hypertension and atherosclerosis.[41]

Some herbal remedies produce adverse and not necessarily publicized side effects on hypertension. Ephedrine, also known as ephedra or ma huang, stimulates adrenergic receptors, and can increase heart rate and peripheral vascular resistance, thus increasing high blood pressure even more.[42] Interestingly, licorice extract is also known to cause increased blood pressure.[25] *Ruscus aculeatus* (butcher's broom) was investigated as a potential treatment for hypotension, but probably would increase rather than lower blood pressure.[43]

Clinical research related to medicinal use of herbal products has grown.[39] Patients are willing to spend their money on herbal and alternative medicines not covered by their insurance if they feel confident about getting a good product. This raises the issue that "the time has come to submit such products to the same rigorous, internationally accepted pharmacoeconomic approach as their synthetic competitors."[39] Herbal remedies are totally unsupervised in the U.S. because of congressional interference with surveillance by the Food and Drug Administration (FDA).[25] The development of patent medicines in the early part of the 20th century caused a decrease in the use of herbal medicines because scientists and physicians touted synthetic and patented medicines as more reliable and effective.[40]

Many dietary treatments have been suggested to slow or reverse the causes of hypertension. One popular program is the DASH (dietary approaches to stop hypertension) diet that calls for 27% calories from fat, 8 to 10 daily fruit and vegetable servings, and limited consumption of meat, including fish and poultry.[9] The DASH diet also recommends that patients stop smoking, lose weight if overweight, reduce daily sodium intake to 2.4 g sodium (or 6 g table salt), maintain adequate dietary intake of potassium, calcium, and magnesium, and limit daily intake of alcohol to less than 1 oz of ethanol (equal to 24 oz beer, 8 oz wine, or 2 oz 100-proof liquor).[25]

The National Cholesterol Education Program (NCEP) recommends reducing total fat intake from the current 36 or 37% of daily caloric intake down to 30%.[44] Another source adds reduction of stress and lower dairy, calcium, and potassium consumption to the list of lifestyle changes.[45] The Third Joint National Committee report recommended nonpharmaceutical treatments that concentrate on weight control, sodium restriction, moderation of alcohol intake, cessation of cigarette smoking, and incorporation of a routine exercise program.[15] A number of studies have shown that a body weight reduction as little as 10 lb is associated with significant reductions in systolic and diastolic arterial blood pressure, serum cholesterol, heart rate, and uric acid concentrations.[15] Blood pressure increases as body weight increases, and excess weight can increase the risk of hypertension two to six times, especially for those with abdominal obesity.[44] Regular aerobic exercise routinely lowers blood pressure. A 30-minute workout at 50% maximum oxygen uptake will lower blood pressure for the remainder of a 24-hour period.[25] A publication of the Joint National Committee V noted a significant reduction in the number of hypertensive patients in the U.S. as a result of these nonpharmaceutical approaches.[15]

In 1999, the World Health Organization's International Society of Hypertension (WHO-ISH) set guidelines for the management of mild hypertension after noticing uncertainty among clinicians and policymakers concerning mild hypertension. The group suggested nonpharmacological lifestyle measures including smoking cessation, weight reduction, moderation of alcohol consumption, reduction of salt intake, dietary changes, increased physical activity, and use of coping skills to manage psychological factors and stress. WHO-ISH found that in controlled dietary trials, the blood pressure lowering effects of vegetarian diets were more dependent on the combined effects of increased consumption of fruits, vegetables, and fiber and the decreased intake of fats than whether meat was consumed.[23] Actions to promote the risks associated with high dietary intake of sodium have met with resistance. Processed foods account for more than 75% of sodium intake in the U.S. diet.[15,25] One source noted that those making and selling snack foods and sodas do not wish to see reductions in their profits and actively resist attempts to reduce dietary fat and salt levels.[25]

For many people, beneficial results can be achieved by reducing intakes of high sodium (Na)/low potassium (K) processed foods while increasing intakes of low Na/high K natural foods in their diets.[25] An increase of fruits and vegetables in daily diet will increase K intake and that will reduce blood pressure[15] and Na intake. The Framingham Heart Study noted that a dietary increase of three servings per day of K-rich fruits and vegetables was associated with a 22% decrease in the risk of stroke.[25]

Fresh fruits and vegetables are important sources of vitamin C, fiber,[46] and magnesium (Mg).[15] While calcium (Ca) supplements or increases of dietary Ca intake exert minimal effects on blood pressure, Mg supplements may cause a small drop in blood pressure. Dietary intake of fruits and vegetables is preferred as a source of Mg.[15,25] Since the causes of hypertension produce long-term effects, a diet high in fruits and vegetables may be preventative.[46] Studies show that a vegetarian diet is associated with low blood pressure[47] and that vegetarians tend to have lower blood pressure overall.[25] When hypertensives go on vegetarian diets, systolic blood pressure falls by an average of about 5 mmHg.[25]

In Norway, an increase of fruits and vegetables proved to decrease stroke mortality.[48] In the Nurses' Health Study, a 12- to 14-year follow-up of the 75,000 female participants indicated a significant reduction in the risk of stroke with increased intake of fruits and vegetables[25] and that a diet including more complex carbohydrates and less refined sugars tends to lower blood pressure.[25] Short- and long-term consumption of black tea was found to regulate endothelial vasomotor abnormalities in coronary artery disease patients.[49] No effect on atherosclerotic risks concerned with plaque on the arteries was discovered in treatments with tea.[49] Other experiments proved that blood pressure in laboratory animals can be lowered by the addition of green tea to water for ingestion.[50,51] The decreases are caused by antioxidants residing in fruits, vegetables, and tea.[46,52] Lowering oxidation levels in spontaneously hypertensive rats has shown physical evidence that antioxidants are antihypertensive.[107]

The effects of grains served as the topic of another study. A total of 88 men and women were divided among 2 groups: 23 males and 22 females consumed an oat cereal over a 12-week period; the remaining 22 males and 21 females were left as a control group. It was noted that 73% of the group given an oat-based diet opposed to 42% of the control group showed decreased blood pressure, took half their recommended doses of hypertension drugs, or even stopped medications completely.[53] Cholesterol levels in the oat group were lowered by 24.2 mg/dl in comparison to the control group, while LDL cholesterol levels decreased by 16.2 mg/dl in the oat group.[53]

In a study conducted with 59 healthy omnivorous subjects at Royal Perth Hospital, the influence of a vegetarian diet on blood pressure was investigated. The 30 women and 29 men, aged 25 to 63 years, and all professional, clerical, or technical employees of the hospital, were divided into 3 groups. The control group ate an omnivorous diet for the entire 14-week period. One experimental group ate an omnivorous diet for 2 weeks, followed by a lacto-ovo-vegetarian diet for 6 weeks, and then resumed the omnivore diet for the final 6 weeks. The second experimental group ate an omnivorous diet for the first 8 weeks, followed by a lacto-ovo-vegetarian diet for the final 6 weeks. On Mondays through Fridays, both groups ate 2 meals per day in the hospital dining room. The participants received instructions about meals eaten outside the hospital.[47]

The systolic, diastolic, and mean blood pressure measurements showed no change in the control group (mean BP = DBP + [(SBP − DBP)/3]).[8,54] All three blood pressure measurements fell significantly in each of the control groups during the time they were on the vegetarian diet. The blood pressure levels of the experimental group that reverted to the omnivorous diet rose significantly at that time. The diet-related decrease measured 5 to 6 mmHg in systolic pressure and 2 to 3 mmHg in diastolic pressure. No correlation was indicated between intakes of Na or K and high blood pressure because the diets were similar in that regard. Furthermore, 52%

of the participants had higher education background, 25% smoked, and 71% ingested moderate amounts of alcohol, so these factors were not indicated as causes for the increase in blood pressure. The blood pressure changes in the experimental groups were most evident during the final week on the vegetarian diet, with the blood pressure returning to previous levels within 5 to 6 weeks of return to the omnivorous diet.[47] Another source indicated that vegetarians tend to have lower blood pressure and that omnivores placed on a vegetarian diet show an average drop of 5 mmHg in systolic blood pressure.[15]

Perhaps the drop in blood pressure was due to increased dietary fiber, polyunsaturated fats, and magnesium; a reduction of dietary saturated fat, cholesterol, and total fat;[47] or ingestion of flavonoids. Another early study concluded "that average flavonoid intake may contribute to differences in mortality from CHD (coronary heart disease) across populations."[55] A study that used a 131-item questionnaire on 34,789 male health professionals aged 40 to 75 years "found a modest but nonsignificant inverse association between intake of flavonols and flavones and subsequent coronary mortality rates." In the conclusion, the researchers admitted the data did "not exclude the possibility that flavonoids have a protective effect in men with established coronary heart disease."[56]

10.5 FLAVONOIDS: TYPES, SOURCES, AND STUDIES

Flavonoids, also called bioflavonoids, are members of a larger group called polyphenols[56,57] and are secondary metabolites extracted from plants and found in numerous foods such as red wine, black tea, onions, and apples.[58] Universally present in vascular plants,[59] they color flowers and fruits to attract pollinators and repel predators.[59] The blue anthocyanins are colored in part by magnesium metal.[60] Flavonoids differ from one plant species to another.[57]

Citrus flavonoids were discovered (and named vitamin P) in 1936 by Rusznyák and Szent-Györgyi, who proposed that their intake strengthens blood vessel walls and decreases capillary fragility seen in scurvy.[57,61,62] The vitamin status was discontinued in 1950 upon recommendation of the Federation of American Societies for Experimental Biology.[61] For the most part, the biologic actions of flavonoids are specific toward activated cells; they exert little or no effect on normal cells.[61] Therefore, "it might be possible to identify a range of flavonoids that could be employed selectively in pharmaceutical use depending on the endpoint desired."[63] Flavonoids are currently under study for potential value in treating allergic reactions, cancer, diabetes, and inflammatory and viral infections.[59] Flavonoids prevent oxidation, chelate or bind metals, stimulate the immune system, prevent the formation of carcinogens, and protect against bacteria and viruses.[64]

More than 4000 flavonoids and many sources have been identified.[57,65] Howard M. Merken and Gary R. Beecher of *Agricultural Research*, a magazine published by the U.S. Department of Agriculture, are reportedly preparing a database of all flavonoids. They previously launched a database of isoflavones in soy foods in 1999.[64]

Flavonoids also have a few nonplant sources. They have been found in the wings and bodies of butterflies in the *Satyridae*, *Lycaenidae*, and *Papilionidae* families.[66] The only reported mammalian source of flavonoids is 4'-methoxyflavan from the scent glands of the Canadian beaver, *Caster fiber*.[66] Flavonoids cannot be synthesized by humans.[65]

Flavonoids have many subclasses including isoflavones, catechins, anthocyanidins, flavonols, flavones, flavanones found in citrus fruits,[56,62,67] biflavone,[68] and biflavonoids.[69] Anthocyanins are found in edible cereals, green and root vegetables, and fruits.[67] Biflavone is also called amentoflavone and is a selective inhibitor of COX.[68] Similarly, bioflavonoids are associated with amentoflavone, bilobetin, morelloflavane, and ginkgetin, and prevent phospholipase A_2.[69] Flavones include chrysin, apigenin, tangeritin, luteolin,[58] and nobiletin. The apigenin flavone is found in parsley and thyme[56] and has been used to treat inflammation.[61] Some common flavonols are kämpferol or kaempferol, quercetin which is found in many Western foods and stops oxidation and cytotoxicity definition of LDLs,[70] myricetin,[58] and rutin. The quercetin and kaempferol flavonols are found predominantly in onions, kale, broccoli, apples, cherries, berries, tea, and red wine.[56] The astilbin (dihydroquercetin 3-rhamnoside) and engeltin (dihydrokaempferol 3- rhamnoside) dihydroflavonols are found in chardonnay grapes and white wines.[67] Flavonones include naringenin, naringin, eriodictyl, hesperetin, and hesperidin. The subclass of dihydroflavonols includes taxifolin or dihydroquercetin. Catechin, gallocatchin, and gallate are flavanes. Isoflavones or phytoestrogens include coumestrol, equol,[58] daidzein, glycitein, and genistein. Coumestrol is one of the coumestanes. Caffeic A (CAFA) is a cinnamate. Alpha-tocopherol (α-TOC) and gamma-tocopherol (γ-TOC) are in the subclass of tocopherols. Another subclass is 3-methyl-cholanthrene.[71]

Flavonoids are composed of benzene rings with multiple hydroxyl groups and as a result are also called polyphenols[62] (see Figure 10.2). Many are also combined molecularly with sugar and called glycosides. Examples are hesperidin, found in oranges, lemons, limes, and tangerines; naringin and narirtin, found in grapefruits; and eriocitrin, found in lemons and limes.[61] It has been suggested that grapefruit juice increases the absorption of several calcium channel blockers.[61] The extreme bitterness of citrus peels is due to naringin.[67] In 1981, Wollenweber and Dietz showed "flavones and flavonols of leaf works and plant extrudes nearly always occur in the free state, without glycosylation, and often in methylated form."[60]

Flavonoids in plants are unaffected by heat, oxygen, dryness, or limited acidity, but they can change in the presence of light.[72] For example, high exposure to light leads to high oxidation.[4] Ultraviolet B rays can encourage accumulation of fla-

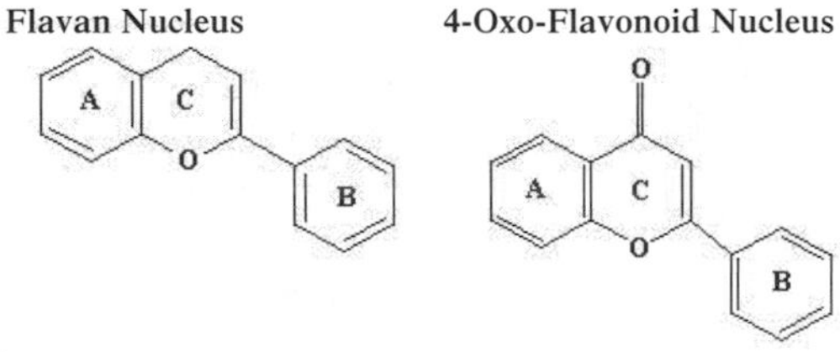

FIGURE 10.2 Chemical structure of nucleus.

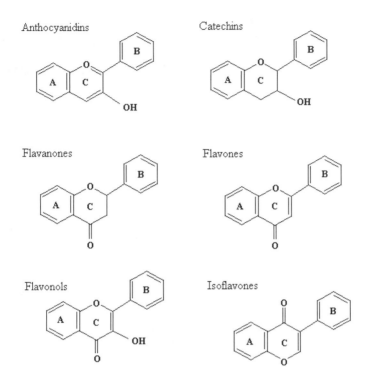

FIGURE 10.3 Nucleus structures of flavonoid classes.

vonoids.[73] Photostability of these molecules is a result of glycosylation or detachment of the hydroxyl group from the C-3 of ring C.[74] Glycosylation causes an increase in the polarity of the flavonoid molecules, which is important for cell vacuole storage in plants.[4]

Most classes of flavonoids, such as flavones and flavanones, are found as glycosides in nearly all plants[72] (see Figure 10.3). Because light can stimulate biosynthesis of 4-oxo-flavonoid, its concentration is greater near the surface of the plant.[4] Vast amounts of quercetin glycosides are found in the skins of red grapes,[75] Spanish cherry tomatoes,[73] and apples.[76] Thus, plants with high skin-to-volume ratios are said to have high flavonol contents.[4] Quercetin content in fruit and vegetables can range from less than 1 mg/100 g (endive) to 147 mg/100 g (cranberries).[77]

Cultivation, preparation, and storage are influential variables as well. Many leafy vegetables including lettuces, endives, and leeks show flavonoid level variations from season to season, whereas red cabbage and pears do not.[77] Grapes grown in warm sunny areas produce wines high in flavonol content compared to grapes grown in colder climates.[75] Boiling can decrease the quercetin content of vegetables and fruits more than microwaving or frying.[78] Storage effects on flavonoid accumulation are not as precisely determined. One study noted that quercetin levels of bilberries and strawberries stored for 9 months at −20°C decreased by 40% and increased by 32%, respectively.[79]

At the Plant Flavonoids in Biology and Medicine meeting held in Buffalo, NY, in 1985, Tony Swain of the Department of Biology at Boston University noted that some of the 6- and 8-hydroxy-substituted flavonoids found in angiosperms did not appear in lower plants. He stated that flavonoids, first, are typical phenolic compounds and thus act as potent antioxidants and metal chelators. It is advantageous to plants to be able to isolate and reduce the activities of oxidant-inducing metals such as iron and copper taken from the soil. Those that include a 4-carbonyl and a 5- (or 3-) hydroxy group are very good metal chelators. Second, flavonoids are conjugated aromatic compounds that screen out ultraviolet light and attenuate visible light. Third, they interfere with the feeding, reproduction, germination, and growth of seedlings, as well as the growth and development of animals, bacteria, fungi, and viruses. Isoflavones particularly simulate steroidal and other growth controllers in predators. Pranthocyanidins, ligans, and biflavonoids (polymeric forms) can bind proteins, enzymes, polysaccharides, nucleic acids, and other polymers. Fourth, flavonoids play a role in strengthening the structures of plant cell walls, especially ligins.[59]

Other sources of flavonoids used to treat a variety of health issues are citrus, extracts of bilberry, hawthorne, horse chestnut (*Aesculus hippocastanum*), gotu kola (*Centella asciatica*), butcher's broom (*Ruscus aculeatus*), and *Ginkgo biloba*. Potentially useful citrus flavonoids were discovered in the peels and leaves of Dancy tangerines.[80] *Achillea wilhelmsii* is an herb that grows wild in Iran and is a rich source of flavonoids.[58] Procyanidins are found in cocoa, red wine, apples, and cranberries.[81] Flavonoids in pomegranates have been associated with anti-aging properties in Israel.[82] Additionally, pycnogenols, complexes of flavonoids or polyphenols found in extracts of grape seeds and the bark of the Landes pine, have been used in the treatment of varicose veins at doses of 150 to 300 mg/day.[13] Grape seeds, pulp, and skins have been used in the treatment of circulatory disorders, as have other proanthocyanidins.[57] Flavonoids have been found in cabbage, beans, radishes, and rhubarb stalks.[67] Flavonoids from pome and stone fruits tend to be concentrated in the peels. Those found in the skins and flesh of soft fruits tend to increase as the fruit ripens. Some raspberries contain hundreds of milligrams of flavonoids per 100 grams of fresh fruit. Blood oranges are colored by glycosides of cyanidin and delphinidin.[67] Flavonoids are also found in grains, legumes, soy, beer, and bourbon.[58]

The low rate of heart disease in France, a high consumer of red wine which is high in flavonoid content, is named the French Paradox. In comparison to Americans, the French have similar levels of serum cholesterol, saturated fat intake, and prevalence of smoking — all considered contributory factors for heart disease.[61]

Flavonols and flavones are subgroups of flavonoids that have antioxidant properties and are most often found in vegetables, fruits, tea, and red wine.[56] The antioxidant properties of flavonols and catechins suggest that they may prevent atherosclerosis. They also inhibit lipoxygenase (LOX).[83] The LOX and cyclooxygenase (COX) enzymes affect blood pressure by increasing aggregation platelets that regulate blood clotting.[84] Individually, LOX mediates pharmacology, while COX increases the production of prostaglandin, a hormone that mediates blood pressure.[20] In general, flavonoids are powerful inhibitors of COX,[83] antioxidants, and tyrosine and kinase blockers.[57] Most attack lipid bilayers[85] and inhibit LDLs[58] and platelets.[86]

Antiplatelet/antioxidant therapy has been accomplished through the actions of flavonoids in red wine and purple grape juice. It is now thought that nitric oxide (NO) is the relaxing factor in coronary and other arteries. NO is secreted by endothelial cells when increased blood flow passes over them.[87] The endothelial cells can be damaged or become dysfunctional through hypertension, increased LDL cholesterol, diabetes, cigarette smoking, free radicals, or elevated plasma homocysteine.[88] This damage would decrease the production of NO. Decreased NO allows platelets and other cells to adhere to arterial walls.[87] This action increases blood pressure as the inner diameters of the arteries decrease. In a dog study, purple grape juice proved better than aspirin as an antiplatelet medication. The dogs were given amounts equal to about 20 oz of purple grape juice for an adult human. The purple grape juice treatment showed no renewed platelet activity, while about 60% renewed activity occurred with aspirin treatment.[87]

Antioxidants include dietary substances and some vitamins that quench free radical reactions and thus lessen oxidation of some cell constituents.[44] An increase in LDL increases the chance of cardiovascular disease (CVD). When LDL is oxidized, "it is more easily taken up by the macrophages, causing foam cell formation in the intima of the arteries, triggering the atherogenic process."[44] Vitamins C and E and beta-carotene appear to play a role in decreasing lipid peroxidation and the oxidization of LDL.[44]

Flavonoids such as quercetin, kaempferol, myristin, epigenin, and luteolin are polyphenolic antioxidants found in fruits, vegetables, and red wines.[44,49] They inhibit oxidation of LDL cholesterol and reduce thrombotic tendencies.[44] Some soy isoflavones are effective in lowering serum cholesterol. Other sources of antioxidant-acting flavonoids revealed in a Japanese study are pine bark — touted as 50 times more powerful than vitamin E — green tea, and persimmons.[57] Persimmon juice has been used as a traditional medicine to treat hypertension and prevent stroke in Japan. Persimmon juice contains various condensed tannins.[89] The mix of proanthocyanidin flavonoids in pine bark varies, and the same is believed true of other flavonoid sources. Researchers studied 6 but only found 1 that was 50 times more powerful than vitamin E. Proanthocyanidins are water-soluble and vitamin E is oil-soluble. Humans require both water- and oil-soluble antioxidants, so pine bark is not a viable replacement for vitamin E.[57] Other sources warn that although antioxidants are popular, their use in the prevention of cardiovascular disease has not yet been proven in trials.[11]

A study was done in Japan to investigate the possible relation between low coronary artery disease and intake of green tea, which is high in flavonoid content, but concluded more study was necessary.[90]

The Caerphilly Study investigating flavonols and ischemic heart disease in Welsh men found that quercetin can inhibit LDL oxidation and therefore prohibit platelet aggregation *in vitro*.[90] The major sources of the flavonols were black and green teas, red wines, and onions.[90]

A separate 6-year study that used a 131-item questionnaire on 34,789 male health professionals aged 40 to 75 years "found a modest but nonsignificant inverse association between the intake of flavonols and flavones and subsequent coronary mortality rates." The biennial follow-up questionnaires were completed and returned via mail by 94% of the original participants in 1988, 1990, and 1992. The participants were questioned about foods and frequencies of intake to determine their intakes of three flavonols and two flavones. The primary food sources of the flavonoids were tea (25%), onions (25%), apples (10%), and broccoli (7%). The study also found that the men with higher intakes of flavonols and flavones were slightly older, drank less alcohol, smoked less, and ate more dietary fiber. These men were also more likely to take vitamin E supplements. In the conclusion, the researchers admitted that the data "do not exclude the possibility that flavonoids have a protective effect in men with established coronary heart disease."[56]

In a Finnish study, an inverse association between flavonols from dietary intake of apples and onions and cardiovascular mortality was reported.[90] Hertog et al. reported an inverse association between the intake of quercetin and coronary mortality of elderly men in Zutphen, the Netherlands.[44,62,99] The major dietary sources of quercetin and related flavonols were tea and onions. However, the study showed heart disease mortality increased with tea and decreased with onion intake. This may be due to the fact that the tea drinkers were more likely to be manual laborers who ate more fat, smoked more, and had lower alcohol intakes. Additionally, metabolic studies indicated that quercetin compounds found in onions had higher bio-availabilities than those from tea.[62] A similar study concluded that although data did not support a strong inverse relationship between flavonoid intake and CHD, it is possible that flavonoids exert a protective effect in men with established CHD.[56]

Rat studies suggest that green tea extract has the ability to lower blood pressure.[92] In humans, blood pressure lowering effects of green tea were noticed in a study comparing the effects of black tea, green tea, and caffeine in water. The subjects consumed equal amounts of one of the liquids, and the caffeinated water was included in order to verify that the blood pressure lowering effects were not results of the caffeine in the teas.[92] Thirty percent of the flavonoids in green tea is epigallocatechin gallate.[57]

Some caution is necessary in regard to isoflavonoids. Unlike other flavonoids, isoflavonoids are plant chemicals whose biosynthesis is dependent on the presence of plant stressors, and therefore may not be consistent in quantity or strength.[93] While flavonoid composition is generally consistent within a plant species, isoflavonoid biosynthesis is particularly dependent on plant pathogens.[93]

Data on the absorption of flavonoids by humans are scarce and sometimes contradictory.[94] One report stated that humans absorb about 52% of the quercetin in onions.[56] Cooking and food preparation account for some loss of flavonoid content. About 20% or less of flavonoid content is believed to be lost through cooking.[94] Flavonoids are more predominant in the peels of pome and stone fruits and in the rinds of citrus fruits rather than in the flesh. They are found in proportion to greenness of the leaves in lettuce, parsley, rosemary, and thyme. The "green tips of asparagus contain enough rutin to react with soluble iron during storage in cans to become discolored."[67]

There is a suggestion that flavonoids may become carcinogenic at high doses. A press release from the School of Public Health of the University of California at Berkeley states that some chemical components from fruits and vegetables that are concentrated and sold in high doses as flavonoid supplements in health food stores can make people sick. Some of these substances are ginkgo pills, quercetin tablets, grape seed extract, and flax seeds. According to a professor of toxicology at Berkeley, these supplements are not regulated by any government agency. They can bind with and damage chromosomes and DNA in cell cultures at high levels, alter the activities of various enzymes, and interfere with hormone metabolism, especially estrogen and thyroid hormones. However, dietary intake could never produce such high levels of flavonoids. For example, people normally ingest 5 to 68 mg of quercetin through food intake daily, whereas one supplement recommends taking 1000 mg daily.[95]

Essential hypertension is usually associated with increased blood viscosity due to erthyrocyte deformability or aggregation. In a study of 20 individuals with moderate hypertension, decreases in blood pressure levels and plasma viscosities were noted following administration of 3 daily doses totaling 3000 mg troxerutin for 4 weeks. Participants' levels of sodium, potassium, glycamia, creatinine, uric acid, cholesterol, triglycerides, and immunoglobulins remained unchanged both over time and compared to the control group of 20 individuals matched for age and sex.[54]

When spontaneously hypertensive rats (SHRs) and normotensive Wistar Kyoto rats were given oral daily doses of quercetin for 5 weeks, the results were reduced blood pressure, plasma, and hepatic malondialdehyde levels and increased glutathione peroxidase activity. Systolic pressure fell by −18%, diastolic by −23%, and mean by 21% in SHRs.[96] None of these effects were noted in the normotensive rats.[97] Similar studies were done using flavonoids extracted from *Spergularia purpurea*. Systolic blood pressure dropped by −17% and diastolic by −24% in SHRs. With the flavonoid substance, the normotensive rats showed decreases of −11% in systolic blood pressure and −16% in diastolic pressure.[98]

The flavonoid compounds responsible for antihypertensive activity are rare, mostly ephedrannins and mahuannis A and B.[99] Four flavonones (5-hydroxy-6,7,3′,4′-tetramethoxyflavone, eupatorin, tetramethylscutellarein, and sinensetin) have been found in the kumis kucing (*Orthosophon aristatus*) leaves used in traditional Javanese medicine to treat hypertension.[100] In tests, these flavones suppressed contractions induced by K ions in endothelium-denuded rat thoracic aorta.[100]

Flavonoids are already used in medical treatments. Daflon® 500 mg is a registered brand name for the purified flavonoid fraction MPFF, and it is used in the treatment of hemorrhoidal and chronic venous insufficiency diseases. It contains 90% diosmin and 10% hesperidine, both derived from flavones.[101] Daflon has been used in cases of venular occlusion associated with elevation in capillary blood pressure and primary venous insufficiency characterized by venous wall dilation and valve dysfunction.[101] It acts favorably by inhibiting the synthesis of prostaglandins and free radicals.[6] Daflon is also known as Ardium, ArVenum 500, Detralex, and Venitol; it is manufactured by Laboratoires Servier in France.[101]

The beta-adrenergic blocking effects of some benzopyrone derivatives, propranolol-type chromone, and flavone derivatives noted in 1986 led to the development of flavodilol as an antihypertensive drug.[102] Flavodilol is a (±) 7-2-hydroxy-3-(propylamino)2-hydroxypropoxy flavone maleate.[102] The flavodilol maleate known as PR 877-530L was synthesized by the organic chemistry department of the Pennwalt Pharmaceutical Division in Rochester, NY, for use in a rat study. SHRs showed about a 26% reduction in systolic blood pressure for 2 to 24 hours after dosing. According to Watkins et al. (1985), flavodilol produced dose-related decreases up to 30% in arterial pressure in SHRs.[103] Interestingly, the same dose did not lower blood pressure or cause hypotension in normotensive Sprague–Dawley rats.[103] Flavodilol was undergoing early phase II clinical trials in 1985.[103] The synthesis and antihypertensive activity of (3-phenyl flavoxy) propanolamines were described by Wu et al (1987). "These active compounds represent a unique series of effective antihypertensive agents that, despite possessing structural characteristics typical of β-blockers, do not have β-adrenergic receptor blocking activity."[102]

Pycnogenol, a mixture of flavonoids in the bark extract from the French maritime pine (*Pinus pinaster*) and used as a dietary supplement, was administered to non-smoking, mildly hypertensive patients. The results showed decreases in systolic blood pressure, but no discernible decreases in diastolic blood pressure.[104] Another study concentrated on pycnogenol's effects on asthma and concluded it could be useful.[105] In a cardiovascular-related study, pycnogenol significantly inhibited platelet aggravation in tobacco smokers without causing increases in bleeding following aspirin use to achieve the same goal.[106]

With so many flavonoids from diverse sources, it is not likely many will appear in tablet form soon. Flavonoids may work better in conjunction with other flavonoids. An added concern is that using isolated flavonoids may be similar to the act of taking beta-carotene and ignoring all the other "mixed" carotenoids.[57] Various laboratory studies are underway to test the effectiveness of flavonoid substances in the treatment of hypertension and other diseases. Research is funded in part by organizations including the National Heart, Lung, and Blood Institute; the Produce for Better Health Foundation;[64] and the Department of Citrus.[71] While we do not yet have any conclusive evidence of success in this area, the hope is for more natural-based remedies with fewer adverse side effects.

10.6 CONCLUSION

Hypertension is prevalent today. Because of the high comorbidity rate associated with this disease, it is costly to treat. Many medical treatments also cause adverse side effects and lead to patient noncompliance with therapy. Alternative therapies include herbal treatments and diet changes concentrating on increased intakes of fruits and vegetables. Flavonoids are considered the active ingredients in fruits and vegetables. Over 4000 flavonoids have been identified and most are active antioxidants. Studies are continuing to test the efficacy of flavonoids as treatments for hypertension, cancer, and cardiovascular and other diseases. Rat studies have shown promising results. Clinical trials with mildly hypertensive humans have begun to test some of the flavonoid substances.

REFERENCES

1. D.B. Bernard, R.R. Townsend, and M.F. Sylvestri (1998), Health and disease management: what is it and where is it going? What is the role of health and disease management in hypertension? *Am. J. Hypertension*, 11, 103S.
2. G.R. Campbell (1996), The enigma of hypertension management, *Pharmacare Econ.*, 11, 16.

3. F.M. Sacks, E. Obarzanek, M.M. Windhauser, et al. (1995), Rationale and design of the dietary approaches to stop hypertension (DASH) trial. *Ann Epidemiol.*, 5, 108. In J. Moline, I.F. Bukharovich, M.S. Wolff, and R. Phillips (2000), Dietary flavonoids and hypertension: is there a link? *Med. Hypoth.*, 55, 306.

4. E. Ambrosioni (2001), Pharmacoeconomics of hypertension management: the place of combination therapy, *Pharmacoeconomics*, 19, 337.

5. E. Ginter (1998), Cardiovascular disease prevention in eastern Europe, *Nutrition*, 14, 452.

6. J.J. Bergan, G.W. Schmid-Schonbein, and S. Takase (2001), Therapeutic approach to chronic venous insufficiency and its complications: place of Daflon 500 mg, *Angiology*, 52 (Suppl. 1), 543.

7. V.L. Burl, P. Whelton, E.J. Rocella, et al. (1995), Prevalence of hypertension in the U.S. adult population: results from the Third National Health and Nutrition Examination Survey, 1988–1991, *Hypertension*, 25, 305.

8. J. Jacobson (2001), Hypertension: update use of angiotensin II receptor blockers, *Geriatrics*, 56, 20 and 25.

9. W.M. Manger and R.W. Grifford, Jr. (2001), *100 Questions and Answers about Hypertension*, Blackwell, Malden, MA.

10. S. MacMahan, R. Peto, J. Cultler, et al. (1990), Blood pressure, stroke, and coronary heart disease, Part 1: prolonged differences in blood pressure: prospective observational studies corrected for the regression dilution bias, *Lancet*, 335, 765. In J. Moline, I.F. Bukharovich, M.S. Wolff, and R. Phillips (2000) Dietary flavonoids and hypertension: is there a link? *Med. Hypoth.*, 55, 306.

11. N. Poulter (2000), Other drug treatments: the evidence, *Proc. Nutr. Soc.*, 59, 425.

12. S. Wood and B. Griffith (1997), *Conquering High Blood Pressure: The Complete Guide to Managing Hypertension*, Plenum Press, New York.

13. J.M. Whitaker (1995), *Dr. Whitaker's Guide to Natural Healing*, Prima Publishing, Rocklin, CA.

14. M. Pagani and D. Lucini (2001), Automatic dysregulation in essential hypertension: insight from heart rate and arterial pressure variability, *Auton. Neurosci. Basic Clin.*, 90, 76.

15. E.D. Frohlich (1998), *Hypertension, Evaluation and Treatment*, Williams & Wilkins, Baltimore.

16. I. Cote, J.P. Gregoire, and J. Moisan (2000), Health-related quality-of-life measurement in hypertension: a review of randomized controlled drug trials, *Pharmacoeconomics*, 18, 435.

17. D. Liao (2000), Arterial stiffness and the development of hypertension, *Ann. Med.*, 32, 383.

18. W.H. Frishman and P. Grewall (2000), Serotonin and the heart, *Ann. Med.*, 32, 195.

19. H.P. Dustan (1990), Obesity and hypertension in blacks, *Cardiovasc. Drug Ther.*, 4 (Suppl. 2), 395. In S. Doll, F. Paccaud, P. Bovet, M. Burnier, and V. Wietlisback (2002), Body mass index, adominal adiposity and blood pressure: consistency of their association across developing and developed countries, *Int. J. Obesity Rel. Metabol. Disorders*, 26, 48.

20. *American Heritage Dictionary of the English Language*, 4th ed. (2000), Houghton Mifflin, New York, <http://www.eref-trade.hmco.com/>

21. M.G.L. Hertog, P.C.H. Hollman, M.B. Katan, and D. Kromhout (1993), Intake of potentially anticarcinogenic flavonoids and their determinants in adults in the Netherlands, *Nutr. Cancer*, 20, 21. In J. Moline, I.F. Bukharovich, M.S. Wolff, and R. Phillips (2000), Dietary flavonoids and hypertension: is there a link? *Med. Hypoth.*, 55, 306.

22. R.L. Ferrer, B.M. Sibai, C.D. Mulrow, E. Chiquette, K.R. Stevens, J. Cornell (2000), Management of mild chronic hypertension during pregnancy: a review, *Obstetr. Gynecol.*, 96, 849.

23. World Health Organization (1999), International Society of Hypertension Guidelines for the Management of Hypertension, *J. Hypertension*, 17, 151.

24. M.M. Muthali, I.F. Benter, Z. Khnadekar, L. Gaber, A. Estes, S. Malik, J.H. Parmentier, V. Manne, and K.U. Malik (2000), Contribution of Ras GTPase MAP kinase and cytochrome P450 metabolites to deoxycorterone-salt-induced hypertension, *Hypertension*, 35, 457.

25. N.M. Kaplan (2002), *Clinical Hypertension*, Lippincott, Philadelphia.

26. C.B. Chapman and T.B. Gibbons (1949), The diet and hypertension, *Medicine*, 29, 26. In D.M. Harlan and G.V. Mann (1982). A factor in food which impairs Na$^+$ K$^+$ATPase *in vitro*, *Am. J. Clin. Nutr.*, 35, 250.

27. M. Weinberger (2001), Sodium and other dietary factors. In *Hypertensive Medicine*, M.A. Weber, Ed., Humana Press, Totowa, NJ.

28. R.F. Furchgott and J.V. Zawadzki. The obligatory role of endothelial cells in the relaxation of arterial smooth muscle by acetylcholine, *Nature*, 288: 373. In S. Taddei and A. Salvetti (1997), Endothelial dysfunction in hypertension, *Hypertension and the Heart: Advances in Experimental Medicine and Biology*, Vol. 432, Plenum Press, New York.

29. R.M.J. Palmer, A.G. Ferrige, and S. Moncada (1987), Nitric oxide release accounts for the biological activity of endothelium-derived relaxing factor, *Nature*, 327, 524. In R.S. Zimmerman (1997), Hormonal and humeral considerations in hypertensive disease, *Med. Clin. N. Amer.*, 81, 1213.

30. M.W. Radomski, R.M.J. Palmer, and S. Moncada (1989), The anti-aggregating properties of vascular endothelium: Interactions between prostacyclin and NO, *Br. J. Pharmacol.*, 92, 639. In S. Taddei and A. Salvetti (1997), Endothelial dysfunction in hypertension, *Hypertension and the Heart: Advances in Experimental Medicine and Biology*, Vol. 432, Plenum Press, New York.

31. S. Taddei and A. Salvetti (1997), Endothelial dysfunction in hypertension, *Hypertension and the Heart: Advances in Experimental Medicine and Biology*, Vol. 432, Plenum Press, New York.

32. A.T. McLellan, D.C. Lewis, C.P. O'Brien, and H.D. Kleber (2000), Drug dependence, a chronic medical illness: implications for treatment, insurance, and outcomes evaluation, *JAMA*, 284, 1689.

33. H. Krum and A. Pellizzer (1998), New and emerging drug treatments for hypertension, *Austr. Fam. Physician*, 27, 235.

34. E.H. Baker (2000), Ion channels and the control of blood pressure, *Br. J. Clin. Pharmacol.*, 49, 185.

35. E. Micheakis, W. Tymchak, D. Lien, L. Webster, K. Hashimoto, and S. Archer (2002), Oral sildenafil is an effective and specific pulmonary vascular in patients with pulmonary arterial hypertension, *Circulation*, 105, 2398.

36. S. Oparil (1999), Arterial hypertension. In *Cecil's Textbook of Medicine,* 20th ed., C.J. Bennet and F. Plum, Eds., W.B. Saunders, Philadelphia, p. 256.

37. J.A. Cutler (1996), High blood pressure and end-organ damage, *J. Hypertension*, 14 (Suppl. 1), 53.

38. C. Kim and Y.S. Kwok (1998), Navajo use of native healers, *Arch. Intern. Med.*, 158, 2303.

39. P.A. DeSmet, G. Bonsel, A. Van der Kuy, Y.A. Hekster, M.H. Pronk, M.J.A. Brorens, J.H.M. Lockefeer, and M.J.C. Nuijten (2000), Introduction to the pharmacoeconomics of herbal medicine, *Pharmacoeconomics*, 18, 1.
40. N.H. Mashour, I. Ling, and W.H. Frishman (1998), Herbal medicine for the treatment of cardiovascular disease: clinical considerations, *Arch. Intern. Med.*, 158, 2225.
41. D. Delioman, I. Calis, F. Ergun, B.S. Dogan, C.K. Buharalioglu, and I. Kanzik (2000), Studies on the vascular effects of the fractions and phenolic compounds isolated from *Viscum album* ssp. album, *J. Ethnopharmacol.*, 72, 323.
42. G.A. Mansoor (2001), Herbs and alternative therapies in the hypertension clinic, *Am. J. Hypertension*, 14, 971.
43. D.A. Redman (2000), *Ruscus aculeatus* (butcher's broom) as a potential treatment for orthostatic hypotension, with a case report, *J. Alt. Compl. Med.*, 6, 539.
44. J. Dwyer (1995), Overview: dietary approaches for reducing cardiovascular disease risks, *J. Nutr.*, 125, 656S.
45. H.A. Twaij, A. Kery, and N.K. Al-Khazraji (1983), Some pharmacological, toxicological and phytochemical investigations on *Centaurea phyllocephala, J. Ethnopharmacol.*, 9, 299.
46. R.M. Acheson and R.R.R. William (1983), Does consumption of fruit and vegetables protect against stroke? *Lancet*, 1, 1191.
47. I.L. Rouse, L.J. Belin, B.K. Armstrong, and R. Vandogen (1983), Blood pressure lowering effect of a vegetarian diet: controlled trial in normotensive subjects, *Lancet*, 1, 5.
48. K.J. Joshipura, A. Ascherio, J.E. Manson, et al. (1999), Fruit and vegetable intake in relation to risk of ischemic stroke, *JAMA*, 282, 1233. In J. Moline, I.F. Bukharovich, M.S. Wolff, and R. Phillips (2000), Dietary flavonoids and hypertension: is there a link? *Med. Hypoth.*, 55, 306.
49. S.J. Duffy, J.F. Keaney, Jr., M. Holbrook, N. Gokce, P.L. Swerdloff, B. Frei, and J.A. Vita (2001), Short- and long-term black tea consumption reverses endothelial dysfunction in patients with coronary artery disease, *Circulation,* 104, 151.
50. Y. Sato, H. Nakatsuka, and R. Qatanabe (1989), Possible contribution of green tea drinking habits to the prevention of stroke, *Tohoku J. Exp. Med.*, 157, 337. In J. Moline, I.F. Bukharovich, M.S. Wolff, and R. Phillips (2000), Dietary flavonoids and hypertension: is there a link? *Med. Hypoth.*, 55, 306.
51. K. Iwata, T. Inayama, S. Miwa, and K. Kawaguchi (1987), Effect of Chinese green tea and oolong tea on blood pressure, plasma and liver lipids in spontaneously hypertensive rats and rats with fructose-induced hyperlipidemia, *J. Jap. Soc. Nutr. Food Sci.*, 40, 469. In J. Moline, I.F. Bukharovich, M.S. Wolff, and R. Phillips (2000), Dietary flavonoids and hypertension: is there a link? *Med. Hypoth.*, 55, 306.
52. S.O. Keli, M.G.L. Hertog, E.J.M. Freskens, and D. Kromhout (1996), Dietary flavonoids, antioxidant vitamins, and incidence of stroke: the Zutphen study, *Arch. Intern. Med.*, 156, 637.
53. J.J. Pins, D. Geleva, J. Keenan, C. Frazel, P.J. O'Conner, and L.M. Cherney (2002), Do whole-grain oat cereals reduce the need for antihypertensive medications and improve blood pressure control? *J. Family Pract.,* 51, 353.
54. M. Gueguen-Duchesne, F. Durand, M.-C. Le Goff, and B. Genefet (1988), Effects of troxerutin on the hemorheological parameters of patients with moderate arterial hypertension. In *Plant Flavonoids in Biology and Medicine II: Biochemical, Cellular, and Medicinal Properties*, V. Cody, E. Middleton, Jr., J. B. Harborne, and A. Beretz, Eds. (1998), Alan R. Liss, New York, p. 401.

55. M.G.L. Hertog, D. Kromhout, C. Aravanis, H. Blackburn, R. Buzina, F. Fidanza, S. Giampaoli, A. Jansen, A. Menotti, S. Nedeljkovic, M. Pekkarinen, S.S. Bozida, H. Toshima, E.J.M. Feskens, P.C.H. Hollman, and M.B. Katan (1995), Flavonoid intake and long-term risk of coronary heart disease and cancer in the Seven Countries Study, *Arch. Intern. Med.*, 155, 381.

56. E.B. Rimm, M.B. Katan, A. Ascherio, M.J. Stampfer, and W.C. Willett (1996), Relationship between intake of flavonoids and risk for coronary heart disease in male health professionals, *Ann. Intern. Med.,* 125, 384.

57. J. Challem (1996), A critical look at the flavonoids and some sound recommendations: the real story behind French pine bark, grape seed extract, green tea, and citrus. In *Nutr. Rep.*, www.nutritionreporter.com/Look_at_Flavonoids.html

58. S. Asgary, G.H. Naderi, N. Sarrafzadegan, N. Mohammadifard, S. Mostafavi, and R. Vakili (2000), Antihypertensive and antihyperlipidemic effects of *Achillea wilhelmsii*, *Drugs Exp. Clin. Res.,* 26, 89.

59. T. Swain (1985), The evolution of flavonoids. In V. Cody, E. Middleton, Jr., and J. Harborne, Eds. (1986), *Plant Flavonoids in Biology and Medicine: Biochemical, Pharmacological, and Structure-Activity Relationships, Progress in Clinical and Biological Research,* Vol. 213, Alan R. Liss, New York, p. 1.

60. J.B. Harborne (1979), Nature, distribution and function of plant flavonoids. In V. Cody, E. Middleton, Jr., and J. Harborne, Eds. (1986), *Plant Flavonoids in Biology and Medicine: Biochemical, Pharmacological, and Structure-Activity Relationships, Progress in Clinical and Biological Research,* Vol. 213, Alan R. Liss, New York, p. 15.

61. J.A. Manthey (1998), Flavonoids in the living system: an introduction. In J.A. Manthey and B.S. Busling, Eds. (1998), *Advances in Experimental Medicine and Biology,* Vol. 439, Plenum Press, New York, p. 1.

62. M.B. Katan (1997), Flavonoids and heart disease, *Am. J. Clin. Nutr.,* 65, 1542.

63. P. M. Fotsist, H. Adlercreutz, T. Hase, R. Montesano, and L. Schweigerer (1995), Genistein: a dietary ingested isoflavonoid inhibits cell proliferation *in vitro* angiogenesis, *J. Nutr.,* 125 (Suppl. 3), 790S.

64. J. McBride, Finessing the flavonoids, *Agric. Res.*, Available at U.S. Department of Agriculture Web site, www.ars.usda.gov/is/AR/archive/febol/flavo201.htm [cited July 2002.]

65. J. Peterson and J. Dwyer (2000), Flavonoids: dietary occurrence and biochemical activity, www.nal.usda.gov/ttic/tektran/data/000011/50/0000115068.html

66. J. Harborne (1985), Nature, distribution and function of plant flavonoids. In V. Cody, E. Middleton, Jr., and J. Harborne, Eds. (1986), *Plant Flavonoids in Biology and Medicine: Biochemical, Pharmacological, and Structure-Activity Relationships, Progress in Clinical and Biological Research,* Vol. 213, Alan R. Liss, New York, p. 15.

67. W.S. Pierpoint (1985), Flavonoids in the human diet. In V. Cody, E. Middleton, Jr., and J. Harborne, Eds. (1986), *Plant Flavonoids in Biology and Medicine: Biochemical, Pharmacological, and Structure-Activity Relationships, Progress in Clinical and Biological Research,* Vol. 213, Alan R. Liss, New York, p. 125.

68. H.P. Kim, I. Mani, L. Iversen, and V.A. Ziboh (1998), Effects of naturally occurring flavonoids and biflavonoids on epidermal cyclooxygenase and lipoxygenase from guinea-pigs, *Prostaglandins Leukor. Essent. Fatty Acids,* 58, 17. In Y.S. Chi, H.G. Jong, K.H. Son, H.W. Chang, S.S. Kang, and H. Pyokim (2001), Effects of naturally occurring prenylated flavonoids on enzymes metabolizing arachidonic acid: cyclooxygenases and lipoxygenase, *Biochem. Pharmacol.,* 62, 1185.

69. H.K. Kim, K.H. Son, H.W. Chang, S.S. Kang, and H.P. Kin (1999), Inhibition of rat adjuvant-induced arthritis by ginkgetin and biflavone, *Planta Med.*, 65, 465. In J.A. Manthey (2000), Biological properties of flavonoids pertaining to inflammation, *Microcirculation*, 7, S29.
70. D. Steinberg, S. Parthasarathy, T.E. Carew, J.C. Khoo, and J.L. Witzum (1989), Beyond cholesterol: modifications of low-density lipoprotein that increase its atherogenicity, *New Engl. J. Med.*, 320, 915. In J. Moline, I.F. Bukharovich, M.S. Wolff, and R. Phillips (2000), Dietary flavonoids and hypertension: is there a link? *Med. Hypoth.*, 55, 306.
71. A.A. Franke, R.V. Cooney, L.J. Custer, L.J. Mordan, and Y. Tanaka (1998), Inhibition of neoplastic transformation and bioavailability of dietary flavonoid agents. In J.A. Manthey and B.S. Buslig, Eds. (1998), *Advances in Experimental Medicine and Biology*, Vol. 439, Plenum Press, New York, p. 237.
72. J. Kühnau (1976), The flavonoids, a class of semi-essential food components: their role in human nutrition, *World Rev. Nutr. Diet.*, 24, 117. In S.A. Aherne and N.M. O'Brien (2002), Dietary flavonoids: chemistry, food content, and metabolism, *Nutrition*, 18, 75.
73. A. Stewart, S. Bozonnet, and W. Mullen. (2000), Occurrence of flavonols in tomato and tomato-based products, *J. Agric. Food Chem.*, 48, 2663.
74. G. Smith, S.J. Thomsen, K.R. Markham, C. Andary, and D. Cardon (2000), The photostabilities of naturally occurring 5-hydroxyflavones, flavonols, their glycosides and their aluminium complexes, *J. Photochem. Photobiol. A*, 136, 87. In S.A. Aherne and N.M. O'Brien (2002), Dietary flavonoids: chemistry, food content, and metabolism, *Nutrition*, 18, 75.
75. K.R. Price, P.J. Breen, M. Valladao, and B.T. Watson. (1995), Cluster sun exposure and quercetin in Pinot noir grape wine, *Am. J. Enol. Vitic.*, 46, 187. In S.A. Aherne and N.M. O'Brien (2002), Dietary flavonoids: chemistry, food content, and metabolism, *Nutrition*, 18, 75.
76. U. Justesen, P. Knuthsen, and T. Leth (1998), Quantitative analysis of flavonols, flavones and flavanones in fruit, vegetables and beverages by high-performance liquid chromatography with photodiode array and mass spectrometric detection, *J. Chromatogr. A*, 799. In S.A. Aherne and N.M. O'Brien (2002), Dietary flavonoids: chemistry, food content, and metabolism, *Nutrition*, 18, 75.
77. M.G.L. Hertog, P.C.H. Hollman, and M.B. Katan. (1992), Content of potentially anticarcinogenic flavonoids of 28 vegetables and 9 fruits commonly consumed in the Netherlands, *J. Agric. Food Chem.*, 40, 2379. In S.A. Aherne and N.M. O'Brien (2002), Dietary flavonoids: chemistry, food content, and metabolism, *Nutrition* 18, 75.
78. A. Crozier, M.E J. Lean, M.S. McDonald, and C. Black (1997), Quantitative analysis of the flavonoid content of commercial tomatoes, onions, lettuce, and celery, *J. Agric. Food Chem.*, 45, 590. In S.A. Aherne and N.M. O'Brien (2002), Dietary flavonoids: chemistry, food content, and metabolism, *Nutrition*, 18, 75.
79. S. Häkkinen and A.R. Törrönen (2000), Content of flavonols and selected phenolic acids in strawberries and *Vaccinium* species: influence of cultivar, cultivation site and technique, *Food Res. Int.*, 33, 517. In S.A. Aherne and N.M. O'Brien (2002), Dietary flavonoids: chemistry, food content, and metabolism, *Nutrition*, 18, 75.
80. A. Montanari, J. Chen, and W. Widmer (1998), Citrus flavonoids: a review of past biological activity against disease: discovery of new flavonoids from Dancy tangerine cold pressed peel oil solids and leaves, *Adv. Exp. Med. Biol.*, 439, 103.

81. J.F. Hammerstone, S.A. Lazarus, and H.H. Schmitz (2000), Procyanidin content and variation in some commonly consumed foods, *J. Nutr.*, 130, 2086S. In T. Schewe, K. Hartmut, and H. Sies (2002), Flavonoids of cocoa inhibit recombinant human 5-lipoxygenase, *J. Am. Soc. Nutr. Sci.*, 132, 1825.

82. www.wholehealthmd.com/refshelf/substances_view/0%2c1525%2c782%2c00.htm

83. M. Weber (1999), Guidelines for assessing outcomes of antihypertensive treatment, *Am. J. Cardiol.*, 84, 2K.

84. *Webster's Revised Unabridged Dictionary* (1998), Micra, Inc. <<ftp://ftp.uga.edu/pup/misc/webster/>>

85. F. Ollila, K. Halling, P. Vuorela, H. Vuorel, and J. P. Slotte (2002), Characterization of flavonoid–biomembrane interactions. *Arch. Biochem. Biophys.*, 399, 103.

86. V.L. McGregor, M. Bellangeon, E. Chignier, L. Lerond, C. Russeelle, and J.L. McGregor (1999), Effect of a micronized purified flavonoid fraction on *in vivo* platelet functions in the rat, *Thromb. Res.*, 94, 235.

87. J.D. Folts (2002), Potential health benefits from the flavonoids in grape products on vascular disease. In B.S. Buslig and J.A. Manthey, Eds. (2002), *Flavonoids in Cell Function*, Plenum, New York.

88. J.A. Vita et al. (1996). In J.D. Folts (2002), Potential health benefits from the flavonoids in grape products on vascular disease. In *Flavonoids in Cell Function*, B.S. Buslig and J.A. Manthey, Eds. (2002), Plenum, New York.

89. S. Uchida, H. Ohta, R. Edamatsu, M. Hiramatsu, A. Mori, G. Nonaka, I. Nishioka, M. Niwa, T. Akashi, and M. Ozaki. (1987), Active oxygen free radicals are scavenged by condensed tannins. In V. Cody, E. Middleton, Jr., J.B. Harborne, and A. Beretz, Eds. (1988), *Plant Flavonoids in Biology and Medicine II: Biochemical, Cellular, and Medical Properties,* Alan R. Liss, New York, p. 135.

90. M.G.L. Hertog, P.M. Sweetnam, A.M. Fehily, P.C. Elwood, and D. Kromhout (1997), Antioxidant flavonols and ischemic heart disease in a Welsh population of men: the Caerphilly Study, *Am. J. Clin. Nutr.*, 65, 1489.

91. M.G.L. Hertog, E.J.H. Fesken, P.C.H. Hollman, M.G. Katin, and P. Kromhart (1993), Dietary antioxidant flavonoids and risk of coronary heart disease: the Zutphen Elderly Study, *Lancet*, 342, 1007.

92. J.M. Hodgson, I.B. Puddey, V. Burke, L.J. Beilin, and N. Jordan (1999), The effects on blood pressure of drinking green and black tea, *J. Hypertension*, 17, 457.

93. P.M. Fotsist, H. Adlercreutz, T. Hase, R. Montesano, and L. Schweigerer (1995), Genistein: dietary ingested isoflavonoid inhibits cell proliferation *in vitro* angiogenesis, *J. Nutr.* 125 (Suppl. 3), 790S.

94. E.B. Rimm, M.B. Katan, A. Ascherio, M.J. Stampfer, and W.C. Willett (1996), Relationship between intake of flavonoids and risk for coronary heart diseases in male health professionals, *Ann. Intern. Med.*, 125, 384.

95. P. McBroom (2000), press release, School of Public Health, University of California at Berkeley. www.berkeley.edu/news/media/releases/2000/09/19_flav.html

96. J. Duarte, R. Pérez-Palencia, F. Vargas, M.A. Ocete, F. Pérez-Vizcaino, A. Zarzuelo, and J. Tamargo (2001), Antihypertensive effects of the flavonoid quercetin in spontaneously hypertensive rats, *Br. J. Pharmacol.*, 133, 117.

97. J. Duarte, M. Galisteo, M.A. Ocete, F. Pérez-Vizcaino, A. Zarzuelo, and J. Tamargo (2001), Effects of chronic quercetin treatment on hepatic oxidative status of spontaneously hypertensive rats, *Mol. Cell. Biochem.*, 221, 155.

98. H. Jouad, M.A. Lacaille-Dubois, B. Lyoussi, and M. Eddoucks. (2001), Effects of the flavonoids extracted from *Spergularia purpurea* Pers. on arterial blood pressure and renal function in normal and hypertensive rats, *J. Ethnopharmacol.*, 76, 159.

99. R. Anton (1988), Flavonoids and traditional medicine. In *Plant Flavonoids in Biology and Medicine II: Biochemical, Cellular, and Medicinal Properties*. V. Cody, E. Middleton, Jr., J.B. Harborne, and A. Beretz, Eds. (1988), Alan R. Liss, New York, p. 42.

100. K. Ohashi, T. Bohgaki, T. Matsubara, and H. Shibuya (2000), Indonesian medicinal plants XXIII: chemical structures of two new migrated pimarane-type diterplenes, neoothosiphols A and B, and suppressive effects on rat thoracic aorta of chemical constituents isolated from the leaves of *Orthosiphon aristatus* (Lamiaceae), *Chem. Pharm. Bull.*, 48, 433.

101. S. Takase, L. Lerond, J.J. Bergan, and G.W. Schmid-Schonbein (2000), The inflammatory reaction during venous hypertension in the rat, *Microcirculation*, 7, 41.

102. A. Beretz and J.P. Cazenave (1988), The effect of flavonoids on blood vessel wall interactions. In *Plant Flavonoids in Biology and Medicine II: Biochemical, Cellular, and Medicinal Properties*, V. Cody, E. Middleton, Jr., J.B. Harborne, and A. Beretz, Eds. (1988), Alan R. Liss, New York, p. 187.

103. C.R. Kensolving, B.E. Watkins, A.R. Barrelli, F.C. Kaiser, and E.S. Wu (1989), Flavodolol: a new antihypertensive agent, *J. Cardiovasc. Pharmacol.*, 14, 127.

104. S. Hosseini, J. Lee, R.T. Sepulveda, P. Rohdewald, and R.R. Watson (2001), A randomized, double-blind, placebo-controlled, prospective, 16-week crossover study to determine the role of pycnogenol in modifying blood pressure in mildly hypertensive patients, *Nutr. Res.*, 21, 1251.

105. S. Hosseini, S. Pishnamazi, S.M.H. Sadrzadeh, F. Farid, R. Farid, and R.R. Watson (2001), Pycnogenol in the management of asthma, *J. Med. Food*, 4, 4.

106. R.R. Watson (1999), Reduction of cardiovascular disease risk factors by French maritime pine bark extract, *CVR&R*, 20, 326.

11 High-Carbohydrate Diets and Lipid Metabolism

Michel Beylot

CONTENTS

11.1 INTRODUCTION

Defining the optimal ratio of fat to carbohydrate in the diet is a major issue in human nutrition.[1] A high proportion of fat in the diet is considered to promote obesity[2] and type II diabetes mellitus and to raise risk factors for the development of atherosclerosis, particularly through an increase in plasma cholesterol level.[3,4] Therefore, dietary recommendations usually given for the prevention of atherosclerosis include a reduction of total fat to $\leq 30\%$ of total energy intake and a reduction of the amount saturated fatty acids (SFAs) to $\leq 10\%$ of energy.[5]

The benefits from eating a low-fat diet and the scientific rationales behind the recommendation have been questioned.[6] Reducing fat in the diet results in an increase in the consumption of carbohydrate (CHO) which can have undesirable side effects such as a decrease in plasma high density lipoprotein (HDL) cholesterol concentration[7,8] and a rise in plasma triglyceride (TG) levels also known as carbohydrate-induced hypertriglyceridemia.[9] Since decreased HDL cholesterol and increased TG concentrations are both risk factors for atherosclerosis, the side effects raised concerns and fuelled a controversy about the use of high-CHO low-fat (HCHO-LF) diets.[3,8] This chapter will focus on the effects of HCHO-LF diets (defined as CHO intake $\geq 55\%$ of energy intake and fat intake $\leq 30\%$ of energy intake) on cholesterol and TG metabolism — a complex issue because these effects appear to depend on both the amount and nature of the CHO ingested and on the population studied.

0-8493-1674-X/04/$0.00+$1.50

11.2 HCHO-LF DIETS AND CHOLESTEROL METABOLISM

Convincing evidence from both cross-sectional and nutritional intervention studies indicates that plasma total cholesterol level is inversely related to CHO intake.[1,10,11] This effect is observed in normolipidemic and hyperlipidemic subjects[12-15] and in subjects with metabolic syndromes.[16] It occurs independently of variations in total energy and cholesterol intake.[11] However, both low density lipoprotein (LDL) and HDL cholesterol participate in this decrease of plasma cholesterol and the HDL over LDL cholesterol ratio is unchanged or sometimes decreased.[10,11,14,15]

This decrease in HDL cholesterol led some authors to question the actual benefits of high-CHO diets compared to diets high in monounsaturated fatty acids with respect to the prevention of atherosclerosis.[8] An important question is whether it is possible to prevent at least in part this fall in HDL cholesterol and achieve a more favorable HDL over LDL cholesterol ratio by carefully choosing the amount and nature of the CHO ingested and by additional modifications of lifestyle. When a reduction in fat intake is associated with increased exercise and decreased body weight, the decrease in HDL cholesterol can be minimized.[3] The studies of Knopp et al.[14,15] suggest that the fall in HDL cholesterol is also limited when the intake in CHO is maintained to <60% of total energy intake.

With respect to the nature of the CHOs ingested, a partial answer came from the MRFIT study[10] that divided CHOs in three components: complex CHOs (mainly starch and animal glycogen), refined and processed sucrose, and simple CHOs other than refined and processed sucrose. Cross-sectional data collected during this study showed that sucrose consumption was inversely related to HDL cholesterol level while starch and other simple CHOs were unrelated. The intervention part of this study (increased intake of starch and simple CHOs other than sucrose and decrease of sucrose intake for 1 to 6 years) concluded that starch and sucrose intakes were inversely related to HDL cholesterol while intake of simple CHOs other than sucrose was directly related to HDL cholesterol and inversely related to total and LDL cholesterol.

The particularly negative effect of sucrose was already noted in the study of Ernst et al.[17] Although the modifications of the concentrations of the various cholesterol fractions were small in the MRFIT study, these data taken together strongly support the recommendation that high-CHO diets should include reduced intakes of refined sucrose and high intakes of sources of CHO such as fruits, vegetables, legumes, and whole grain products. However, studies aimed at investigating specifically the effects of various simple CHOs are needed.

The mechanisms behind these modifications of cholesterol metabolism and the differences between the effects of complex and simple CHOs are unclear and may differ between control and hypercholesterolemic subjects. Moreover, it is difficult to differentiate the specific effects of raised CHO intake and reduced fat, particularly saturated fat intake. Stacpoole et al.[12] found a decrease in cholesterol synthesis in hypercholesterolemic subjects fed high-CHO diets. Vidon et al.[11] found on the contrary that cholesterol synthesis increased when control subjects were shifted from high-fat to high-CHO diets. HMG-CoA reductase messenger ribonucleic acid (mRNA) concentrations in circulating mononuclear cells were increased by the high-CHO diet. Both studies suggested an increased clearance rate of LDL cholesterol. This could be explained by the decreased intake of saturated fatty acid (SFA) during ingestion of high-CHO diets since SFA decreases LDL receptor expression and LDL receptor-mediated catabolism.[18,19]

Vidon et al. found no increase of LDL receptor mRNA in circulating mononuclear cells with high-CHO diets. LRP mRNA concentrations were decreased.[11] However, whether circulating mononuclear cells are representative of other tissues, especially liver, with respect to the expression of key regulatory genes of cholesterol metabolism is uncertain. The modifications of HDL cholesterol may be explained by the decrease in the intake of saturated fat with a high-CHO diet. Saturated fatty acids have been shown to increase HDL cholesterol through a reduced clearance of HDL-Apo-AI from plasma[3] and reduced dietary intake of SFAs decreases HDL apo-AI production.[20] Reverse cholesterol transport is dependent on the amounts of apo-AI in the plasma and of key proteins controlling the efflux of excess cholesterol from peripheral cells (transporter ABCA1),[21] the uptake of HDL cholesterol by the liver (mainly SR-B10),[22] and cholesterol excretion in the bile as cholesterol or bile acids (mainly cholesterol-7-alpha hydroxylase).[23]

Much attention has been paid to the molecular mechanisms regulating the expression of these key proteins by nuclear factors such as LXR, FXR and PPAR.[21,23] We know of no data available about the potential role of the fat-to-carbohydrate ratio in the diet in the regulation of the expression and activity of these key regulatory proteins of reverse cholesterol transport.

11.3 HCHO-LF DIETS AND TRIGLYCERIDE METABOLISM

The concept of carbohydrate-induced hypertriglyceridemia emerged as soon as the first studies comparing plasma lipid concentrations during high-fat and high-CHO diets were performed in the 1950s.[9,24] Since high TG level appears as an independent risk factor for coronary heart disease (CHD),[25] this possible adverse effect raised, in addition to the decrease in HDL cholesterol, concerns about using high-CHO diets for the prevention of atherosclerosis.[1,3]

These concerns are increased by the demonstration that the CHO-induced increase in TG occurs in the postprandial and postabsorptive states,[7,26–28] and, despite initial evidence that the effect is only transient,[29] persists on a long-term basis.[16] The impact of increased CHO consumption on TG metabolism has been the subject of extensive research aimed at understanding the mechanisms responsible for the rise in TG concentrations and defining the factors modulating TG response to high-CHO diet.

An increase in postabsorptive TG concentrations may result from enhanced secretion of VLDL-TG, impaired clearance, or both phenomena (experimental evidence points to both). A defect in TG clearance was postulated as early as 1964 by Knittle and Ahrens.[30] This possibility was supported by Mancini et al.[31] who found via an intravenous fat tolerance test that feeding HCHO diets to normal subjects increased the half-life of plasma TG. Parks et al.[32] found decreased clearance rates of VLDL-TG in normo- and moderately hypertriglyceridemic subjects fed HCHO diets (68% CHO, mainly complex) for 5 weeks compared to a control diet (50% CHO). Conversely, Huff and Nestel[33] found increased clearance rates after HCHO feeding; the type of CHO (simple or complex) was not stated and may play a role in the difference in responses. Blades and Garg[34] found no modifications of TG clearance rate after a HCHO diet despite a large increase in TG concentrations. Their study was conducted in type II diabetic patients and the responses may differ in diabetic and control subjects.

The epuration of TG is dependent on the activity of lipoprotein lipase (LPL) that acts mainly on VLDL-TG and chylomicron TG and of hepatic lipase (HL) that acts on the remnants of VLDL and chylomicrons. Few data are available on the possible effects of HCHO diets on LPL and HL activities. Fredrickson et al.[35] reported a decrease in postheparin plasma lipolytic activity after a HCHO diet but did not separate LPL and HL activities. Jackson et al. reported that HCHO diets lowered postheparin LPL activity; the effect was transient in men and persisted only in women.[36] Campos et al. found a decreased plasma LPL activity after 6 weeks of HCHO diet in healthy men.[37] Different results were obtained in type II diabetic patients: the HCHO diet induced no modification of HL activity[28,34] and induced either an increase[28] or no modification[34] of postheparin LPL activity. This was not explained by lower values of lipase activities preceding the HCHO diet because the basal levels were similar to basal values obtained in control subjects. The divergent responses of control and diabetic subjects may play a role in their different TG clearance responses to HCHO diets.

LPL is located on the surfaces of capillary endothelial cells mainly in the heart, skeletal muscle, and adipose tissue. The regulation of its activity in muscles and adipose tissue appears different.[38] Some data suggest that HCHO diets can lower skeletal muscle LPL activity,[39,40] although no such decrease was found by Yost et al.[41] However, a decrease in muscle skeletal muscle LPL activity may be compensated by an increase in adipose tissue LPL activity. Further studies should investigate the effect of HCHO diet on LPL activity, particularly the individual contributions of muscle and adipose tissue. Since LPL is activated by apoprotein CII and inhibited by apo-CIII, studies on the concentration of these apoproteins would also be useful. Huff and Nestel[33] found that CHO feeding induced an increase in the concentration of apo-CIII in VLDL.

Raised TG levels may also result from increased VLDL secretion through an increase in the number of VLDL particles secreted, an increase in the amount of TG contained by each particle, or both phenomena. Since there is only one apo-B100 protein per VLDL particle, the number of circulating VLDL particles and their turnover rates can be appreciated, respectively, by measuring the concentration of apo-B100 and the incorporation of a labelled amino acid such as leucine into apo-B100 of VLDL.[42,43] Measuring the turnover rate of the TG part of VLDL needs either the intravenous injection of VLDL previously labelled on the TG moiety or following the kinetics of the incorporation of intravenously injected glycerol or fatty acid in the TG part of VLDL.[44] With the exception of Ginsberg et al. who found no modification of apo-B100 turnover rate,[45] most studies using liquid formula or mainly simple carbohydrate to raise dietary CHO intake found an increase in apo-B100 or TG secretion rates.[12,33,46–48] Studies of high-CHO diet with whole food and mainly complex CHOs revealed no modifications of TG or apo-B100 kinetics,[32,49] and showed major differences in metabolic effects induced by simple or complex CHOs.

Four potential sources for hepatic TG synthesis are available and could therefore contribute to the CHO-induced increase in VLDL-TG secretion: (1) fatty acids taken from the plasma pool of nonesterified fatty acids (NEFAs) that originate in the fasting state mainly from adipose tissue, (2) fatty acids provided by *de novo* hepatic lipogenesis, (3) fatty acids provided by the degradation of TG-rich lipoproteins taken up by the liver, mainly remnants of chylomicrons and VLDL, and (4) fatty acids stored in the liver in TG droplets. Only the first two candidate sources have been investigated; the two others are awaiting appropriate methods.

Enhanced flow of plasma NEFA to the liver contributes to high TG levels in patients with endogenous, genetically controlled hypertriacylglycerolemia.[50] No evidence points to such a mechanism during high CHO-induced hypertriglyceridemia. To our knowledge, the only reported comparison of plasma NEFA turnover rates in subjects receiving low- or high-CHO diets are by Schwarz et al.[51] and Mittendorfer and Sidossis who found decreased whole body plasma NEFA flux after high-CHO diets and a trend of lower splanchnic NEFA uptake.[51] Parks et al. found no modifications of the contribution of plasma NEFA reesterification to TG secretion rate in normo- or moderately hypertriglyceridemic subjects fed high-CHO diets.[32] Mittendorfer and Sidossis[52] showed that high-CHO diets decrease splanchnic fatty acid oxidation, suggesting that the percent of plasma fatty acids taken up by liver for hepatic reesterification was increased. Such a modification of liver fatty acid metabolism would be consistent with increased *de novo* hepatic lipogenesis. Indeed, a high-CHO diet could increase *de novo* lipogenesis through an increased flow of glucose through glycolysis and into the lipogenic hepatic acetyl-CoA pool through a stimulation of the expression of lipogenic genes.[53] This has been examined since methods of measuring *de novo* liver lipogenesis in humans were developed.[54–57] In normal subjects consuming moderately high fat diets, *de novo* lipogenesis contributes usually about 5% or less to the fatty acid pool of circulating TG[44,56,58] and represents a synthetic lipid rate of only 1 to 2 g/day. Increasing CHO intake can increase this contribution of *de novo* lipogenesis to about 30%,[51,59,60] but this represents only few grams per day of lipid synthesized. The effect was observed during a large CHO overfeeding.

When the effects of raised CHO consumption are tested in an isoenergetic setting, a clear and large stimulation of *de novo* lipogenesis is observed only in subjects fed liquid formula rich in mono- or disaccharides.[61–63] No stimulation[32,63] or only moderate stimulation (unpublished data) was observed in subjects fed high-CHO diets rich in complex CHOs. All these studies investigated mainly control subjects. It is important to know whether subjects at risk of developing hyperlipidemia, e.g., obese people, have increased hepatic lipogenesis and are more responsive to the effects of high-CHO diets.

Increased basal (in the postabsorptive state) hepatic lipogenesis was found in *ad libitum*-fed obese subjects[58,64] and was directly related to BMI.[58] This was also observed in obese subjects receiving isoenergetic diets for 3 days,[65] but not when obese subjects received euenergetic diets for 2 weeks.[61] This last observation and the normal decrease of hepatic lipogenesis in obese subjects during energy restriction[64] suggest that there is no intrinsic, perhaps genetically determined, increased hepatic lipogenesis activity in obese patients. The acute response increase of liver lipogenesis to a high-CHO meal was more important in obese men than in lean men in a study by Marques-Lopes et al.[65] This difference between lean and obese subjects during acute stimulation was not found during more prolonged over-feeding (96-h overfeeding with sucrose or glucose[66] or 2 weeks of high-CHO diet).[61] No clear evidence indicates enhanced sensitivity of hepatic lipogenesis to high-CHO intake in obese subjects.

In a study of Hudgins et al.,[61] plasma TG levels were increased by a high-CHO diet and were directly correlated with hepatic lipogenesis. This suggests that the increased lipogenesis may play a role in the rise of TG concentration; however, the increased lipogenesis may be related simply to another metabolic process that plays a more important role such as diversion of the metabolism of plasma fatty acids taken up by the liver toward reesterification rather than oxidation.[52]

Lastly, the effect of high-CHO diets on adipose tissue lipogenesis should be investigated because a stimulating effect may on a long-term basis promote the development of excessive fat mass. Adipose tissue lipogenesis is usually considered less active than hepatic lipogenesis and therefore a minor metabolic pathway in humans.[67,68] Recent studies suggest that human adipose tissue lipogenesis may become significant with a high-CHO diet.[60,69] However, this was observed in subjects massively overfed with CHO. We found no evidence for such stimulation in subjects receiving moderately high CHO diets (unpublished data).

11.4 EFFECTS OF NONDIGESTIBLE CARBOHYDRATES

Nondigestible CHOs (NDCs) such as inulin and oligofructose[70] are fermentable in the colon and produce short chain fatty acids (acetic acid, propionid, and butyric acids). A large body of evidence indicates that NDCs can decrease in rodent TG and cholesterol concentrations.[71–76] The decrease in TG levels has been ascribed to inhibition of hepatic lipogenesis,[74,77] decreased reesterification of fatty acids by the liver,[73] and a reduction of VLDL-TG secretion.[74] Liver lipogenesis may be inhibited by propionic acid.[78]

Wolever et al. showed that propionate decreased the incorporation of ^{13}C labelled colonic acetate in plasma TG in humans; the effect on the incorporation in plasma cholesterol was not significant.[79] Several studies showed that NDCs reduce TG con-centrations in control humans, particularly while on high-CHO diets,[80–82] and can also reduce cholesterol levels.[82] Negative results have also been reported in normal subjects, probably because of low doses of CHOs and relatively high fat diets.[83,84]

Hepatic lipogenesis was decreased by inulin[80] and the decrease probably participated in the reduction of plasma TG concentrations. Unlike liver lipogenesis, neither cholesterol synthesis nor concentrations of mRNA for lipogenic enzymes in adipose tissue were modified by inulin. More conflicting results were reported in type II diabetic patients and in subjects with moderate hyperlipidemias. NDCs decreased plasma cholesterol but had no effect on plasma TG[85–87] or plasma lipids.[88,89] These discrepancies suggest that the metabolic effects of NDCs on lipid metabolism may be different in normal subjects and in pathological situations. NDC administration in obese Zucker rats did not decrease circulating TG levels, contrary to findings in control rats, and decreased only malic enzyme activity among all the lipogenic enzymes.[90]

11.5 PRACTICAL CONSIDERATIONS OF HIGH-CHO DIETS

Since high-CHO diets exert both favorable (reduction in total and LDL cholesterol) and potentially adverse (decrease in HDL cholesterol and increase in TG concentrations) effects on lipid metabolism, one is left to wonder whether the sum of these CHO-induced changes provides net benefits to a patient or population. No definitive answer yet exists, but some guidelines can help reduce the unfavorable effects of high-CHO diets:

1. Weight loss should be advised for individuals on high-CHO diets because it would have beneficial effects on TG and HDL cholesterol concentrations. Such weight losses occur frequently because subjects spontaneously reduce their energy intake as a result of the increased volume of a low-fat diet. Otherwise, reduction of total energy intake should be advised.
2. Since evidence does not clearly show that increasing CHO intake above 60% of total energy provides any additional advantage and may produce more pronounced adverse effects, very high CHO (or very low fat) diets do not appear more useful than moderately high CHO diets. Moreover, the increase in CHO intake should be progressive.
3. Diets should contain mainly complex CHOs; simple CHO, especially refined and processed sucrose, should be avoided as should alcohol consumption. Increased fiber intake should also be recommended to reduce risk of hypertriglyceridemia.

REFERENCES

1. Grundy, S., The optimal ratio of fat to carbohydrate in the diet, *Annu. Rev. Nutr.,* 19, 325, 1999.
2. Bray, G. and Popkin, B., Dietary fat intake does affect obesity, *Am. J. Clin. Nutr.,* 68, 1157, 1998.
3. Schaefer, E., Lipoproteins, nutrition and heart disease, *Am. J. Clin. Nutr.,* 75, 191, 2002.
4. Grundy, S. and Denke, M., Dietary influence on serum lipids and lipoproteins, *J. Lipid Res.,* 31, 1149, 1990.
5. World Health Organization Study Group on Diet, Nutrition and the Prevention of Noncommunicable Diseases, Geneva, 1991.
6. Taubes, G., The soft science of dietary fat, *Science,* 291, 2536, 2001.
7. Abbasi, F., McLaughlin, T., Lamemdola, C. et al., High carbohydrate diets, triglyceride-rich lipoproteins, and coronary heart disease risk, *Am. J. Cardiol.,* 85, 45, 2000.

8. Katan, M., Effect of low fat diet on plasma high-density lipoprotein concentrations, *Am. J. Clin. Nutr.,* 67 (Suppl.), 573S, 1998.
9. Parks, E. and Hellerstein, M., Carbohydrate-induced hypertriglyceridemia: historical perspective and review of biological mechanisms, *Am. J. Clin. Nutr.,* 71, 412, 2000.
10. Tillotson, J., Grandits, G., Bartsch, G. et al., Relation of dietary carbohydrates to blood lipids in the special intervention and usual care groups in the Multiple Risk Factor Intervention Trial, *Am. J. Clin. Nutr.,* 65 (Suppl.), 314S, 1997.
11. Vidon, C., Boucher, P., Cachefo, A. et al., Effects of isoenergetic high-carbohydrate compared with high-fat diets on human cholesterol synthesis and expression of key genes of cholesterol metabolism, *Am. J. Clin. Nutr.,* 73, 878, 2001.
12. Stacpoole, P., Von Bergmann, K., Kilgore, L. et al., Nutritional regulation of cholesterol synthesis and apolipoprotein B kinetics: studies in patients with familial hypercholesterolemia and normal subjects treated with a high carbohydrate low fat diet, *J. Lipid Res.,* 32, 1837, 1991.
13. Starc, T., Shea, S., Cohn, L. et al., Greater dietary intake of simple carbohydrate is associated with lower concentrations of high-density-lipoprotein cholesterol in hypercholesterolemic children, *Am. J. Clin. Nutr.,* 67, 1147, 1998.
14. Knopp, R., Walden, C., Retzlaff, B. et al., Long-term cholesterol-lowering effects of four fat-restricted diets in hypercholesterolemic and hyperlipidemic men: the Dietary Alternatives Study, *JAMA,* 278, 1509, 1997.
15. Knopp, R., Retzlaff, B., Walden, C. et al., One-year effects of increasingly fat-restricted, carbohydrate-enriched diets on lipoprotein levels in free-living subjects, *Proc. Soc. Exp. Biol. Med.,* 225, 191, 2000.
16. Poppitt, S., Keogh, G., Prentice, A. et al., Long-term effects of *ad libitum* low-fat, high-carbohydrate diets on body weight and serum lipids in overweight subjects with metabolic syndrome, *Am. J. Clin. Nutr.,* 75, 11, 2002.
17. Ernst, N., Fisher, M., and Smith, W., The association of plasma high-density lipoprotein cholesterol with dietary intake and alcohol consumption, *Circulation,* 62 (Suppl. IV), 41, 1980.
18. Woollett, L., Spady, D., and Dietschy, J., Saturated and unsaturated fatty acids independently regulate low density lipoprotein receptor activity and production rate, *J. Lipid Res.,* 33, 77, 1992.
19. Woollett, L., Spady, D., and Dietschy, J., Regulatory effects of the saturated fatty acids 6:0 to 18:0 on hepatic low density lipoprotein receptor activity in the hamster, *J. Clin. Invest.,* 89, 1133, 1992.
20. Velez-Carrasco, W., Lichtenstein, A., Welhy, F. et al., Dietary restriction of saturated fat and cholesterol decrease HDL apo-AI secretion, *Arterioscler. Thromb. Vasc. Biol.,* 19, 918, 1999.
21. Santamarina-Fojo, S., Remaley, A., Neufeld, E. et al., Regulation and intracellular trafficking of the ABCA1 transporter, *J. Lipid Res.,* 42, 1339, 2001.
22. Trigatti, B., Rigotti, A., and Braun, A., Cellular and physiological roles of SR-BI, a lipoprotein receptor which mediates selective lipid uptake, *Biochim. Biophys. Acta,* 1529, 276, 2000.
23. Davis, R., Miyake, J., Hui, T. et al., Regulation of cholesterol-7-alpha hydroxylase: barely missing a SHP, *J. Lipid Res.,* 43, 533, 2002.
24. Parks, E., Dietary carbohydrates: effects on lipogenesis and the relationship of lipogenesis to blood insulin and glucose concentrations, *Brit. J. Nutr.,* 87 (Suppl. 2), S247, 2002.

25. Hokanson, J., Plasma triglyceride level is a risk factor for cardiovascular disease independent of high-density lipoprotein cholesterol level: a meta-analysis of population-based prospective studies, *J. Cardiovasc. Risk,* 3, 213, 1996.
26. Van Wijk, J., Cabezas, M., Halkes, C. et al., Effects of different nutrient intakes on daytime triacylglycerolemia in healthy, normolipemic, free-living men, *Am. J. Clin. Nutr,* 74, 171, 2001.
27. Jeppesen, L., Chen, Y., Zhou, M. et al., Effect of variations in oral fat and carbohydrate load on post-prandial lipemia, *Am. J. Clin. Nutr.,* 62, 1201, 1995.
28. Chen, Y., Coulston, A., Zhou, M. et al., Why do low-fat diet high-carbohydrate diets accentuate post-prandial lipemia in patients with NIDDM? *Diabetes Care,* 18, 10, 1995.
29. Antonis, A. and Bersohn, I., Serum triglyceride levels in South African Europeans and Bantu and in ischaemic heart disease, *Lancet,* 1, 998, 1960.
30. Knittle, J. and Ahrens, E., Carbohydrate metabolism in two forms of hyperglyceridemia, *J. Clin. Invest.,* 43, 485, 1964.
31. Mancini, M., Mattock, M., Rabaya, F. et al., Studies of the mechanisms of carbohydrate induced lipaemia in normal man, *Atherosclerosis,* 17, 445, 1973.
32. Parks, E., Krauss, R., Christiansen, M. et al., Effects of a low-fat, high-carbohydrate diet on VLDL-triglyceride assembly, production and clearance, *J. Clin. Invest.,* 104, 1087, 1999.
33. Huff, M. and Nestel, P., Metabolism of apolipoproteins CII, CIII and VLDL-B in human subjects consuming high carbohydrate diets, *Metabolism,* 31, 493, 1982.
34. Blades, B. and Garg, A., Mechanisms of increase in plasma triacylglycerol concentrations as a result of high carbohydrate intakes in patients with non-insulin-dependent diabetes mellitus, *Am. J. Clin. Nutr.,* 62, 996, 1995.
35. Fredrickson, D., Ono, K., and Davis, L., Lipolytic activity of post-heparin plasma in hyperglyceridemia, *J. Lipid Res.,* 4, 21, 1963.
36. Jackson, R., Yates, M., McNermey, C. et al., Relationship between post-heparin plasma lipases, triglycrides and high density lipoproteins in normal subjects, *Horm. Metab. Res.,* 22, 289, 1990.
37. Campos, H., Dreon, D., and Krause, R., Associations of hepatic and lipoprotein lipase activities with changes in dietary composition and low density lipoprotein subclasses, *J. Lipid Res.,* 36, 462, 1995.
38. Braun, J.E. and Severson, D.L., Regulation of the synthesis, processing and translocation of LPL, *Biochem. J.,* 287, 337, 1992.
39. Lithell, H., Jacobs, I., Vessby, B. et al., Decrease in lipoprotein lipase activity in skeletal muscle in man during a short term carbohydrate rich regime. with special reference to HDL-cholesterol, apolipoprotein and insulin concentrations. *Metabolism,* 31, 994, 1982.
40. Kiens, B., Essen-Guvstasson, B., Gad, P. et al., Lipoprotein lipase activity and intramuscular triglyceride stores after long-term high-fat and high-carbohydrate diets in physically trained men, *Clin. Physiol.,* 7, 1, 1987.
41. Yost, T., Jensen, D., Haugen, B. et al., Effect of dietary macronutrient composition on tissue specific lipoprotein lipase activity and insulin action in normal weight subjects, *Am. J. Clin. Nutr.,* 68, 296, 1998.
42. Lichtenstein, A.H., Cohn, J.S., Hachey, D.L. et al., Comparison of deuterated leucine, valine and lysine in the measurement of human apolipoprotein A-I and B-100 kinetics, *J. Lipid Res.,* 31, 1693, 1990.

43. Cohn, J., Wagner, D., Cohn, S. et al., Measurement of very low density and low density lipoprotein apoprotein (apo)B-100 and high density lipoprotein Apo A-I production in human subjects using deuterated leucine, *J. Clin. Invest.,* 85, 804, 1990.

44. Diraison, F. and Beylot, M., Role of human liver lipogenesis and reesterification in triglyceride secretion and in FFA reesterification, *Am. J. Physiol.,* 274, E321, 1998.

45. Ginsberg, H., Le, N., Melish, J. et al., Effect of a high carbohydrate diet on apoprotein-B catabolism in man, *Metabolism,* 30, 347, 1981.

46. Quarfordt, S., Frank, A., Shames, D. et al., Very low density lipoprotein triglyceride transport in type IV hyperlipoproteinemia and the effects of carbohydrate-rich diets, *J. Clin. Invest.,* 49, 2281, 1970.

47. Melish, J., Le, N., Ginsberg, H. et al., Dissociation of the rates of production of apoprotein-B and TG of very-low-density lipoproteins during high carbohydrate feeding in man, *Am. J. Physiol.,* 239, E354, 1980.

48. Reaven, G., Hill, D., Gross, R. et al., Kinetics of triglyceride turnover of very low density lipoproteins in human plasma, *J. Clin. Invest.,* 44, 1826, 1965.

49. Abbott, W., Swinburn, B., Ruotolo, G. et al., Effect of a high-carbohydrate diet on apolipoprotein B and triglyceride metabolism in Pima Indians, *J. Clin. Invest.,* 86, 642, 1990.

50. Kissebah, A.H., Alfarsi, S., and Adams, P.W., Integrated regulation of very low density lipoprotein triglyceride and apoprotein-B kinetics in man: normolipemic subjects, familial hypertriglyceridemia and familial combined hyperlipidemia, *Metabolism,* 30, 856, 1981.

51. Schwarz, J., Neese, R., Turner, S. et al., Short term alterations in carbohydrate energy intake in humans: striking effects on hepatic glucose production, *de novo* lipogenesis, lipolysis and whole body fuel selection in humans, *J. Clin. Invest.,* 96, 2735, 1995.

52. Mittendorfer, B. and Sidossis, L., Mechanism for the increase in plasma triacylglycerol concentrations after consumption of short-term high carbohydrate diets, *Am. J. Clin. Nutr.,* 73, 892, 2001.

53. Girard, J., Perdereau, P., Foufelle, F. et al., Regulation of lipogenic enzyme genes expression by nutrients and hormones, *FASEB J.,* 8, 36, 1994.

54. Jones, P., Tracing lipogenesis in humans using deuterated water, *Can. J. Physiol. Pharmacol.,* 74, 755, 1996.

55. Hellerstein, M., Kletke, C., Kaempfer, S. et al., Use of mass isotopomer distribution in secreted lipids to sample lipogenic acetyl CoA pool *in vivo* in humans, *Am. J. Physiol.,* 261, E479, 1991.

56. Hellerstein, M., Christiansen, M., Kaempfer, S. et al., Measurement of *de novo* lipogenesis in humans using stable isotopes, *J. Clin. Invest.,* 87, 1841, 1991.

57. Diraison, F., Pachiaudi, C., and Beylot, M., Measuring lipogenesis and cholesterol synthesis in humans with deuterated water: use of simple gas chromatography mass spectrometry techniques, *J. Mass Spectrom.,* 32, 81, 1997.

58. Faix, D., Neese, R., Kletke, C. et al., Quantification of menstrual and diurnal periodocities in rates of cholesterol and fat synthesis in humans, *J. Lipid Res.,* 34, 2063, 1993.

59. Neese, R., Benowitch, N., Hoh, R. et al., Metabolic interactions between surplus dietary energy intake and cigarette smoking or its cessation, *Am. J. Physiol.,* 237, E1023, 1994.

60. Aarsland, A., Chinkes, D., and Wolfe, R., Hepatic and whole body fat synthesis in humans during carbohydrate overfeeding, *Am. J. Clin. Nutr.,* 65, 1174, 1997.

61. Hudgins, L., Hellerstein, M.K., Seidman, C. et al., Relationship between carbohydrate-induced hypertriglyceridemia and fatty acid synthesis in lean and obese subjects, *J. Lipid Res.*, 41, 595, 2000.
62. Hudgins, L.C., Hellerstein, M.K., Seidman, C. et al., Human fatty synthesis is stimulated by a eucaloric low fat high carbohydrate diet, *J. Clin. Invest.*, 98, 2081, 1996.
63. Hudgins, L., Seidman, C., Diakun, J. et al., Human fatty acid synthesis is reduced after the substitution of dietary starch for sugar, *Am. J. Clin. Nutr.*, 67, 631, 1998.
64. Diraison, F., Dusserre, E., Vidal, H. et al., Increased hepatic lipogenesis but decreased expression of lipogenic gene in adipose tissue in human obesity, *Am. J. Physiol.*, 282, E46, 2002.
65. Marques-Lopes, I., Ansorena, D., Astiasaran, I. et al., Postprandial *de novo* lipogenesis and metabolic changes induced by a high-carbohydrate, low-fat meal in lean and overweight men, *Am. J. Clin. Nutr.*, 73, 253, 2001.
66. McDevitt, R., Bott, S., Harding, M. et al., *De novo* lipogenesis during controlled overfeeding with sucrose or glucose in lean and obese women, *Am. J. Clin. Nutr.*, 74, 737, 2001.
67. Marin, P., Rebuffe-Scrive, M., Smith, U. et al., Glucose uptake in human adipose tissue, *Metabolism*, 36, 1154, 1987.
68. Marin, P., Hogh-Christiansen, I., Jansson, S. et al., Uptake of glucose carbon in muscle glycogen and adipose tissue triglycerides *in vivo* in humans, *Am. J. Physiol.*, 263, E473, 1992.
69. Acheson, K.J., Flatt, J.P., and Jequier, E., Glycogen synthesis versus lipogenesis after a 500-g carbohydrate meal, *Metabolism*, 31, 1234, 1982.
70. Niness, R., Inulin and oligofructose: what are they? *J. Nutr.*, 129, 1402S, 1999.
71. Delzenne, N. and Kok, N., Effects of fructans-type prebiotics on lipid metabolism, *Am. J. Clin. Nutr.*, 73, 456S, 2001.
72. Delzenne, N., Kok, N, Fiordaliso, M. et al., Dietary fructo-oligosaccharides modify lipid metabolism in rats, *Am. J. Clin. Nutr.*, 57, 820S, 1993.
73. Fiordaliso, M., Kok, N., Desager, F. et al., Oligofructose-supplemented diet lowers serum and VLDL concentrations of triglycerides, phospholipids and cholesterol in rats, *Lipids*, 30, 163, 1995.
74. Kok, N., Roberfroid, M., Robert, A. et al., Involvement of lipogenesis in the lower VLDL secretion induced by oligofructose in rats, *Br. J. Nutr.*, 76, 881, 1996.
75. Kok, N., Roberfroid, M., and Delzenne, N., Dietary oligofructose modifies the impact of fructose on hepatic triacylglycerol metabolism, *Metabolism*, 45, 1547, 1996.
76. Trautwein, E., Rieckhoff, D., and Erbersdobler, H., Dietary inulin lowers plasma cholesterol and triacylglycerols and alters biliary bile acid profile in hamsters, *J. Nutr.*, 128, 1937, 1998.
77. Delzenne, N. and Kok, N., Biochemical basis of oligofructose-induced hypolipidemia in animal models, *J. Nutr.*, 129, 1467S, 1999.
78. Nishina, P. and Freeland, R., Effects of propionate on lipid biosynthesis in isolated rat hepatocytes, *J. Nutr.*, 120, 669, 1990.
79. Wolever, T., Spadafora, P., Cunnane, S. et al., Propionate inhibits incorporation of colonic [1,2-13C] acetate into plasma lipids in humans, *Am. J. Clin. Nutr.*, 61, 1241, 1995.
80. Letexier, D., Diraison, F., and Beylot, M., Addition of inulin to a moderately high carbohydrate diet reduces hepatic lipogenesis and plasma triacylglycerol concentration in humans, *Am. J. Clin. Nutr.*, 77, 559, 2003.
81. Williams, C., Effects of inulin on lipid parameters in humans, *J. Nutr.*, 129, 1471S, 1999.

82. Brighenti, F., Casiraghi, M., Canzi, E. et al., Effect of consumption of a ready-to-eat breakfast cereal containing inulin on the intestinal milieu and blood lipids in healthy male volunteers, *Eur. J. Clin. Nutr.,* 53, 726, 1999.

83. Pedersen, A., Sandstrom, B., and Van Amelsvoort, J., The effect of ingestion of inulin on blood lipids and gastrointestinal symptoms in healthy females, *Br. J. Nutr.,* 78, 215, 1997.

84. Luo, L., Rizkalla, S., Alamowitch, C. et al., Chronic consumption of short-chain fructo-oligosaccharides by healthy subjects decreased basal hepatic glucose production but had no effect on insulin-stimulated glucose metabolism, *Am. J. Clin. Nutr.,* 63, 939, 1996.

85. Yamashita, K., Kawai, K., and Itakura, M., Effects of fructo-oligosaccharides on blood glucose and serum lipids in diabetic subjects, *Nutr. Res.,* 4, 961, 1984.

86. Jackson, K., Taylor, G., Clohessy, A. et al., The effect of the daily intake of inulin on fasting lipid, insulin, and glucose concentrations in middle-aged men and women, *Br. J. Nutr.,* 82, 23, 1999.

87. Davidson, M., Maki, K., Synecki, C. et al., Effects of dietary inulin on serum lipids in men and women with hypercholesterolemia, *Nutr. Res.,* 18, 503, 1998.

88. Hollenbeck, C., Coulston, A., and Reaven, G., To what extent does increased dietary fiber improve glucose and lipid metabolism in patients with noninsulin-dependent diabetres mellitus? *Am. J. Clin. Nutr.,* 43, 16, 1986.

89. Alles, M., De Roos, N., Baks, J. et al., Consumption of fructo-oligosaccharides does not favorably affect blood glucose and serum lipid concentrations in patients with type 2 diabetes, *Am. J. Clin. Nutr.,* 69, 64, 1999.

90. Daubioul, C., Taper, H., De Wispelaere, L. et al., Dietary oligofructose lessens hepatic steatosis, but does not prevent hypertriglyceridemia in obese Zucker rats, *J. Nutr.,* 130, 1314, 2000.

12 Vasculoprotective Effects of Olive Oil: Epidemiological Background and Direct Vascular Antiatherogenic Properties

Marika Massaro, Maria Annunziata Carluccio, Maria Assunta Ancora, Egeria Scoditti, and Raffaele De Caterina

CONTENTS

12.1 INTRODUCTION

Early in this new millennium, atherosclerotic vascular disease continues to be the main cause of death in Western countries and is spreading throughout the world despite the use of newer drugs and interventions. Epidemiological evidence emphasizes the need for preventive approaches to cope with the recently termed atherosclerotic "pandemy."

One of the emerging strategies gaining particular credit is the dietary preventive approach designated the Mediterranean Diet or — a more accurate description — Mediterranean Diets. The strategy is based on the observations since the late 1950s of very low incidences of coronary artery disease (CAD) in residents of Mediterranean countries (e.g., Greece and southern Italy) and the role of the "alimentary factor" in protection afforded by their diets. Among other components, Mediterranean Diets are very rich in extra-virgin olive oil as the main alimentary fat. It is now clear that olive oils composed mainly of oleic acid exert relatively minor effects on cholesterol levels but directly interfere with the inflammatory responses characterizing early atherogenesis.

Similar or even stronger anti-inflammatory properties are shared by other typical, although quantitatively minor, components of olive oils, namely a number of structurally diverse antioxidant phytochemicals such as hydroxytyrosol and oleuropein that also share strong antioxidant properties. This review summarizes our current understanding of direct vascular atheroprotective effects of oleic acid and olive oil phytochemicals involving reduced surface expression of endothelial leukocyte adhesion molecules, largely explained by the reduced activation of the nuclear κB transcription factor and the generation of reactive oxygen species (ROS).

Possibly in concert with more highly unsaturated fatty acids and folate largely available through such dietary patterns, olive oils, especially extra-virgin oils that are the richest in antioxidant compounds, seem to contribute to the prevention of atherosclerosis through direct modulation of inflammatory gene expression.

12.2 EVIDENCE OF CARDIOPROTECTION BY MEDITERRANEAN DIETS

For years, serum cholesterol has been accepted as a major risk factor for coronary artery disease (CAD).[1] This view led to the hypothesis that reduction of plasma cholesterol by dietary means might reduce cardiovascular risk. It must be noted, however, that among all the many dietary trials conducted, only those reproducing Mediterranean or Asian-vegetarian types of diets have shown significant reduction of CAD morbidity and mortality.[2] The phenomenon occurred independent of dietary effects on plasma cholesterol.[3-5]

Typical traditional diets in Mediterranean countries (Table 12.1) are characterized by large intakes of cereals, vegetables, and vegetable-derived foods rich in complex carbohydrates and fiber, fresh fruit rich in natural antioxidants, and marine foods rich in polyunsaturated omega-3 fatty acids; moderate wine consumption; very small intakes of meat, dairy foods, eggs and sweets; and high consumption of olive oil rich in omega-9 monounsaturated fatty acid oleate and antioxidant polyphenols as the main source of fat.[6-7]

The basic observation that spurred interest in the Mediterranean dietary style, at least until the early 1960s, was that adults living in certain regions around the Mediterranean Sea had rates of chronic diseases among the lowest in the world and life expectancies among the highest. Such favorable statistics could not be

TABLE 12.1
Percent of Total Energy Contributed by Major Food Groups in the Diet of Crete Compared with Their Availability in the Food Supplies of Greece and the United States in 1948–1949

Food Group	Crete	Greece	U.S.
Energy (kcal/day)	2547	2477	3129
Foods (%)			
Cereals	34	61	25
Pulses, nuts, and potatoes	11	8	6
Vegetables and fruits	11	5	6
Meat, fish, and eggs	4	3	19
Dairy products	3	4	14
Oils and fats	29	15	15
Sugar and honey	2	4	15

Source: Nestle, M., Mediterranean diet: historical and research overview. *Am. J. Clin. Nutr.*, 61, 1313s, 1995.

explained by educational level, financial status, or health care because all socio-economic indicators in those regions were often lower than those in more indus-trialized countries where, conversely, the incidence of coronary artery disease was higher.[7]

Such preliminary observations led to the start of a cooperative investigation of the epidemiology of coronary heart disease (CHD), named the "Seven Countries Study," involving 12,770 men aged 40 through 59 years in Finland, Greece, Italy, Japan, the Netherlands, the U.S., and Yugoslavia.[8] At entry, large differences among cohorts in age-standardized prevalence rates of CHD were inferred from electrocar-diographic evidence of previous myocardial infarction, which was many times more frequent in the U.S. and Finland than in Yugoslavia, Greece, Italy, and Japan. Among 12,529 men judged free of CHD at the entry examination, age-standardized CHD incidence rates differed largely among study cohorts in a 5-year experience. The uppermost and lowermost extremes were Finland on the one hand, and Japan and Greece on the other (Figure 12.1).

The examination of the most important risk factors known at that time showed that cigarette smoking, sedentary lifestyles, and body weight did not explain the intercohort differences in the incidence of CHD. Such differences were marginally related to the prevalence of hypertension in the cohorts, but strongly related to values of serum cholesterol and dietary calories provided by saturated fats. Surprisingly, a negative correlation between CHD incidence rates and the average percentage of calories from monounsaturated fatty acids was also found (Figure 12.2).

In particular, the identification of monounsaturated fatty acids as "dietary pro-tective factors" was also supported by the observation that in Crete (Greece), a change from traditional toward more Westernized dietary habits coincided with a

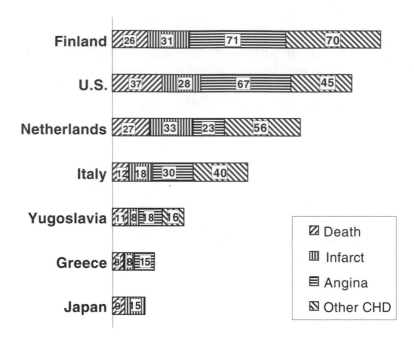

FIGURE 12.1 Age-standardized average yearly CHD incidence rates per 10,000 of 12,529 men aged 40 to 59 judged free of CHD at the start of the study and followed for 5 years in 7 countries. Rates differed largely among study cohorts; the extremes were Finland (top) and Greece and Japan (bottom). (Modified from Keys, A., *Circulation*, 41, 1, 1970. With permission.)

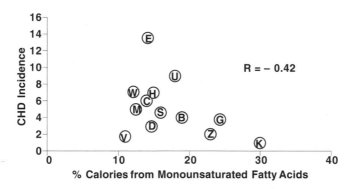

FIGURE 12.2 Correlation of CHD incidence rates and average percentages of calories from monounsaturated fatty acids in the Seven Countries Study. Age-standardized 5-year incidence rate of CHD among men deemed CHD-free at entry is plotted against the average percentage of total dietary calories provided by monounsaturated fatty acids. A negative correlation between CHD incidence rates and percentages of calories from monounsaturated fatty acids was found (r = –0.42). B = Belgrade faculty. C = Crevalcore, Italy. D = Dalmatia. E = East Finland. G = Corfu, Greece. K = Crete, Greece. N = Zutphen, the Netherlands. M = Monte-giorgio, Italy. S = Slavonia. U = U.S. V = Velika Krsna, Serbia. W = West Finland. Z = Zrenjanin, Serbia. (Modified from Keys, A., *Circulation*, 41, 1, 1970. With permission.)

rapid increase in the incidence of chronic diseases. The increase was apparently related to a significant decrease in the consumption of monounsaturated fatty acids, particularly oleic acid, in addition to the increase in consumption of saturated fatty acids and total serum cholesterol, which increased from 4.7 mmol/L in 1962 to 6.4 mmol/L in 1988.[9]

Experimental studies demonstrated that one of the most important cardioprotective effects of dietary oleic acid is the quantitative and qualitative regulation of serum cholesterol levels. While high consumption of food rich in saturated fat increases plasma cholesterol concentrations, controlled metabolic studies on fat metabolism have shown that dietary replacement of saturated fatty acids with monounsaturated or polyunsaturated fatty acids results in a significant hypocholesterolemic effect.[10–12] In particular, consumption of diets relatively high in monounsaturated — compared to polyunsaturated — fatty acids apparently has the advantage of selectively decreasing low density lipoprotein (LDL) cholesterol without lowering high density lipoprotein (HDL) cholesterol,[10] which is considered a good marker of the abundance of lipoproteins (HDLs) instrumental in removing excess cholesterol from extrahepatic tissues and transporting it to the liver and steroidogenic organs.[13]

Moreover, because the atherogenicity of LDL is increased by postsecretory oxidation of LDL particles,[14–15] LDL enrichment in monounsaturated fatty acids less prone to oxidation by reducing LDL oxidation makes them significantly less atherogenic.[16–17]

12.3 ANTIOXIDANT POTENTIAL OF MEDITERRANEAN DIETS

Interest in the antioxidant contents of Mediterranean diets has increased with the recognition that oxidative damage is an important factor in the pathogenesis of chronic and degenerative diseases.[18] Fruits and vegetables are rich in natural antioxidant nutrients such as vitamin C, vitamin E, beta-carotene, lycopene (in tomatoes), organic sulfides (in garlic and onions), glucosinolates, dithiothiones, ubiquinone, and polyphenols such as quercitin, anthocyanines, procyanidines, and tannins. Their consumption has been shown to be associated with low risk for CHD.[19]

Few prospective studies have specifically examined the role of dietary antioxidants on CHD risk. In a Finnish study examining the association of fiber, vegetable and fruit intake, and CHD mortality, a strong inverse association was found between vegetable and fruit intake and CHD risk in both men and women, and vitamins A and E appeared particularly protective.[20] These results are consistent with other prospective studies conducted in female nurses[21] and male health professionals.[22] In those studies, high intakes of vitamin E (more than 100 IU/day for more than 2 years) were associated with a decreased risk of developing CHD.

In the Cambridge Heart Antioxidant Study,[23] 2002 patients with coronary atherosclerosis were randomly assigned to receive 400 to 800 IU of vitamin E per day (or placebo). After a median follow-up of 1.4 years, a large reduction in the number of patients with nonfatal myocardial infarction was observed (relative risk = 0.60).

However, many other studies also reported no clear association with dietary antioxidants.[24-25] In the Alpha-Tocopherol–Beta-Carotene Cancer Prevention Study (ATBC Study),[24] the effects of daily supplementation of 50 mg alpha-tocopherol or 20 mg beta-carotene on 29,133 male smokers were examined. After a 6-year follow-up, the overall net effect was that neither supplement produced a significant change in the risk of death from CHD.

These findings are supported by the results of the GISSI Prevenzione Study[26] and the Heart Outcomes Prevention Evaluation (HOPE).[27] Patients who had myocardial infarctions were randomly assigned to receive 300[26] and 400[27] mg of vitamin E per day, respectively. After 3.5 (GISSI) and 4.5 (HOPE) years of follow-up, the results indicate that such treatments had no effects on the risk of death or cardiovascular event. Because higher vitamin E consumption was associated with higher intakes of other antioxidants[20] in the epidemiological studies that found an association between higher vitamin E intake and lower rates of CHD, it is possible that vitamin E supplementation requires cofactors to have beneficial effects on CHD risk. This may explain the discrepancies observed among the various epidemiological studies. The effects of supplementation of multivitamins on the risk of myocardial infarction and death was investigated in the Heart Protection Study.[28] Here too results were negative, leaving unproven the hypothesis that antioxidants are related to atherosclerosis.[29] One possibility is that other antioxidants present in the diet were not supplemented in the trials.[29]

12.4 PATHOGENESIS OF ATHEROSCLEROSIS AND POTENTIAL SITES OF ACTION OF NEWLY DISCOVERED COMPOUNDS

Atherosclerosis, the main cause of CAD, is a process that includes inflammatory components.[30-31] In most animal models, atherosclerosis begins with the accumulation of monocyte-derived macrophages in the arterial intima. These cells, by taking up lipid droplets (mostly oxidized or other modified LDL), become foam cells that are typical cellular elements of the earliest detectable atherosclerotic lesion (the "fatty streak").[32-33] Animal observations have also shown that fatty streaks precede the development of "intermediate lesions"[34-35] composed of macrophages and smooth muscle cells. Activation of these cell types leads to a release of hydrolytic enzymes, cytokines, chemokines, and growth factors that can induce focal necrosis or apoptosis.

Cycles of mononuclear cell accumulation, migration and proliferation of smooth muscle cells, and formation of fibrous tissue lead to the enlargement and restructuring of the lesion, the formation of a fibrous cap, and other morphological changes. Plaques range from those with prevalent lipid components (fatty plaques) to those with prevailing fibrous tissue (fibrous plaques) that increase in size and may cause ischemia in the myocardium or peripheral muscles. Most sudden deaths and myocardial infarcts are due to ruptures or fissures of the fibrous cap, particularly at the macrophage-rich shoulder of the lesion, resulting in plaque hemorrhage, thrombosis, and arterial occlusion.[36]

12.5 ENDOTHELIAL ACTIVATION AS MAIN TARGET FOR ANTIATHEROGENIC PROPERTIES OF OLIVE OIL COMPONENTS

The earliest morphologically detectable cellular event in atherogenesis is the adherence of circulating blood monocytes to the arterial endothelium.[37–39] This occurs because of a modification of the normal functional state of the arterial endothelium consisting of the appearance of new antigenic and functional properties, in general termed "endothelial activation."[40] Possible causes of endothelial activation include elevated levels of oxidized and minimally modified low density lipoproteins (LDLs), free radicals caused by cigarette smoking, diabetes mellitus and hypertension, elevated plasma homocysteine concentrations, and infectious microorganisms.

In normal conditions, vascular endothelium does not support the adhesion of leukocytes. However, when vascular endothelium is chronically exposed to the above-mentioned stimuli, leukocyte adhesion to the endothelium occurs because of the selective expression of endothelial leukocyte adhesion molecules and endothelial chemoattractants. These slow the leukocyte run in the circulation, determine leukocyte rolling over endothelial cells, tether leukocytes in a labile and then stable fashion, and subsequently induce their transendothelial migration.[41]

The specific molecules thought to play pivotal roles in monocyte recruitment are vascular cell adhesion molecule-1 (VCAM-1), intercellular adhesion molecule-1 (ICAM-1), and E-selectin.[30] The expression of VCAM-1, ICAM-1, and E-selectin on cultured endothelial cells can be triggered by a variety of stimuli. These include inflammatory cytokines such as interleukin (IL)-1 and tumor necrosis factor (TNF), which are products of activated macrophages, bacterial endotoxins (lipopolysaccharides or LPS), and phorbol myristate acetate (PMA). Some of these activators such as the inflammatory cytokines may be relevant *in vivo*, possibly by involvement in the amplification of the local inflammatory response once monocytes/macrophages have been recruited.

These agents induce the *in vitro* expression of the entire variety of products of endothelial activation including VCAM-1 and various chemoattractants such as macrophage-colony stimulating factor (M-CSF). As a consequence of this broad activation, the adhesion of polymorphonuclear cells, monocytes, and lymphocytes is induced in a relatively unselective fashion. Possibly more relevant pathophysiological stimuli triggering the initial events in atherogenesis are minimally oxidized LDLs and the advanced glycation endproducts of diabetes.[30]

The detection and quantitation of increased adhesion molecule expression and the subsequent monocyte adhesion after stimulation of cultured endothelial cells with cytokines allows the establishment of an *in vitro* system suitable to study the molecular machinery involved in endothelial activation. This system allows an assessment of how external interventions modulate the response to a given constant amount of stimulation, having therefore the potential of identifying new triggers and detecting and comparing external interventions. This has proven useful to identify the inhibitory action of nitric oxide,[42] n-3 polyunsaturated fatty acids,[43] and some antioxidants[44] in early atherogenesis. We devised a series of experiments to investigate whether oleate and natural antioxidants obtained from extra-virgin olive oil influence the endothelial responses to pro-inflammatory stimuli triggering endothelial activation.

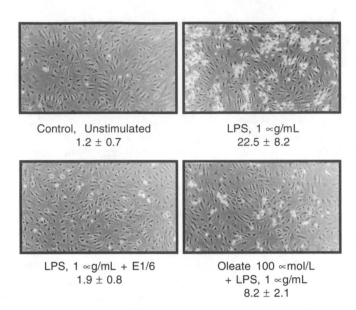

Control, Unstimulated
1.2 ± 0.7

LPS, 1 ∝g/mL
22.5 ± 8.2

LPS, 1 ∝g/mL + E1/6
1.9 ± 0.8

Oleate 100 ∝mol/L
+ LPS, 1 ∝g/mL
8.2 ± 2.1

FIGURE 12.3 Oleate decreases monocytoid cell adhesion to human umbilical vein endothelial cells. Cells from the monocytoid U937 line (largely behaving like monocytes as to adhesion features) do not normally adhere to unstimulated monolayers when added to endothelial cells and are easily removed by washing (upper left). Adhesion is dramatically increased by the addition of bacterial lipopolysaccharide (upper right). This increased adhesion is to a large extent abolished by the blocking monoclonal antibody E1/6 directed against the adhesion molecule VCAM-1, demonstrating partial VCAM-1-dependence of the phenomenon. Oleate decreases U937 cell adhesion by more than 50% (lower right). Cell counts are shown (mean ± standard deviation, n = 6 for each condition) within a grid area at high power field (0.16 mm^2). LPS vs. unstimulated condition: $P < 0.001$; oleate + LPS vs. LPS: $P < 0.01$; LPS + E1/6 vs. LPS: $P < 0.01$. (From Carluccio, M.A., *Arterioscler. Thromb. Vasc. Biol.*, 19, 220, 1999. With permission.)

12.5.1 Anti-Inflammatory Properties of Oleic Acid

To test for antiatherogenic properties of oleic acid — the most representative component of olive oil — we first assessed the direct effect of oleate on the stimulated adhesion of a monocytoid cell line (U937) to an endothelium activated by LPS. Preincubation of human umbilical vein endothelial cell (HUVEC) with oleate (100 μmol/L) for 48 h before the stimulation with LPS significantly reduced the adhesion of U937 monocytoid cells to the endothelium (Figure 12.3).[45] Because U937 cell adhesion is mostly due to VCAM-1 expression, we then proceeded to specifically investigate the effects of oleate on the endothelial expression of VCAM-1. This was carried out in several types of cultured endothelia including aortic and venous endothelial cells.

Using HUVEC as a cellular model, we observed that the exposure to oleate (50 μmol/L) for 48 h before the stimulation with several kinds of stimuli, namely LPS, IL-1, and PMA, always inhibited the expression of VCAM-1 compared to an unsupplemented medium and a medium supplemented with the saturated stearate fatty acid (Figure 12.4 and Figure 12.5), as well as the release of M-CSF in the culture medium (Table 12.2).[46] Concentrations of oleate found active in this system are

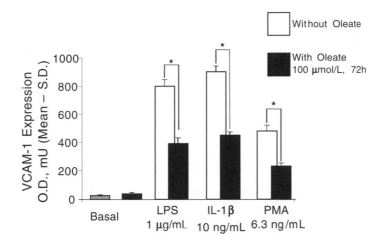

FIGURE 12.4 Inhibition of stimulated expression of VCAM-1 in HUVEC. Oleate and sodium salt were dissolved in culture medium 199 containing 10% serum and incubated with endothelial monolayers in 96-well plates for 48 h, after which various stimuli were added for an additional 16 h to induce surface expression of VCAM-1. Values of expression are shown as percent of maximum response (without oleate) ± standard deviation. Data are based on 3 experiments for each cell type, with 16 repeats for each stimulus used. *P < 0.01 vs. stimulated condition. (From Carluccio, M.A., *Arterioscler. Thromb. Vasc. Biol.*, 19, 220, 1999. With permission.)

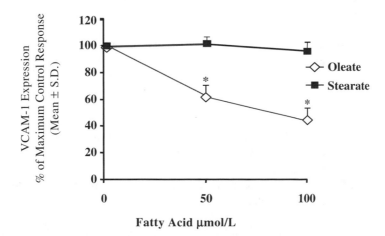

FIGURE 12.5 Oleate, but not the saturated fatty acid stearate, reduces stimulated VCAM-1 expression. Sodium oleate and stearate were added to tissue culture medium for 48 h, after which VCAM-1 expression was induced by adding lipopolysaccharide (LPS) at 1 μg/mL for a further 16 h. VCAM-1 expression was assessed by cell-surface EIA. Only oleate inhibits VCAM-1 expression in a concentration-dependent fashion. *P < 0.01 for oleate vs. stearate effect.

TABLE 12.2
The Effect of Stearate and Oleate (all at 25 μmol/L) on the Release of M-CSF in Culture Medium

Treatment	Basal	IL-1, 10 ng/ml	Stearate/IL-1	Oleate/IL-1
M-CSF released, pg/mL (mean ± SD)	45 ± 2	505 ± 30[a]	463 ± 20	406 ± 10[b]

Note: Fatty acids were added to HUVEC for 48 h before the addition of IL-1 (for further 6 h), after which aliquots of culture medium were removed for the assay. Experiments were performed in triplicate in each experiment, with $n = 10$ for each condition. Data are expressed as mean ± S.D.

M-CSF = macrophage-colony stimulating factor

[a] $P < 0.05$ vs. control
[b] $P < 0.01$ vs. IL-1

nutritionally achievable in consideration of the high abundance of oleic acid in Mediterranean diets.[47–48]

Under the same experimental conditions, we also noted that the inhibition of VCAM-1 expression was accompanied by a concomitant decrease in the corresponding messenger RNA (mRNA) on Northern analysis, thus suggesting a pretranslational interference of oleate[45] (Figure 12.6). Oleate-mediated inhibition of VCAM-1 expression was paralleled by oleate incorporation in total cellular lipids. The comparative monitoring of fatty acids in total cell lipids and of VCAM-1 expression revealed that significant inhibition of VCAM-1 expression was only found after a substantial oleate incorporation, which occurred at the expense of saturated fatty acids and only minimally altered the amounts or relative proportions of more highly unsaturated fatty acids[46] (Figure 12.7).

12.5.2 ANTI-INFLAMMATORY PROPERTIES OF POLYPHENOLIC ANTIOXIDANTS

Olive oil is obtained from the fruits (drupes) of *Olea europea,* a tree that is best grown between the 30° and 45° parallels. Drupes are therefore continuously exposed to substantial environmental stresses due to ultraviolet radiation and relatively high temperatures, and need compounds such as polyphenolic antioxidants to preserve their integrity from oxidative insults. Olive oil obtained by means of physical pressure, without the use of chemicals, retains the lipophilic polyphenolic antioxidants of the drupe.

High-quality olive oil is particularly rich in oleuropein (a secoiridoid) and hydroxytyrosol (a phenolic alcohol). Both are polyphenolic compounds with very strong antioxidant properties due to their orthodiphenolic structures[49] (Table 12.3). These compounds are dose-dependently absorbed in humans[50] and show several remarkable antiatherogenic activities including inhibition of LDL oxidation,[51] inhibition of platelet aggregation,[52] and enhancement of nitric oxide production by LPS-challenged murine macrophages.[53]

We first assessed the direct effects of olive oil polyphenols on the stimulated adhesion of a monocytoid cells line (U937) to LPS-activated endothelium. Preincubation of

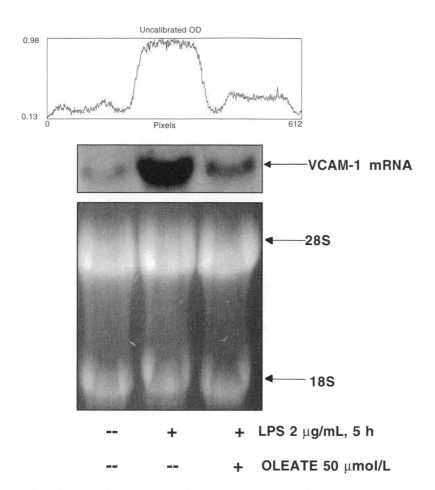

FIGURE 12.6 Oleate decreases VCAM-1 mRNA steady state levels. Northern analysis of VCAM-1 mRNA (middle) and ethidium bromide staining for total RNA (bottom, as control for equal loading of lanes during Northern analysis) at time 0 h (left band), 6 h after LPS (1 μg/mL) stimulation (middle band), and 6 h after LPS stimulation preceded by incubation with 100 μmol/L oleate for 72 h (right band). Oleate treatment is associated with a 65% reduction of VCAM-1 mRNA by densitometric analysis, the plot of which is shown at the top. (From Carluccio, M.A., *Arterioscler. Thromb. Vasc. Biol.*, 19, 220, 1999. With permission.)

HUVEC with polyphenols (15 μmol/L) for 0.5 h before LPS stimulation significantly reduced the adhesion of U937 cells to the endothelium (Figure 12.8). Since redox-sensitive mechanisms are implicated in the endothelial expression of VCAM-1, E-selectin, and ICAM-1,[54] we investigated the effects of oleuropein and hydroxytyrosol on the stimulated expression of these adhesion molecules. Both oleuropein and its derivative hydroxytyrosol reduced the stimulated expression of each adhesion molecule tested (Figure 12.9). The importance of the antioxidant ortodiphenolic structure in the modulating action of these compounds was confirmed by the lack of activity by tyrosol, a phenol with only one hydroxyl group. Table 12.3 shows the structure and properties of some biologically relevant olive oil phenolic compounds.

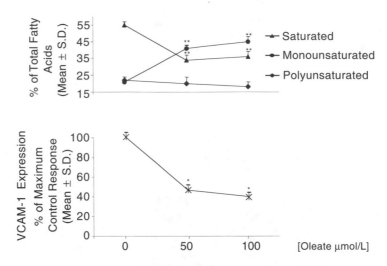

FIGURE 12.7 Comparison of oleate inhibitory effect on stimulated adhesion molecule expression and modification of lipid composition of HUVEC induced by oleate treatment. VCAM-1 expression as assessed by cell surface EIA is shown as percent of LPS (1 μg/mL)-stimulated response and is correlated with modification of saturated, monounsaturated, and polyunsaturated fatty acids induced by the exposure of HUVEC to 50 and 100 μmol/L oleate for 48 h. Each fatty acid group is expressed as percent of total fatty acids as determined by gas–liquid chromatography. * $P < 0.01$ vs. stimulated condition. ** $P < 0.05$ vs. control condition. (From Massaro, M., *Thromb. Haemost.*, 88, 176, 2002. With permission.)

TABLE 12.3
Structure, Name, and Physico-Chemical Characteristics of Olive Oil Phenols

Structure	Name	Solubility	Antioxidant Properties
	Tyrosol (4-hydroxy-phenyl-ethanol)	Ethanol/water	None[67]
	Hydroxytyrosol 2-(3,4-dihydroxy-phenyl)ethanol	Ethanol/water	Strong antioxidant[67]
	Oleuropein	Ethanol	Strong antioxidant[67]

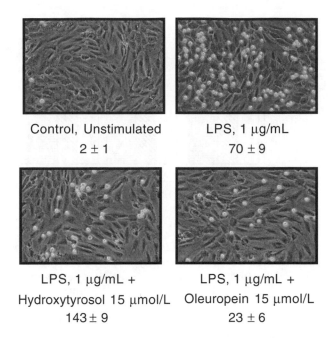

Control, Unstimulated
2 ± 1

LPS, 1 μg/mL
70 ± 9

LPS, 1 μg/mL +
Hydroxytyrosol 15 μmol/L
143 ± 9

LPS, 1 μg/mL +
Oleuropein 15 μmol/L
23 ± 6

FIGURE 12.8 Olive oil antioxidant polyphenols decrease monocytoid cell adhesion to HUVEC. U937 cells added in suspension to HUVEC do not normally adhere to unstimulated monolayers and are easily removed with washing (control, no stimulation), while adhesion is dramatically increased by the addition of LPS (1 μmol/L). U937 cell adhesion is reduced about 50% (lower panels) in HUVEC treated with hydroxytyrosol and oleuropein at 15 μmol/L for 30 min and then stimulated with LPS. Cell counts shown (mean ± SD, n = 6 for each condition) within a grid area at high power field (0.16 mm^2). This experiment was repeated four times with similar results.

Because VCAM-1 is the adhesion molecule principally and specifically involved in the initiation and progression of atherosclerotic lesions,[55] we focused our interest on its modulation by olive oil polyphenols. We assessed and compared the inhibition of stimulated VCAM-1 expression by polyphenols in response to structurally unrelated agonists such as LPS, cytokines, and PMA, which served as a stimulus for endothelial activation that bypasses membrane receptors. We observed that both oleuropein and hydroxytyrosol inhibited stimulated VCAM-1 expression to the same extent with all stimuli, independent of the relative potency of the stimuli tested (Figure 12.10).

The observation that olive oil polyphenols decrease VCAM-1 protein expression regardless of the agonist suggests that olive oil polyphenols act downstream of membrane receptors, possibly through interference with ROS production and redox-sensitive transcription factor activation involved in VCAM-1 induction.[44] Most relevant, such effects occurred at low micromolar concentrations within the plasma concentration range expected to be achieved with a classical Mediterranean diet.[50] It is likely that such beneficial effects would be amplified *in vivo* because of the continuous exposure of vascular endothelia to these compounds.

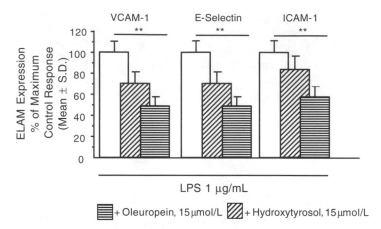

FIGURE 12.9 Olive oil polyphenols inhibit LPS-stimulated expression of various endothelial adhesion molecules. HUVEC were treated with polyphenols (15 µmol/L) for 30 min and then stimulated with LPS. Adhesion molecule expression was assessed by cell-surface EIA by specific monoclonal antibodies. All data are plotted as percentage of maximum control response (percent of stimulated response without polyphenols). Control vehicles (ethanol 0.05% vol/vol or methanol 0.005% vol/vol) had no effect on stimulated expression of VCAM-1. Data are based on six different experiments, each consisting of eight or more repeats for each condition. ** $P < 0.01$ vs. LPS alone.

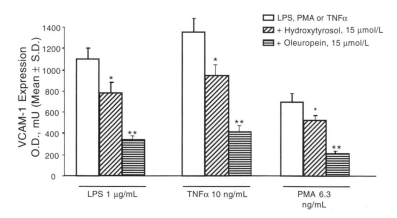

FIGURE 12.10 Effects of olive oil antioxidant polyphenols on VCAM-1 expression are independent of stimuli used to elicit endothelial activation. Olive oil antioxidant polyphenols similarly reduce VCAM-1 expression induced by LPS, TNFα, or PMA in HUVEC as assessed by cell-surface EIA. Antioxidants (15 µmol/L) were all added 30 min before the addition of the stimulus. OD mU denotes milliunits of optical density. Data are based on four different experiments, each consisting of eight or more repeats for each condition. *$P < 0.05$. ** $P < 0.01$ vs. LPS, TNFα, or PMA alone.

12.6 CLUES TO POSSIBLE MECHANISMS OF OLIVE OIL COMPONENTS ON ENDOTHELIAL ACTIVATION: INFLUENCE ON INTRACELLULAR REDOX STATUS

The concerted expression of VCAM-1, ICAM-1, E-selectin, and soluble inducible products such as M-CSF expressed and/or released by activated endothelial cells is regulated by a few transcription factors including the early response genes (c-*jun*, c-*fos*), GATA, and nuclear factor-κB (NF-κB).[56] Recent evidence suggests that some overproduction of reactive oxygen species (ROS) is involved in the endothelial activation of NF-κB and consequently in the induced expression of NF-κB-dependent genes such as VCAM-1 and E-selectin.[57–58]

Although multiple transduction pathways are involved in the activation of NF-κB by different triggers, it appears that all of them lead to the activation of protein kinases with subsequent phosphorylation-dependent proteolytic degradation of the NF-κB inhibitory subunit IκB. This would allow the translocation of NF-κB heterodimers into the nucleus where, in concert with other transcription factors, they promote the expression of genes having specific consensus sequences for NF-κB in their promoters. There is evidence that NF-κB activation can be effectively blocked by antioxidants.[44–58] It has therefore been proposed that the induction of ROS is the common mechanism of NF-κB activation, regardless of the type of stimuli.[59] Interference with the generation of ROS, ultimately leading to decreased intracellular concentration of H_2O_2, is a plausible mechanism of action for many agents inhibiting endothelial activation.

Against this background, the antioxidant properties of olive oil polyphenols may very well explain their *in vitro* anti-inflammatory properties. However, this is not an obvious explanation that fits the observed anti-inflammatory properties of oleic acid. Therefore, we attempted to explain the effects of oleic acids on endothelial activation and hypothesized an interference with NF-κB activation, possibly through inhibition of ROS production. In agreement with this hypothesis, pre-incubation of endothelial cells with oleate and with antioxidant polyphenols from olive oil reduced the activation of NF-κB, as demonstrated by electrophoretic mobility shift assays (EMSA).[45]

Under the same experimental conditions we also observed that the same stimuli able to induce endothelial activation, such as TNFα, were able to increase intracellular ROS concentrations. Pretreatment of cells with oleate, besides reducing NF-κB activation, also partially prevented TNFα-induced increases in intracellular ROS[46] (Figure 12.11).

Because this reduced concentration of intracellular ROS, as a consequence of oleate treatment, might in turn depend on the increased activity of the main cellular enzymes governing the scavenging of ROS (superoxide dismutase and catalase) or regulating glutathione levels (glutathione peroxidase, glutathione reductase, and glutathione S-transferase),[60–62] we also tested under the same conditions the activities of these enzymes. None of the above activities was altered by oleate treatment (Table 12.4).

Unsaturated fatty acids recently emerged as possible physiological regulators of the endothelial responsiveness to activating cytokines.[63] We previously

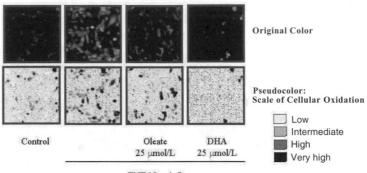

FIGURE 12.11 Representative example of the effect of oleate and DHA on ROS production induced by TNFα as measured by dichlorofluorescein (DCF) fluorescence emission. Subconfluent HUVEC were pretreated with 25 μmol/L oleate for 48 h and then stimulated with 10 ng/mL TNFα for 1 h. Monolayers were then washed and loaded with reduced DCF for 30 min and imaged as described in the reference. Upper panels depict original microphotographs; sides of each square are 300 μm long. Lower panels depict corresponding pseudocolor transformations of digitalized images; lighter areas indicate low generation of ROS and darker areas indicate increased ROS generation proportional to color intensity. (From Massaro, M., *Thromb. Haemost.*, 88, 176, 2002. With permission.)

TABLE 12.4
The Effect of 50 μmol/L Oleate Incubation for 48 h ± LPS for Further 60 min on the Activity of Some Antioxidant Enzymes in HUVEC

Treatment	GSH-px	GSH-S-ts	GSSG-red	SOD	CAT
Oleate	85 ± 10	113 ± 20	98 ± 14	100 ± 20	87 ± 23
LPS	75 ± 16	95 ± 19	135 ± 49	105 ± 35	74 ± 15
Oleate/LPS	82 ± 2	97 ± 3	117 ± 21	103 ± 20	89 ± 37

Experiments performed in quadruplicate. Values are expressed as percentage of control for each enzyme ± S.D. Legend: GSP-px = glutathione peroxidase; GSH-S-ts = glutathione transferase; GSSG-red = glutathione reductase; SOD = superoxide dismutase; CAT = catalase. All figures reported are insignificantly different from controls.

reported that highly unsaturated n-3 fatty acids such as docosahexanoic acid (22:6 n-3) are inhibitors of endothelial activation, thus decreasing the expression of VCAM-1, E-selectin, ICAM-1, IL-6, and IL-8.[43] Structure-activity analysis of the effects of unsaturated fatty acids on endothelial activation revealed that the inhibitory potency of an unsaturated fatty acid is roughly proportional to the number of double bonds accommodated in the carbon chain length. Thus, the n-3 polyunsaturated docosahexaenoic fatty acid that has six double bonds was found to be roughly six times more potent than oleate.[64] Although oleic acid has only one double bond, the analysis of fatty acid incorporation in total cellular lipids pointed out that its addition to culture medium significantly increased the unsaturation index, an indicator of the number of double bonds present in the total cellular lipid pool.[45] This happens because of a relatively selective replacement of saturated fatty acids by oleate, leaving higher unsaturated fatty acid pools relatively unaffected.[46] These results led us to hypothesize a direct physical interference of oleate with generated ROS.[64] This is in agreement with physio–chemical demonstrations of the possible reaction of superoxide anion even with the single double bond present in oleate[65] involving the original formation of hydroperoxyl groups.

A current working hypothesis is therefore that oleate oxidation would scavenge superoxide anion. This perhaps increases the formation of hydroperoxides on the one hand, but also leads to a reduced probability for unmatched superoxide to be dismutated to hydrogen peroxide on the other. If hydrogen peroxide or some of its downstream products are directly responsible for NF-κB activation, then the interaction of oleate with superoxide anion, independent of any interference with enzyme activities controlling ROS levels, would be sufficient to explain the observed downstream effects of oleate as well as antioxidant olive oil polyphenols on endothelial activation (Figure 12.12).

12.7 CONCLUSIONS

Many epidemiological and experimental studies have supported the notion of health benefits of Mediterranean dietary patterns. Traditional Mediterranean diets were based mainly on plant foods, contained only small amounts of animal foods, and used olive oil as the principal daily fat. Our findings revealed a new molecular mechanism by which olive oil components, oleic acid, and antioxidant polyphenols — abundant components of the Mediterranean diet — may favorably affect the early phases of atherogenesis, preventing the formation of fatty streaks. They act directly at the vascular surface, reducing monocyte attachment and the formation of fatty streaks.

These findings allow a new understanding of how nutrients may affect human diseases and add new items to the now long list of examples of how nutritional interventions may affect gene expression.[66,67] They also suggest the possibility of preventive interventions in atherosclerosis based on the modulation of vascular response to classical triggers (high levels of cholesterol and advanced glycation endproducts of diabetes) through a strategy fundamentally different — and thereby complementary — to those now in fashion and based on drugs.

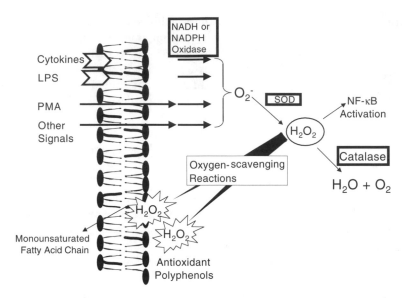

FIGURE 12.12 Possible mechanism for the effect of olive oil components on endothelial activation. The intracellular mediators of NF-κB activation, i.e., ROS produced by NADH or NADPH oxidase activation after cytokine stimulation, are preferentially scavenged by the double bonds, more abundant after cell exposure to oleate.

REFERENCES

1. Brown, M.S. and Goldstein J.L., Heart attacks: gone with the century? [editorial], *Science,* 272, 629, 1996.
2. Corr, L.A. and Oliver M.F., The low fat/cholesterol diet is ineffective, *Eur. Heart J.,* 18, 18, 1997.
3. Burr, M.L. et al., Effect of changes in fat, fish, and fibre intakes on death and myocardial reinfarction: diet and reinfarction trial (DART), *Lancet,* II, 757, 1989.
4. Singh, R.B. et al., Randomised controlled trial of cardioprotective diet in patients with recent myocardial infarction: results of one year follow-up, *Br. M. J.,* 304, 1015, 1992.
5. de Lorgeril, M. et al., Mediterranean alpha-linoleic acid-rich diet in secondary prevention of coronary heart disease, *Lancet,* 343, 1454, 1994.
6. Keys, A., Mediterranean diet and public health: personal reflections, *Am. J. Clin. Nutr.,* 61 (Suppl.), 1321S, 1995.
7. Nestle, M., Mediterranean diet: historical and research overview, *Am. J. Clin. Nutr.,* 61, 1313S, 1995.
8. Keys, A., Coronary heart disease in seven countries, *Circulation,* 41, 1, 1970.
9. Kafatos, A. et al., Coronary-heart-disease risk factor status of the Cretan urban population in the 1980s, *Am. J. Clin. Nutr.,* 54, 591, 1991.
10. Mattson, F.H. and Grundy S.M., Comparison of effects of dietary saturated, monounsaturated, and polyunsaturated fatty acids on plasma lipids and lipoproteins in men, *J. Lipid Res.,* 26, 194, 1985.

11. Mensink, R.P. and Katan M.B., Effect of dietary fatty acids versus complex carbo-hydrates on high-density lipoprotein in healthy men and women, *Lancet,* I, 122, 1987.

12. Mensink, R.P. and Katan M.B., Effect of dietary fatty acids on serum lipids and lipoproteins: a meta-analysis on 27 trials, *Arterioscler. Thromb.,* 12, 911, 1992.

13. Rigotti, A. et al., Scavenger receptor BI: a cell surface receptor for high density lipoprotein, *Curr. Opin. Lipidol.,* 8, 181, 1997.

14. Steinberg, D., Parthasarathy S., and Witztum J., Beyond cholesterol: modifications of low-density lipoprotein that increase its atherogenicity, *New Engl. J. Med.,* 320, 915, 1989.

15. Steinberg, D. and Witztum J.L., Lipoproteins and atherogenesis: current concepts, *JAMA,* 264, 3047, 1990.

16. Parthasarathy, S. et al., Low density lipoprotein rich in oleic acid is protected against oxidative modification: implications for dietary prevention of atherosclerosis, *Proc. Natl. Acad. Sci. USA,* 87, 3894, 1990.

17. Reaven, P. et al., Effects of oleate-rich and linoleate-rich diets on the susceptibility of low density lipoprotein to oxidative modification in mildly hypercholesterolemic subjects, *J. Clin. Invest.,* 91, 668, 1993.

18. Halliwell, B., Oxidant and human disease: some new concepts, *FASEB J.,* 1, 358, 1987.

19. Ness, A.R. and Powles, J.W., Fruit and vegetables, and cardiovascular disease: a review, *Int. J. Epidemiol.,* 26, 1, 1997.

20. Knekt, P. et al., Antioxidant vitamin intake and coronary mortality in a longitudinal population study, *Am. J. Epidemiol.,* 139, 1180, 1994.

21. Stampfer, M.J. et al., A prospective study of vitamin E consumption and risk of coronary heart disease in women, *New Engl. J. Med.,* 1993, 1444, 1993.

22. Rimm, E.B. et al., A prospective study of vitamin E consumption and risk of coronary heart disease men, *New Engl. J. Med.,* 328, 1450, 1993.

23. Stephens, N.G. et al., Randomised controlled trial of vitamin E in patients with coronary disease: Cambridge Heart Antioxidant Study, *Lancet,* 781, 1996.

24. Alpha-Tocopherol–Beta-Carotene Cancer Prevention Study Group, The effect of vita-min E and beta-carotene on the incidence of lung cancer and other cancers in male smokers, *New Engl. J. Med.,* 330, 1029, 1994.

25. Leppala, J.M. et al., Controlled trial of α-tocopherol and β-carotene supplements on stroke incidence and mortality in male smokers, *Arterioscler. Thromb.Vasc. Biol.,* 20, 230, 2000.

26. Gruppo Italiano per lo Studio della Sopravivenza nell' Infarto Miocardico, Dietary supplementation with n-3 polyunsaturated fatty acids and vitamin E after myocardial infarction: results of the GISSI Prevenzione trial, *Lancet,* 354, 447, 1999.

27. Yusuf, S. et al., Vitamin E supplementation and cardiovascular events in high-risk patients: the Heart Outcomes Prevention Evaluation Study Investigators, *New Engl. J. Med.,* 342, 154, 2000.

28. MRC/BHF Heart Protection Study, Antioxidant vitamin supplementation in 20,536 high-risk individuals: a randomised placebo-controlled trial, *Lancet,* 360, 23, 2002.

29. Steinberg, D. and Witztum J.L., Is the oxidative modification hypothesis relevant to human atherosclerosis? Do the antioxidant trials conducted to date refute the hypoth-esis?, *Circulation,* 105, 2107, 2002.

30. De Caterina, R. and Libby P., Towards an understanding of the molecular pathogenesis of acute coronary syndromes, *Cardiologia,* 42, 359, 1997.

31. Ross, R., Atherosclerosis: an inflammatory disease, *New Engl. J. Med.,* 340, 115, 1999.

32. Gimbrone, M.A., Kume N., and Cybulsky M.I., Vascular endothelium dysfunction and the pathogenesis of atherosclerosis, in *Atherosclerosis Reviews*, Reaven Press, New York, 1993.

33. De Caterina, R. and Gimbrone, M.A., Leukocyte–endothelial interactions and the pathogenesis of atherosclerosis, in *n-3 Fatty Acid: Prevention and Treatment in Vascular Disease*, Kristensen, S., Ed., Springer-Verlag, London, 1995, p. 9.

34. Masuda, J. and Ross R., Atherogenesis during low level hypercholesterolemia in the nonhuman primate II: fatty streak conversion to plaque fibers, *Arteriosclerosis*, 10, 187, 1990.

35. Masuda, J. and Ross R., Atherogenesis during low level hypercholesterolemia in the nonhuman primate I: Fatty streak formation, *Arteriosclerosis*, 10, 178, 1990.

36. Falk, E., Shah P., and Fuster V., Coronary plaque distruption, *Circulation*, 92, 657, 1995.

37. Gerrity, R., The role of monocyte in atherogenesis I: transition of blood–bone monocytes into foam cells in fatty lesions, *Am. J. Pathol.*, 103, 181, 1981.

38. Joris, T. et al., Studies on the pathogenesis of atherosclerosis I: adhesion and emigration of mononuclear cell in the aorta of hypercolesterolemic rats, *Am. J. Pathol.*, 113, 341, 1983.

39. Faggiotto, A., Ross R., and Harker L., Studies of hypercholesterolemia in nonhuman primates I: changes that lead to fatty streak formation, *Arteriosclerosis*, 4, 323, 1984.

40. Pober, J.S. and Cotran R.S., Cytokines and endothelial cell biology, *Physiol. Rev.*, 70, 427, 1990.

41. Springer, T.A., Traffic signals for lymphocyte recirculation and leukocyte emigration: the multistep paradigm, *Cell*, 76, 301, 1994.

42. De Caterina, R. et al., Nitric oxide decreases cytokine-induced endothelial activation, *J. Clin. Invest.*, 96, 60, 1995.

43. De Caterina, R. et al., The omega-3 fatty acid docosahexaenoate reduces cytokine-induced expression of proatherogenic and proinflammatory proteins in human endothelial cells, *Arterioscler. Thromb. Vasc. Biol.*, 14, 1829, 1994.

44. Marui, N. et al., Vascular cell adhesion molecule-1 (VCAM-1) gene transcription and expression are regulated through an antioxidant-sensitive mechanism in human vascular endothelial cells, *J. Clin. Invest.*, 92, 1866, 1993.

45. Carluccio, M.A. et al., Oleic acid inhibits endothelial cell activation, *Arterioscler. Thromb. Vasc. Biol.*, 19, 220, 1999.

46. Massaro, M. et al., Quenching of intracellular ROS generation as a mechanism for oleate-induced reduction of endothelial activation and early atherogenesis, *Thromb. Haemost.*, 88, 176, 2002.

47. Rao, C., Zang E., and Reddy B., Effect of high fat corn oil, olive oil and fish oil on phospholipids fatty acid composition in male F344 rats, *Lipids*, 28, 441, 1993.

48. Yaqoob, P. et al., Comparison of the effects of a range of dietary lipids upon serum and tissue lipid composition in the rat, *Int. J. Biochem. Cell Biol.*, 27, 297, 1995.

49. Galli, C. and Visioli F., Antioxidant and other activities of phenolics in olives/olive oil, typical components of the Mediterranean diet, *Lipids*, 34, S23, 1999.

50. Visioli, F. et al., Olive oil phenolics are dose-dependently absorbed in humans, *FEBS Lett.*, 468, 159, 2000.

51. Visioli, F. et al., Low density lipoprotein oxidation is inhibited *in vitro* by olive oil constituents, *Atherosclerosis*, 117, 25, 1995.

52. Petroni, A. et al., Inhibition of platelet aggregation and eicosanoid production by phenolic components of olive oil, *Thromb. Res.*, 78, 151, 1995.

53. Visioli, F., Bellosta S., and Galli C., Oleuropein, The bitter principle of olives, enhances nitric oxide production by mouse macrophages, *Life Sci.,* 62, 541, 1998.

54. Sen, C.K. and Paker L., Antioxidant and redox regulation of gene transcription, *FASEB J.,* 10, 709, 1996.

55. Dansky, H. et al., Adhesion of monocytes to arterial endothelium and initiation of atherosclerosis are critically dependent on vascular cell adhesion molecule-1 gene dosage, *Arterioscler. Thromb. Vasc. Biol.,* 21, 1662, 2001.

56. Collins, T., Endothelial nuclear factor-κB and the initiation of the atherosclerotic lesion, *Lab. Invest.,* 68, 499, 1993.

57. Lo, S.K. et al., Hydrogen peroxide-induced increase in endothelial adhesiveness is dependent on ICAM-1 activation, *Am. J. Physiol.,* 264, 406, 1993.

58. Thanos, D. and Maniatis T., NF-κB: a lesson in family values, *Cell,* 80, 529, 1995.

59. Schreck, R., Albermann K., and Baeuerle P.A., Nuclear Factor -κB: an oxidative stress-responsive transcription factor of eukariotic cells, *Free Rad. Res. Commun.,* 17, 221, 1992.

60. Harlan, J. M. et al., Glutathione redox cycle protects cultured endothelial cells against lysis by extracellularly generated hydrogen peroxide, *J. Clin. Invest.,* 73, 706, 1984.

61. Buckley, B.J., Tanswell A.K., and Freeman B.A., Liposome-mediated augmentation of catalase in alveolar type II cells protects against H_2O_2 injury, *J. Appl. Physiol.,* 63, 359, 1987.

62. Visner, G.A. et al., Regulation of manganese superoxide dismutase by lipopolysaccharide, interleukin-1, and tumor necrosis factor: role in acute inflammatory response, *J. Biol. Chem.,* 265, 2856, 1990.

63. De Caterina, R., Liao J.K., and Libby P., Fatty acid modulation of endothelial activation, *Am. J. Clin. Nutr.,* 71 (Suppl. 1), 213S, 2000.

64. De Caterina, R. et al., Structural requirements for inhibition of cytokine-induced endothelial activation by unsaturated fatty acids, *J. Lipid Res.,* 39, 1062, 1998.

65. Porter, N.A., Caldwell, S.E., and Mills, K.A., Mechanism of free radical oxidation of unsaturated lipids, *Lipids,* 30, 277, 1995.

66. De Caterina, R. et al., Nutrients and gene expression, in *Nutrition and Fitness: Diet, Genes, Physical Activity and Health,* Simopoulos, A. and Pavlou, K., Eds., Karger, Basel, 2001, p. 23.

67. Visioli, F., Bellomo G., and Galli C., Free radical-scavenging properties of olive oil polyphenols, *Biochem. Biophys. Res. Commun.,* 247, 60, 1998.

13 Cardiovascular Effects of Dietary Soy

Thomas B. Clarkson and Susan E. Appt

CONTENTS

13.1 INTRODUCTION

Interest in soy protein, both as a dietary supplement and as a component of diet, has increased rapidly based on the assumption that it may provide certain health benefits, particularly the reduction of coronary heart disease. The putative cardiovascular benefits of soy protein are related in part to the observation that Asian populations consuming diets rich in soy protein have lower rates of cardiovascular disease (CVD) than Western populations. Mortality rates due to CVD are eight times higher for men and women living in the U.S. than for Japanese men and women living in Asia. However, Japanese men and women who have migrated to the U.S. have risks of CVD similar to Western populations.[1]

In 1999, the U.S. Food and Drug Administration (FDA) authorized a health claim stating that "25 grams of soy protein per day, as a part of a diet low in saturated fat and cholesterol, may reduce the risk of heart disease."[2] To carry this claim, a soy product must contain a minimum of 6.25 g of soy protein per serving and state the level of protein per serving and its proportion of the recommended 25 g/day total protein. The FDA was persuaded to approve this health claim largely by results of a meta-analysis by Anderson et al. (1995)[3] that reported reductions in plasma low density lipoprotein (LDL) of ~13% and triglycerides (TG) of ~10%, and modest increases in high density lipoprotein (HDL) concentrations of ~2%. In July 2002, this claim was adopted in Europe by the Joint Health Claims Initiative as its first generic health claim for soy.[4]

The magnitude of soy's beneficial effects on plasma lipids and lipoproteins predicted by the meta-analysis have come into question recently. Nestel (2002)[5] pointed out that "about half of the quoted studies showed minor or no cholesterol-lowering effects and three of every four trials included in the meta-analysis had such wide confidence limits that an alternative conclusion might have been reached with equal validity."

The bioactive components of soy responsible for its cardiovascular health benefits are the subjects of much ongoing research. Components studied include intact proteins, individual amino acids, peptides, globulins, and non-nutritive components: saponins, phytic acid, protease inhibitors, and isoflavones (phytoestrogens).[6] Current data indicate that soy protein and isoflavones are the most likely components to provide cardiovascular benefits. Isoflavones are compounds present naturally in soy protein matrices that have structures similar to estradiol and have been reported to have both estrogenic and antiestrogenic properties.[7] Soybeans contain three isoflavones (genistein, daidzein, and glyceitin) present in the beans as glycosides; they are converted to aglycones during absorption from the small intestine. Soy protein from which isoflavones have been extracted [soy (−)] may have different health benefits from intact soy [soy (+)]. In this chapter, we review the effects of soy (with and without isoflavones) on cardiovascular risk markers including plasma lipids, vascular function, blood pressure, and atherosclerosis extent. We also explore potential beneficial interactions of soy and estrogen and their subsequent health implications.

13.2 LIPIDS AND LIPOPROTEINS

It seems clear, based on current evidence, that soy protein as a part of a diet or as a supplement exerts beneficial effects on plasma lipids and lipoproteins, but the magnitude of the beneficial effects is uncertain. The uncertainty probably relates to a number of poorly understood variables that relate to differences in metabolism among human and nonhuman primates and lower animals, and the effects of intervening variables, such as stage of the menstrual cycle and perhaps plasma concentrations of nonovarian-derived estrogens. In this brief review we attempt to put these various issues in the context that is possible based on current knowledge. Since soy supplements are more widely used by postmenopausal females than by males, the majority of the studies have focused on females.

Our group conducted and reported on several studies comparing the effects of diets containing casein/lactalbumin (C/L) and isolated soy protein on the plasma lipids and lipoproteins of surgically postmenopausal monkeys. Compared to C/L, soy protein resulted in reductions in low density lipoprotein plus very low density lipoprotein (LDL + VLDL) cholesterol of 30 to 40% and increases in high density lipoprotein (HDL) cholesterol of 20 to 50%.[8–10]

Using the cynomolgus monkey model, our group also sought to determine how much of the plasma lipid lowering effect of soy protein relates to the presence of the isoflavones and how much relates to soy peptides.[11–13] Monkeys fed intact soy (+) protein generally had higher HDL concentrations (~12%) than those fed soy (–) protein that had been alcohol washed to remove the isoflavones. The LDL + VLDL cholesterol concentrations of monkeys fed soy (+) were about 16% lower than those fed soy (–).

Studies of human patients consuming intact soy protein, however, showed only modest changes in plasma lipoprotein concentrations. Human subjects consuming intact soy protein had reductions in plasma LDL cholesterol of 2.6 to 6.5%, with no effect seen on HDLC concentrations.[14–16] A comparison of soy's effects on plasma lipids of postmenopausal monkeys[11] and women[15] is depicted in Figure 13.1. In a recent and carefully controlled nutritional study,[17] very small reductions in LDL cholesterol (2%) and increases in HDL (3%) were reported when soy/soy isoflavones were administered to postmenopausal women in amounts comparable to those used in monkey studies.

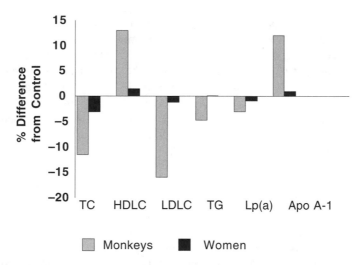

FIGURE 13.1 Effect of soy isoflavones on total cholesterol (TC), high density lipoprotein cholesterol (HDLC), low density lipoprotein cholesterol (LDLC), triglycerides (TG), lipoprotein (a) [Lp(a)], and apolipoprotein A-1 (Apo A-1) in postmenopausal monkeys (grey bars = 129 mg/day isoflavones, women's equivalent) and women (black bars = 132 mg/day isoflavones). Data expressed as percent differences from controls. (From Clarkson, T.B., Anthony M.S., and Morgan T.M., *J. Clin. Endocrinol. Metab.*, 186, 41, 2001 and modified from Wangen, K.E. et al., *Am. J. Clin. Nutr.*, 73, 225, 2001. With permission.)

While the monkey studies comparing soy (−) and soy (+) have suggested the probable importance of the isoflavones in mediating changes in plasma lipoprotein concentrations, the issue is far from settled. We have been unable to show that the addition of purified soy isoflavones to C/L diets or back to soy (−) restores the lipid lowering effectiveness of intact soy (+) protein.[12,18]

Clinical studies of purified isoflavones have also failed to show an effect on plasma lipids and lipoproteins. In a study with peri- and postmenopausal women treated for 5 weeks with 80 mg/day of soy isoflavone extract, improved systemic arterial compliance was observed but there were no changes in plasma concentrations of HDL and LDL cholesterols.[19] That observation was confirmed in another study of postmenopausal women that found no effects of soy isoflavone extracts on plasma lipoproteins concentrations.[20] It would be premature to reach a firm conclusion about the lipoprotein effects of purified soy isoflavones. While no effects of isoflavone extracts can be seen based on current clinical and monkey studies, we lack a clear understanding of dose, timing of administration, effect of aglycone or glycoside form, and other intervening variables that should be considered in such evaluations.

The reasonably intense international research effort resulting in large numbers of recent publications has made it possible to gain some insights into the complexities of differences in soy protein effects on lipids and lipoproteins in various human and nonhuman primate studies. It seems appropriate to discuss some of them.

13.2.1 OPTIMUM DOSES OF SOY AND SOY ISOFLAVONES

Current studies of effects of soy/soy isoflavones on plasma lipids and lipoproteins makes clear that we have no good idea about optimum dose. Crouse et al. (1999)[14] reported an increasing reduction in LDL cholesterol concentration with increasing isoflavone content (from 3 to 62 mg of isoflavones/day) in 25 g of soy protein. Among normocholesterolemic premenopausal women, soy protein with the highest isoflavone content (129 mg/day) had a more robust effect on lowering LDL cholesterol than did the same amount of soy protein with about half the isoflavone content (65 mg).[21] Similarly, among postmenopausal women, consumption of soy protein with 132 mg isoflavone lowered LDL cholesterol more than the same amount of soy protein with about half as much isoflavone.[15]

Somewhat surprisingly, some recent studies have found cardiovascular benefits with much lower intakes of soy isoflavones. De Kleijn et al. (2002)[22] reported on the favorable metabolic cardiovascular risk profiles of postmenopausal women in the Framingham study in relation to their dietary intakes of isoflavones. Among the Framingham subjects, dietary isoflavone consumption was quite low compared to other studies reported with various supplements. On average, the total isoflavone intake was only about 0.78 mg/day. Despite these low dietary intakes, there was a favorable dose response relationship in the metabolic cardiovascular risk profile, particularly among those subjects defined as having the metabolic syndrome.

Van der Schouw et al. (2002)[23] also reported beneficial cardiovascular effects of dietary isoflavones consumed by postmenopausal women, again in very low amounts. Their patients on average consumed 0.57 mg/day of isoflavones. Despite these low intakes, they concluded that the isoflavones had a protective effect on the risk of atherosclerosis through an effect on the artery walls. In another study of postmenopausal women, Goodman-Gruen and Silverstein (2001)[24] reported on the cardiovascular benefits of low dietary intakes of soy isoflavones. The highest tertile of intake in their study was about 6 mg isoflavones/day. They reported that the total isoflavone intake was positively associated with plasma HDL cholesterol concentrations ($p = 0.05$).

Our finding that postmenopausal monkeys fed the same soy diet containing a single "dose" of isoflavone (equivalent to 120 mg/day/women) vary widely in their plasma isoflavone concentrations and that these genotypic/phenotypic differences were associated with large differences in lipoprotein profiles and atherosclerosis protective benefits of soy, led us to conclude that an optimum dose for all individuals may not exist. Monkeys with total plasma isoflavones below 400 nmol/L had increased HDLCs, lower LDLCs, and marked inhibition of coronary artery atherosclerosis progression. On the other hand, monkeys whose total plasma isoflavone concentration was greater than about 700 nmol/L showed no improvement in their plasma lipoprotein profiles nor any protection against progression of coronary artery atherosclerosis.[25] The finding prompted us to speculate that the optimum dose of isoflavones may vary from individual to individual based on genotypic/phenotypic differences in isoflavone metabolism. Furthermore, there may be an optimum plasma isoflavone concentration that must be maintained in order to provide cardiovascular benefits which may only be possible through individual patient dosing and measurement of plasma isoflavone concentrations.

13.2.2 DIFFERENCES IN ISOFLAVONE METABOLISM

As we mentioned earlier, soy has three isoflavones (genistein, daidzein, and glyceitin) that undergo metabolism in the intestinal tract prior to absorption. The isoflavones in most soy foods are conjugated to sugars (glycoside form) that are hydrolyzed by the intestinal brush border membrane and bacterial glucosidase enzymes to the active aglycone form. Figure 13.2 illustrates that under certain circumstances daidzein is converted by specific bacterial reactions in the cecum and large intestine to a compound known as equol. Three strains of bacteria that convert daidzein to equol *in vitro* have been identified by Ueno et al. (2001).[26] Approximately 30% of people (equol producers) and nearly 100% of the animals studied (monkeys, rats, and mice) that consume soy isoflavones produce equol.

The biological properties of equol are not well understood. A study in ovariectomized mice by Marrian and Haselwood (1932)[28] suggested that it had no estrogenic activity. Further investigation using bioassays indicated that equol may be a weak estrogen.[29] Increased uterine weights of rats given equol subcutaneously has been reported, and recently equol was found to have a similar binding affinity to estrogen receptor alpha (ERα) and estrogen receptor beta (ERβ) as genistein.[27,30] Our group has had an opportunity to evaluate endometrial and mammary gland proliferation rates of monkeys with very high plasma equol concentrations for a 3-year period (equivalent to 9 years of human experience). There was no indication of increased proliferation at either site (based on personal communication with Mark Cline).

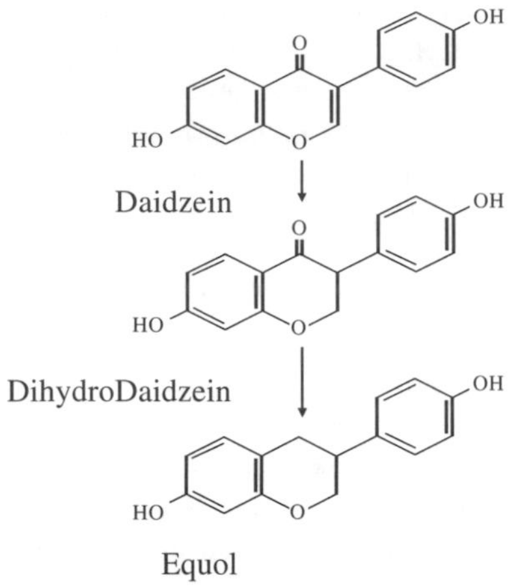

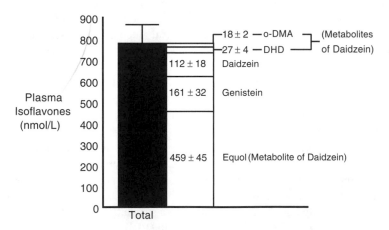

FIGURE 13.2 Conversion of the soy isoflavone daidzein to equol by intestinal brush border enzymes. (Modified from Setchell, K.D.R., Brown, N.M., and Lydeking-Olsen, E., *J. Nutr.,* 132, 3577, 2002.)

While virtually all cynomolgus monkeys have high plasma equol concentrations when fed soy containing diets (Figure 13.3), only about a third of human subjects consuming soy are equol producers and they apparently produce only about half as much equol as cynomolgus monkeys (Figure 13.4).[27,31] We found no evidence for gender differences among human subjects that determine whether they are equol or nonequol producers. Understanding of the clinical importance of equol is at an early stage, although the potential clinical implications have been described well by Setchell et al. (2002).[27]

FIGURE 13.3 Distribution of individual isoflavones and metabolites measured in plasma of cynomolgus monkeys fed soy protein. Data expressed as mean individual isoflavone concentration relative to total isoflavone concentration (nmol/L). (From Clarkson, T.B., Anthony M.S., and Morgan T.M., *J. Clin. Endocrinol. Metab.,* 186, 41, 2001 and modified from Wangen, K.E. et al., *Am. J. Clin. Nutr.,* 73, 225, 2001. With permission.)

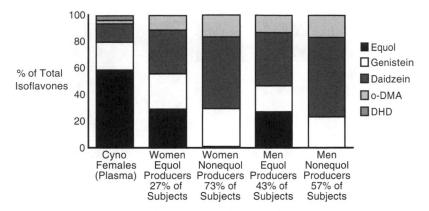

FIGURE 13.4 Isoflavone metabolite profile of cynomolgus monkey females and humans. Data expressed as mean percent of total isoflavones. (From Clarkson, T.B., Anthony M.S., and Morgan T.M., *J. Clin. Endocrinol. Metab.*, 186, 41, 2001 and modified from Lampe, J.W. et al., *Proc. Soc. Exp. Biol. Med.*, 217, 335, 1998. With permission.)

We concur with Setchell et al. (2002)[27] about appropriate interest in the possibility that the conversion or lack of conversion of daidzein to equol may be an important modulator of the effect, or lack of effect, of soy on changes in plasma lipid/lipoprotein concentrations. They report on a reevaluation of a randomized placebo-controlled crossover lipid-lowering study of 23 mildly hypercholesterolemic women who initially had no significant changes in plasma lipids when soy foods were compared with dairy foods. It was found that consuming 5 servings per day of soy for 5 weeks significantly lowered plasma concentrations of cholesterol (8.5%), LDLC (10.0%), TG (21%), and lipoprotein (a) (11%), but only in the equol producers. Although the issue remains speculative, it seems increasingly likely that the very beneficial effects of soy diets on plasma lipoprotein profiles of monkeys may relate to their plasma equol concentrations. The mixed effectiveness observed in studies with humans may be due to failure to separate equol producers from nonequol producers.

13.2.3 LDL Oxidation

Evidence is accumulating to suggest that soy/soy isoflavones may inhibit atherosclerosis progression through a mechanism independent of their plasma lipoprotein concentration effects. One of the primary events in the early formation of atherosclerosis is the accumulation of oxidized LDL within artery walls.[32] The presence of oxidized LDL in artery walls enhances the accumulation of macrophage-derived foam cells within the atherosclerotic plaques resulting in more complicated and possibly less stable plaques.[33] Several studies reported reductions of markers of LDL oxidation (conjugated diene concentration, copper-induced oxidation lag time) in humans consuming soy protein with isoflavones or isoflavone pills.[34–38]

In a crossover study by Jenkens and coworkers[35] depicted in Figure 13.5, hyperlipidemic men and women who ate soy-containing cereal (168 mg/day isoflavones)

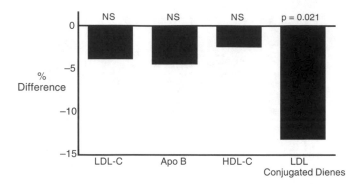

FIGURE 13.5 Effect of consuming soy-containing cereal (36 g/day soy protein compared with control of 8 g/day wheat protein) on hyperlipidemic human subjects. Data expressed as mean difference from baseline. Note lack of effect on plasma lipoproteins and beneficial effect on preventing LDL oxidation. (Modified from Jenkens, D.J.A. et al., *Metabolism*, 49, 1496, 2000. With permission.)

had lower LDL-conjugated diene concentrations (~12%) than those who ate the control diet (8 g/day wheat bran), despite no significant effect on plasma LDLC, HDLC, or ApoB concentrations. Yamakoshi et al. (2000) reported the effect on atherosclerosis progression of feeding aglycone-rich soy extract to male New Zealand white rabbits.[39] Similar to Jenkens and colleagues, they found no effect of the low isoflavone (0.33 g/100 g diet) or high isoflavone (1 g/100 g diet) diet on plasma lipid concentrations, but both diets resulted in reduced atherosclerosis extent (60 and 80%) and plasma cholesterol ester hydroperoxide (30 and 90%) when compared to controls (Figure 13.6).

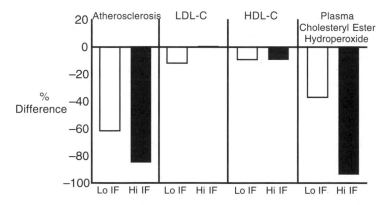

FIGURE 13.6 Effects on atherosclerosis extent (thoracic aorta), low density lipoprotein cholesterol (LDL-C), high density lipoprotein cholesterol (HDL-C), and cholesteryl ester hydroperoxide on rabbits fed atherogenic diet, containing low (0.33 g/100 g diet) or high (1 g/100 g diet) isoflavone extract. Data expressed as mean difference from control. Note lack of effect on LDL-C and HDL-C and reductions in cholesteryl ester hydroperoxide (indication of plasma oxidation) that parallel reductions in atherosclerosis extent. (Modified from Yamakoshi, J. et al., *J. Nutr.*, 130, 1887, 2000. With permission.)

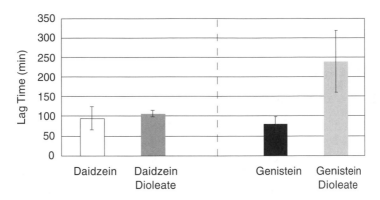

FIGURE 13.7 Antioxidant effects of free versus esterified soy isoflavones incorporated into low density lipoproteins *in vitro*. Data expressed as lag time (minutes) to copper-induced oxidation. (Modified from Meng, Q.H. et al., *Biochim. Biophys. Acta.*, 1438, 369, 1999. With permission.)

The mechanism for the effect of soy/soy isoflavones on LDL oxidation is not clear. The antioxidant activity appears to be related consistently to the isoflavone component of soy protein and several *in vitro* studies have shown reductions of LDL oxidation by genistein.[33,40] Tikkanen et al. (1998) reported that soy consumption (60 mg isoflavones) reduced LDL oxidation by ~15%.[36] This reduced oxidation potential could not be related to incorporation of the isoflavones or their metabolites into the LDL particles because they were present in such small amounts. The phenomenon is likely due to their hydrophilic nature, while the LDL particle is lipid rich. Estrogens can be incorporated into lipoproteins *in vitro* in the form of lipophilic fatty acid esters.[41] Since isoflavones share a structural resemblance with estrogen, Meng et al. (1999) suggested that a similar mechanism of esterification may allow incorporation of isoflavones into LDL, thereby increasing antioxidant potential.[42] *In vitro* data (Figure 13.7) was reported to support this hypothesis for genistein.[42] It seems likely that fatty acid esters of soy isoflavones, particularly of genistein, may be an important new research direction for soy effects on atherosclerosis.

13.2.4 LIPOPROTEIN (A)

The contribution of elevated plasma concentrations of lipoprotein (a) [(Lp(a)] to cardiovascular disease remains unclear. The literature suggests that elevated concentrations of lipoproteins contribute very little, if at all, to the conversion from fatty streaks to plaques and then to larger plaques.[43] On the other hand, reasonable data support the conclusion that elevated concentrations of Lp(a) contribute to increased rates of coronary heart disease events, probably by facilitating the development of plaque-associated mural thrombi.[43]

Nevertheless, much interest focuses on whether and how soy and/or its isoflavones affect plasma concentrations of Lp(a). The literature is more or less divided about whether soy protein causes small increases or decreases in plasma concentrations of Lp(a).[6] What seems clear from recent research is that while the soy peptides may reduce Lp(a) concentrations slightly, the concentrations are in fact increased by the soy isoflavones.[44]

13.3 ARTERIAL FUNCTION

13.3.1 VASCULAR REACTIVITY

Normal coronary arterial function is important in the prevention of myocardial ischemia. Evaluation of arterial function falls into two categories: (1) **active** dilation or constriction of arteries (vascular reactivity) and (2) measurement of arterial stiffness or **passive** dilation (arterial compliance). In this section, we discuss what is known about the effects of soy/soy isoflavones on both measures of arterial function.

Vascular reactivity is used as a marker of endothelial function and is evaluated using one of two methods. In the first, intravascular perfusion of acetylcholine causes an artery to release substances (i.e., nitric oxide) that result in dilation. Constriction or lack of dilation following acetylcholine perfusion is considered an indication of abnormal vascular function. In the second approach, flow through the artery is mechanically restricted, causing the normal endothelium to release substances that result in dilation of the vessel when flow is reestablished (flow-mediated dilation). Studies of vascular reactivity in animal models and human subjects consuming soy/soy isoflavones produced mixed results with respect to gender and menopausal status. For this reason, we will discuss soy's effects on premenopausal, postmenopausal, and male subjects separately.

13.3.1.1 Premenopausal Subjects

Premenopausal monkeys were fed either a soy protein diet with isoflavones [soy (+)] or one from which the isoflavones had been extracted [soy (−)] for 6 months. Vascular reactivity of the proximal left circumflex coronary artery was evaluated. Figure 13.8 depicts the finding that arteries from females in the soy (+) group

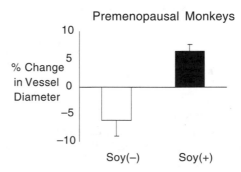

FIGURE 13.8 Effect of diet with isoflavones extracted [soy (−)] versus soy containing isoflavones [soy (+)] on coronary artery dilation in premenopausal female monkeys. Data expressed as percent change in vessel diameter from baseline +/− SEM. (Modified from Honoré, E.K. et al., *Fertil. Steril.*, 67, 148, 1997. With permission.)

dilated (~6% change in diameter) after acetylcholine infusion while arteries of those fed soy (−) constricted (~−6% change in diameter).[45] Interestingly, intravenous administration of genistein into the left main coronary arteries of the monkeys fed soy (−) caused arterial dilation. A similar finding in premenopausal women was reported by Walker et al. (2001); intravenous administration of genistein into the brachial artery caused dilation.[46]

13.3.1.2 Postmenopausal Subjects

Our group observed that arterial dilation following acetylcholine perfusion could not be demonstrated in postmenopausal monkeys with low plasma estrogen concentrations (<5 pg/ml; unpublished data). However, as depicted in Figure 13.9, Williams et al. (2001) reported that when postmenopausal monkeys were treated with estradiol (equivalent to a woman's dose of 1 mg/day), their arteries dilated (~5%).[47] Furthermore, when a combined treatment of estradiol and soy (129 mg/day equivalent to woman's dose) was given, the arteries responded with greater degrees of dilation (~12%) than with either treatment alone, indicating a significant ($p < 0.05$) interactive effect of soy and estradiol on vascular reactivity.

Soy's effects on vascular reactivity in postmenopausal women, as measured by flow-mediated dilation (FMD) of the brachial artery, appear to be minimal. In a comprehensive study by Teede et al. (2001), there was no significant increase in brachial artery flow mediated dilation in postmenopausal women consuming soy

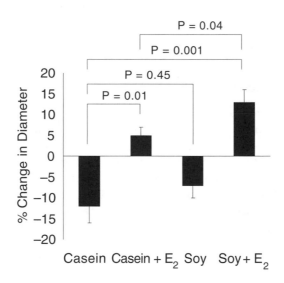

FIGURE 13.9 Coronary artery vascular response of surgically postmenopausal cynomolgus monkeys after intracoronary infusion with acetylcholine. Monkeys were fed one of four treatment diets: casein control, casein + E_2 (1 mg estradiol/day, women's equivalent), soy (129 mg isoflavones/day, women's equivalent), and soy + E_2. Data expressed as mean percent change in diameter +/− SEM. Soy × E_2 interaction is significant ($p < 0.05$). (Modified from Williams, J.K., Anthony, M.S., and Herrington, D.M., *Menopause*, 8, 307, 2001. With permission.)

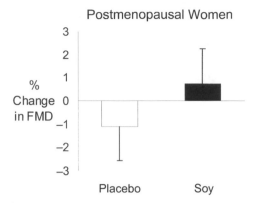

FIGURE 13.10 Effects of soy containing isoflavones on brachial artery vascular reactivities of postmenopausal women. Data expressed as percent change in flow mediated dilation (FMD) from baseline +/− SEM. (From Teede, H.J. et al., *J. Clin. Endocrinol. Metab.*, 86, 3053, 2001. With permission.)

protein (118 mg isoflavones/day) compared to placebo (Figure 13.10).[48] Similarly, it has been reported that consumption of an isoflavone extract had no effect on endothelial function in perimenopausal and postmenopausal women.[19,20] A recent report by Hale and coworkers (2002) found no difference in brachial FMD between postmenopausal women who consumed a soy isoflavone concentrate (80 mg/day) for 2 weeks and those taking the placebo.[49] It remains to be determined whether the lack of effect of isoflavones on postmenopausal women relates to their low plasma estradiol concentrations, as was the case for postmenopausal monkeys.

13.3.1.3 Male Subjects

Soy protein containing isoflavones has potential adverse effects on vascular reactivity in males. Arteries of male monkeys fed soy (+) constricted in response to acetyl-choline perfusion (~7%), whereas males fed soy (−) constricted only minimally (<2%) (Figure 13.11A).[45] Similarly, soy protein treatment (118 mg isoflavones/day) worsened brachial artery dilation in men (Figure 13.11B).[48] In contrast, Yildirir et al. (2001) observed an improvement in brachial artery dilation in hypercholester-olemic men who replaced 60% of their usual animal protein intake with soy protein.[50] Likewise, intravenous administration of genistein caused brachial artery dilation.[46]

In summary, the evidence regarding vascular reactivity suggests that soy protein may enhance the vasodilatory effects of estrogens (endogenous or exogenous) in women and most likely are not beneficial to men.

13.3.2 ARTERIAL COMPLIANCE

A second and perhaps more reliable predictor of normal arterial function is the measurement of **passive** changes in diameter of the artery due to increased pressure in the lumen (arterial compliance). These changes in diameter relate to components of the artery wall, such as elastin and collagen, that give arteries their properties of

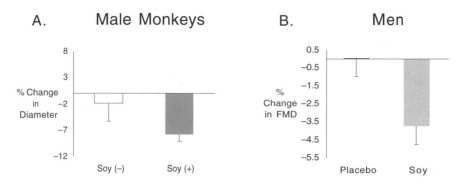

FIGURE 13.11 (A) Effect of dietary soy with isoflavones removed [soy (–)] versus soy containing isoflavones [soy (+)] on coronary artery dilation in response to acetylcholine infusion in male monkeys. Data expressed as percent change in vessel diameter from baseline +/– SEM. (Modified from Honoré, E.K. et al., *Fertil. Steril.*, 67, 148, 1997. With permission.) (B) Effect of soy on brachial artery vascular reactivity of men. Data expressed as percent change in flow mediated dilation (FMD) from baseline +/– SEM. (From Teede, H.J. et al., *J. Clin. Endocrinol. Metab.*, 86, 3053, 2001. With permission.)

stretchiness and/or stiffness. Arterial compliance measurement is often done directly with MRI or ultrasound imaging of the artery in question. Pulse wave velocity and peripheral vascular resistance are also used as indirect measures of arterial compliance. Several studies have reported that decreased arterial compliance is a significant predictor of coronary heart disease.[51–54] From the Rotterdam study (population-based), van Popele et al. (2001) found a strong association between arterial compliance and atherosclerosis extent.[55]

Evidence is accumulating to suggest that supplementation of soy protein in human subjects increases arterial compliance. Peri- and postmenopausal women treated with 80 mg isoflavones/day for 5 weeks had improved arterial compliance (26%) compared with placebo.[19] Although total systemic arterial compliance was not improved with soy treatment in men and postmenopausal women studied by Teede et al. (2001), pulse wave velocity of femoral dorsalis arterial segments were significantly improved ($p = 0.02$) compared with casein placebo.[48]

Recently, van der Schouw and coworkers (2002) reported on the effects of isoflavone and lignan intake (recorded by food frequency questionnaires) on aortic stiffness as measured by pulse wave velocity.[23] Isoflavone intake was associated with decreased aortic stiffness and the effect was most pronounced in older women. It appears that soy may exert beneficial effects on arterial compliance by some unknown mechanism, despite its lack of effect on current measures of vascular reactivity.

13.4 BLOOD PRESSURE

Hypertension is a primary contributor to cardiovascular disease in men and women. However, the incidence is much lower in premenopausal women than in men of similar age. It has been suggested that estrogen is responsible for this disparity between men and women and is therefore protective against hypertension. This is further supported by the observation that after menopause, when plasma estrogen concentrations are low, a woman's risk for hypertension is equal to that of men at a similar age.[56] It follows then that natural plant estrogens such as soy isoflavones may have similar beneficial effects on blood pressure. In this section, we discuss the few published studies about the effects of soy and soy isoflavones on blood pressure.

Five studies of humans provide evidence that consumption of soy containing isoflavones has beneficial effects on blood pressure.[14,48,57–59] Reductions in systolic[48,58] and diastolic[57] blood pressure were reported in healthy men and post-menopausal and perimenopausal women consuming soy with isoflavones (34 to 118 mg). Burke and coworkers reported a significant ($p < 0.006$) decrease in systolic (5.9 mmHg) and diastolic (2.6 mmHg) blood pressure in treated hypertensive subjects who consumed soy (66 g/day containing 23 mg isoflavones).[59] Crouse and colleagues (1999) gave moderately hypertensive men and women soy with increasing amounts of isoflavones (3 to 62 mg isoflavones/25 g diet).[14] A significant trend (p for trend = 0.04) for lower diastolic blood pressure with increasing isoflavone dose was observed in that study. In contrast, consumption of soy cereal containing 136 mg of isoflavones for 3 weeks had no effect on blood pressure in hypercholesterolemic men or women.[35]

Whether the observed antihypertensive effects of soy are due to its isoflavone content is unclear. Two clinical studies of healthy postmenopausal women reported no effects on blood pressure after supplementation with 80 to 100 mg of soy isoflavones for 8 to 16 weeks.[20,60] On the other hand, a study by Karamsetty and coworkers (2001) demonstrated enhanced pulmonary arterial relaxation in chronically hypoxic rats treated with genistein (30 μM) and daidzein (30 μM) isoflavones.[61] No response was seen in the normoxic rats. Isoflavones were also found to have a beneficial effect on blood pressure in NaCl-induced hypertensive ovariectomized rats.[62] Further study in this area is required to determine whether and by what mechanism isoflavones may be responsible for soy's beneficial effect on blood pressure.

13.5 ATHEROSCLEROSIS EXTENT

Several approaches are used to quantify atherosclerosis extent in animal models. Measurements of total arterial cholesterol (or cholesterol ester) may be adequate in some experiments. However, cholesterol content does not provide detailed information about atherosclerotic plaque size, chronicity of lesions, or stenosis. This information can be obtained via morphometric analyses of artery walls at necropsy. Because the coronary and cerebral arteries are the arterial sites most often associated with clinical events, they are given the most attention.

Evidence in several animal models (nonhuman primates, mice, and rabbits) indicates that substitution of animal protein with soy protein results in reduced atherosclerosis extent when the animals are fed diets with added cholesterol.[63] Current research is focused mainly on the role of soy isoflavones in this process. Our group studied the effects of isoflavones on atherosclerosis extent in surgically postmenopausal and male cynomolgus monkeys.[8,11] Figure 13.12 shows that the

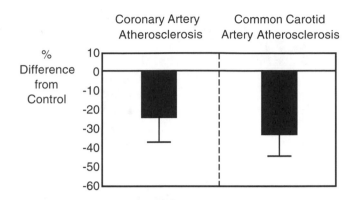

FIGURE 13.12 Effects of soy containing isoflavones on common carotid and coronary artery atherosclerosis extent in postmenopausal cynomolgus monkeys. Data expressed as percent difference from the control group (fed soy with phytoestrogens removed) +/- SEM. (From Clarkson, T.B., Anthony, M.S., and Morgan, T.M., *J. Clin. Endocrinol. Metab.*, 186, 41, 2001. With permission.)

postmenopausal monkeys fed the diet containing isoflavones [soy (+)] had significant reductions in internal carotid artery atherosclerosis ($p = 0.02$) and reduced amounts of coronary artery atherosclerosis (although not statistically significant, $p = 0.12$) compared to the group fed soy with isoflavones removed [soy (−)]. This study lacked a group fed an animal protein (e.g., casein or lactalbumin) diet so we cannot speculate about the degree, if any, of the antiatherogenic effect of the soy (−) or the component(s) of the soy (+) that provided atherosclerosis protection. In the second study, the males fed soy (+) had atherosclerotic lesions 90% smaller than those fed the control (casein and lactalbumin) diet. An intermediate reduction (50%) in atherosclerosis extent was seen in those fed the soy (−) diet.

The use of the mouse as a model of atherosclerosis has increased rapidly since the introduction of transgenic and receptor knockout models that develop atherosclerotic lesions more reliably than wild type mice. Studies using mice in which the LDL receptor or apolipoprotein E (ApoE) receptor has been knocked out showed a decrease in atherosclerosis extent in mice fed soy (+) compared to soy (−) or casein.[64–66] These studies suggest that soy's effects on atherosclerosis are mediated, at least in part, by these receptors. The reduction of atherosclerosis in the soy (+)-fed mice appears to be independent of soy's effects on plasma lipids in two of these studies.[64,66]

Yamakoshi and coworkers fed two doses (0.78 g and 2.33 g/100 g diet) of soy isoflavone extract along with cholesterol (1 g/100 g diet) to rabbits.[39] Despite the fact that no effects on plasma lipid concentrations were noted, the rabbits had significantly less atherosclerosis in their aortic arches when fed either the low- or high-isoflavone diet [26.3% ($P < 0.05$) and 36.9% ($P < 0.01$), respectively], compared with those fed cholesterol alone. An indication of the mechanism of the atheroprotective effect of the isoflavones was their observation that LDL antioxidant effects paralleled the decreases in atherosclerosis extent. Both doses of isoflavones used in this study are several-fold higher than doses used in previous animal studies.

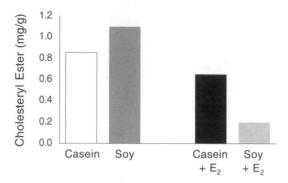

FIGURE 13.13 Effect of casein control, soy (148 mg/day/1800 cal), casein + E_2 (1 mg estradiol/day, women's equivalent), and soy + E_2 on aortic cholesteryl content of postmenopausal cynomolgus monkeys. Data expressed as means adjusted for baseline. Note significant E_2 ($p = 0.001$) main effect and significant soy × E_2 interaction ($p = 0.02$). (Modified from Wagner, J.D. et al., *Metab. Clin. Exp.*, 46, 698, 1997. With permission.)

After reviewing the evidence, it appears that soy protein containing isoflavones [soy (+)] has more antiatherogenic potential than soy that has had isoflavones removed [soy (–)]. Whether this difference between soy (+) and soy (–) is due to the isoflavones is still uncertain.

13.6 SOY INTERACTIONS WITH ESTROGENS: IMPLICATIONS FOR SOY AS A COMPLEMENTARY HORMONE REPLACEMENT THERAPY

Accumulating evidence suggests that significant interactions occur between plasma estradiol and soy isoflavones that may decrease risk factors for cardiovascular disease. In 1997, Wagner and coworkers reported on a study with cynomolgus macaque females with preexisting diet-induced coronary artery atherosclerosis.[67] Both soy and estradiol reduced aortic cholesterol ester content but more importantly, as shown in Figure 13.13, the soy and estradiol combination resulted in a greater reduction in cholesterol ester concentration than with either treatment alone (soy protein × estradiol interaction, $p = 0.02$). Similarly, as mentioned earlier in the chapter, a significant ($p < 0.05$) interactive effect of soy and estradiol on vascular reactivity of postmenopausal monkeys has also been reported.[47]

Important interactions have also been described between changing plasma estradiol concentrations of premenopausal women and the extent to which relatively high doses of soy isoflavones (129 mg/day) reduced plasma LDLC concentrations. Merz-Demlow and coworkers (2000) compared the reductions in plasma LDLC concentration among women consuming moderate doses of soy isoflavones (65 mg/day) and higher soy isoflavone doses (129 mg/day) across their menstrual cycles.[21] In the same subset of women, Duncan et al. (1999) reported on the plasma estradiol concentrations of the women in each of the cycle stages evaluated by Merz-Demlow and colleagues.[68] As seen in Figure 13.14, the only significant reductions in LDLC occurred at the soy isoflavone 129 mg/day dose and the magnitude of the response

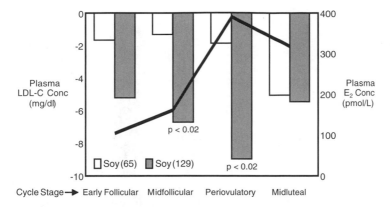

FIGURE 13.14 Effect of stage of menstrual cycle and plasma estradiol concentrations on changes in plasma LDL-C concentrations of premenopausal women administered soy with low isoflavone amounts (65 mg/d) or higher amounts (129 mg/d). Data expressed as difference from control; alcohol-washed soy with residual isoflavones of 10 mg/d. (Modified from Merz-Demlow, B.E. et al., *Am. J. Clin. Nutr.*, 71, 1462, 2000 and Duncan, A.M. et al., *J. Clin. Endocrinol. Metab.*, 84, 3479, 1999. With permission.)

was directly related to increasing plasma estradiol concentration; no significant effects were seen in the early follicular and midluteal stages.

Clinical investigators must consider the stage of the menstrual cycle in timing of samples for lipoprotein analyses. For example, based on the data of Merz-Demlow et al. (2000), by collecting samples at random across the menstrual cycle, one would have only a 50% chance of finding a significant effect ($p < 0.02$).[21] Since nonovarian-derived plasma estradiol concentrations of postmenopausal women vary widely from 1 to 2 pg/ml up to 50 pg/ml, it may also be important to consider estradiol concentration as a potential modifier of the magnitude of soy effects on LDL concentrations in that age group.

Recently our group observed an interaction between soy and tibolone, a synthetic steroid hormone-replacement drug.[69] Tibolone is metabolized into three steroids with estrogenic, progestogenic, and androgenic activities and is used in several countries to treat menopausal symptoms and osteoporosis. Concern has arisen about its cardiovascular safety due to reductions in plasma high density lipoprotein cholesterol (HDLC) reported in women taking the drug. Since soy has been shown to increase plasma HDLC, we sought to determine whether coadministration of soy with tibolone would attenuate the tibolone-induced reductions in HDLC and reduce the risk for coronary heart disease.

Surgically postmenopausal cynomolgus macaques were randomly assigned to one of four treatment diets. The diets contained either casein/lactalbumin (C/L) or soy containing isoflavones with or without tibolone (women's equivalent, 1.25 mg/day). As expected, HDLC concentration was significantly ($p < 0.01$) reduced with tibolone treatment and increased slightly (nonsignificant) with soy. However, as seen in Figure 13.15, when soy was combined with tibolone, there was no reduction in HDLC concentration when compared to controls. Further study is required to determine the mechanism responsible for this soy/tibolone interaction.

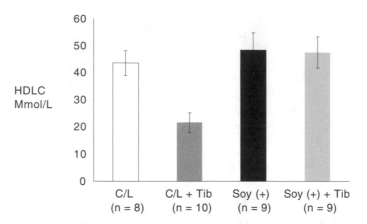

FIGURE 13.15 Effect of soy on tibolone-associated decreases on high density lipoprotein cholesterol concentration (HDLC) in surgically postmenopausal cynomolgus monkeys. Soy diets contained 137 mg isoflavones/1800 cal diet. Tibolone was added to soy and casein at 1.25 mg/1800 cal diet. Data expressed as mean +/– SEM HDLC concentration (mg/dL) and adjusted for pretreatment differences in HDLC (From Appt, S.E. et al., *FASEB J.*, in press. With permission.)

13.7 CONCLUSIONS

Based on increasing evidence, soy supplementation provides some protection against the progression of cardiovascular disease. Male and postmenopausal female cynomolgus monkeys had reduced amounts of coronary and cerebral artery atherosclerosis when fed soy protein containing isoflavones as a part of their moderately atherogenic diets. Some, but not likely all, of the mechanisms that provide atheroprotection involve beneficial changes in plasma lipids and lipoproteins, reductions in blood pressure, antioxidant effects (particularly the protection of LDL particles from oxidative changes), and improvement in arterial compliance.

Whether the cardiovascular beneficial effects of soy protein are due to its isoflavones appears likely but has not been proven. Current national and international research should clarify this complex enigma in the near future.

A challenging current research problem concerns whether and to what extent the cardiovascular benefits of soy relate to the conversion of daidzein to equol. Monkeys have high plasma concentrations of equol and robust effects on plasma lipid profiles. Only women who are equol producers have comparable plasma lipid benefits from soy supplementation.

Another unexplored research challenge concerns the optimum dose of soy to achieve cardiovascular benefits. Evidence suggests that genotypic/phenotypic differences may make it necessary to define an optimum dose for each individual, with *optimum* defined as a particular plasma isoflavone concentration rather than a given amount of soy.

Soy supplementation is widely used by postmenopausal women as an alternative to traditional hormone replacement therapy. For most women it proves inadequate to control some key postmenopausal disorders, i.e., hot flushes, vaginal dryness, and bone loss. For that reason, it seems likely that many women will consider soy as a complementary approach to hormone therapy. Fortunately, increasing evidence indicates that soy interacts favorably with exogenous estrogens to provide greater cardiovascular benefits than either soy or estrogens alone.

REFERENCES

1. Vitolins, M.Z., Anthony, M.S., and Burke, G.L., Epidemiology of soy isoflavones and cardiovascular disease, in *Phytoestrogens and Health*, Gilani, G.S. et al., Eds., American Oil Chemists Society, Champaign, IL, 2002, p. 260.

2. Food and Drug Administration, Food labeling health claims: soy protein and coronary heart disease, 21 CFR part 101, *Fed. Regist.*, 64, 577700, 1999.

3. Anderson, J.W., Johnstone, B.M., and Cook-Newell, M.E., Meta-analysis of the effects of soy protein intake on serum lipids, *New Engl. J. Med.*, 333, 276, 1995.

4. Joint Health Claims Initiative, Generic health claim for soya and blood cholesterol: generic claims assessment, Leatherhead, Surrey, U.K., November 29, 2002.

5. Nestel, P.J., Role of soy protein in cholesterol lowering: how good is it? *Arterioscler. Thromb. Vasc. Biol.*, 22, 1743, 2002.

6. Anthony, M.S., Soy/isoflavones and risk factors for cardiovascular disease, in *Phytoestrogens and Health*, Gilani, G.S. et al., Eds., American Oil Chemists Society, Champaign, IL, 2002, p. 268.

7. Setchell, K.D.R., Soy isoflavones: benefits and risks from nature's selective estrogen receptor modulators (SERMs), *J. Am. Coll. Nutr.*, 20, 354S, 2001.

8. Anthony, M.S. et al., Soy protein versus soy phytoestrogens in the prevention of diet-induced coronary artery atherosclerosis of male cynomolgus monkeys, *Arterioscler. Thromb. Vasc. Biol.*, 17, 2524, 1997.

9. Anthony, M.S. et al., Soybean isoflavones improve cardiovascular risk factors without affecting the reproductive system of peripubertal rhesus monkeys, *J. Nutr.*, 126, 43, 1996.

10. Anthony, M.S. and Clarkson, T.B., Association between plasma isoflavone and plasma lipoprotein concentrations, *J. Medicinal Food*, 2, 263, 1999.

11. Clarkson, T.B., Anthony, M.S., and Morgan, T.M., Inhibition of postmenopausal atherosclerosis progression: a comparison of the effects of conjugated equine estrogens and soy phytoestrogens, *J. Clin. Endocrinol. Metab.*, 186, 41, 2001.

12. Anthony, M.S., Blair, R.M., and Clarkson, T.B., Neither isoflavones nor the alcohol-extracted fraction added to alcohol-washed soy protein isolate restores the lipoprotein effects of soy protein isolate, *J. Nutr.*, 132, 583S, 2002.

13. Anthony, M.S., Clarkson, T.B., and Williams, K.J., Effects of soy isoflavones on atherosclerosis: potential mechanisms, *Am. J. Clin. Nutr.*, 68, 1390S, 1998.

14. Crouse, J.R. et al., A randomized trial comparing the effect of casein with that of soy protein containing varying amounts of isoflavones on plasma concentrations of lipids and lipoproteins, *Arch. Intern. Med.*, 159, 2070, 1999.

15. Wangen, K.E. et al., Soy isoflavones improve plasma lipids in normocholesterolemic and mildly hypercholesterolemic postmenopausal women, *Am. J. Clin. Nutr.*, 73, 225, 2001.

16. Baum, J.A., Teng, H., and Erdman, J.W., Long-term intake of soy protein improves blood lipid profiles and increases mononuclear cell low-density-lipoprotein receptor messenger RNA in hypercholesterolemic postmenopausal women, *Am. J. Clin. Nutr.*, 68, 545, 1998.

17. Lichtenstein, A.H. et al., Lipoprotein response to diets high in soy or animal protein with and without isoflavones in moderately hypercholesterolemic subjects, *Arterioscler. Thromb. Vasc. Biol.*, 22, 1852, 2002.

18. Greaves, K.A. et al., Intact dietary soy protein, but not adding an isoflavone-rich soy extract to casein, improves plasma lipids in ovariectomized cynomolgus monkeys, *J. Nutr.*, 129,1585, 1999.

19. Nestel, P.J. et al., Soy isoflavones improve systemic arterial compliance but not plasma lipids in menopausal and perimenopausal women, *Arterioscler. Thromb. Vasc. Biol.*, 7, 3392, 1997.

20. Simons, L.A. et al., Phytoestrogens do not influence lipoprotein levels or endothelial function in healthy, postmenopausal women, *Am. J. Cardiol.*, 85, 1297, 2000.

21. Merz-Demlow, B.E. et al., Soy isoflavones improve plasma lipids in normocholesterolemic, premenopausal women, *Am. J. Clin. Nutr.*, 71, 1462, 2000.

22. De Kleijn, M.J. et al., Dietary intake of phytoestrogens is associated with a favorable metabolic cardiovascular risk profile in postmenopausal U.S. women: the Framingham study, *J. Nutr.*, 132, 276, 2002.

23. van der Schouw, Y.T. et al., Higher usual dietary intake of phytoestrogens is associated with lower aortic stiffness in postmenopausal women, *Arterioscler. Thromb. Vasc. Biol.*, 22, 1316, 2002.

24. Goodman-Gruen, D. and Silverstein, D.K., Usual dietary isoflavone intake is associated with cardiovascular disease risk factors in postmenopausal women, *J. Nutr.*, 131, 1202, 2001.

25. Clarkson, T.B. et al., A paradoxical association between plasma isoflavone concentration on a soy-containing diet, and both plasma lipoproteins and atherosclerosis, *J. Nutr.*, 132, 583S, 2002.

26. Ueno, T. and Uchiyama, S., Identification of the specific intestinal bacteria capable of metabolizing soy isoflavone to equol, *Ann. Nutr. Metab.*, 45, 114 (Abstr.), 2001.

27. Setchell, K.D.R., Brown, N.M., and Lydeking-Olsen, E., The clinical importance of the metabolite equol: a clue to the effectiveness of soy and its isoflavones, *J. Nutr.*, 132, 3577, 2002.

28. Marrian, G. and Haslewood, G., A new active phenol isolated from the ketohydroxyoestrin fraction of mares' urine, *Biochem. J.*, 26, 1227, 1932.

29. Shutt, D. and Braden, A., The significance of equol in relation to the oestrogenic response in sheep ingesting clover with a high formonentin content, *Aust. J. Agric. Res.*, 19, 545, 1968.

30. Morito, K. et al., Interaction of phytoestrogens with estrogen receptors α and β, *Biol. Pharm. Bull.*, 24, 351, 2001.

31. Lampe, J.W. et al., Urinary equol excretion with soy challenge: influence of habitual diet, *Proc. Soc. Exp. Biol. Med.*, 217, 335, 1998.

32. Woolf, N., Pathology of atherosclerosis, in Betteridge, J., Illingworth, R., Shepherd, J., Eds., *Lipoproteins in Health and Disease*, Hodder & Stoughton, London, 1999, p. 533.

33. Patel, R.P. et al., Antioxidant mechanisms of isoflavones in lipid systems: paradoxical effects of peroxyl radical scavenging, *Free Radic. Biol. Med.*, 31, 1570, 2001.

34. Jenkens, D.J.A. et al., Effect of soy protein foods on low density lipoprotein oxidation and *ex vivo* sex hormone receptor activity: a controlled crossover trial, *Metabolism*, 49, 537, 2000.

35. Jenkens, D.J.A. et al., Effect of soy-based breakfast cereal on blood lipids and oxidized low density lipoprotein, *Metabolism*, 49, 1496, 2000.

36. Tikkanen, M.J. et al., Effect of soybean phytoestrogen intake on low density lipoprotein oxidation resistance, *Proc. Natl. Acad. Sci. USA*, 95, 3106, 1998.

37. Wiseman, H. et al., Isoflavone phytoestrogens consumed in soy decrease F2-isoprostane concentrations and increase resistance of low density lipoprotein to oxidation in humans, *Am. J. Clin. Nutr.*, 72, 395, 2000.

38. Samman, S. et al., The effect of supplementation with isoflavones on plasma lipids and oxidisability of low density lipoprotein in premenopausal women, *Atherosclerosis*, 147, 277, 1999.

39. Yamakoshi, J. et al., Isoflavone aglycone-rich extract without soy protein attenuates atherosclerosis development in cholesterol-fed rabbits, *J. Nutr.*, 130, 1887, 2000.

40. Kim, H., Peterson, T.G., and Barnes, S., Mechanisms of action of the soy isoflavone genistein: emerging role for its effects via transforming growth factor beta signaling pathways, *Am. J. Clin. Nutr.*, 68, 1418, 1998.

41. Hochberg, R.B., Biological esterification of steroids, *Endocr. Rev.*, 19, 331, 1998.

42. Meng, Q.H. et al., Incorporation of esterified soybean isoflavones with antioxidant activity into low density lipoprotein, *Biochim. Biophys. Acta*, 1438, 369, 1999.

43. Hopkins, P. N. et al., Lipoprotein (a) interactions with lipid and non lipid risk factors in early familial coronary artery disease, *Arterioscler. Thromb. Vasc. Biol.*, 17, 2783, 1997.

44. Mienertz, H., Nilausen, K., and Hilden, J., Alcohol-extracted, but not intact dietary soy protein lowers lipoprotein (a) markedly, *Arterioscler. Thromb. Vasc. Biol.*, 22, 312, 2002.

45. Honoré, E.K. et al., Soy isoflavones enhance coronary vascular reactivity in atherosclerotic female macaques, *Fertil. Steril.*, 67, 148, 1997.

46. Walker, H.A. et al., The phytoestrogen genistein produces acute nitric oxide-dependent dilation of human forearm vasculature with similar potency to 17β-estradiol, *Circulation*, 103, 258, 2001.

47. Williams, J.K., Anthony, M.S., and Herrington, D.M., Interactive effects of soy protein and estradiol on coronary reactivity in atherosclerotic, ovariectomized monkeys, *Menopause*, 8, 307, 2001.

48. Teede, H.J. et al., Dietary soy has both beneficial and potential adverse cardiovascular effects: a placebo-controlled study in men and postmenopausal women, *J. Clin. Endocrinol. Metab.*, 86, 3053, 2001.

49. Hale, G. et al., Isoflavone supplementation and endothelial function in menopausal women, *Clin. Endocrinol.*, 56, 693, 2002.

50. Yildirir, A. et al., Soy protein diet significantly improves endothelial function and lipid parameters, *Clin. Cardiol.*, 24, 711, 2001.

51. Guerin, A.P. et al., Impact of aortic stiffness attenuation on survival of patients in end-stage renal failure. *Circulation*, 103, 987, 2001.

52. Blacher, J. et al., Aortic pulse wave velocity as a marker of cardiovascular risk in hypertensive patients, *Hypertension*, 33, 1111, 1999.

53. Kingwell, B.A. et al., Large artery stiffness predicts ischemic threshold in patients with coronary artery disease, *J. Am. Coll. Cardiol.*, 40, 773, 2002.

54. Cameron, J.D., Jennings, G.L., and Dart, A.M., Systemic arterial compliance is decreased in newly diagnosed patients with coronary heart disease: implications for predictors of risk, *J. Cardiovasc. Risk*, 6, 495, 1996.

55. van Popele, N.M. et al. Association between arterial stiffness and atherosclerosis, *Stroke*, 32, 454, 2001.

56. Kotchen, J.M., Mckean, H.E., and Kotchen, T.A. Blood pressure trends with aging, *Hypertension*, 4, 128, 1982.

57. Washburn, S. et al., Effect of soy protein supplementation on serum lipoproteins, blood pressure, and menopausal symptoms in perimenopausal women, *Menopause*, 6, 7, 1999.

58. Vigna, G.B. et al., Plasma lipoproteins in soy-treated postmenopausal women: a double-blind placebo-controlled trial, *Nutr. Metab. Cardiovasc. Dis.*, 10, 315, 2000.

59. Burke, V. et al., Dietary protein and soluble fiber reduce ambulatory blood pressure in treated hypertensives, *Hypertension*, 38, 821, 2001.

60. Han, K.K. et al., Benefits of soy isoflavone therapeutic regimen on menopausal symptoms, *Obstet. Gynecol.*, 99, 389, 2002.

61. Karamsetty, M.R., Klinger, J.R., and Hill, N.S., Phytoestrogens restore nitric oxide-mediated relaxation in isolated pulmonary arteries from chronically hypoxic rats. *J. Pharmacol. Exp. Ther.*, 297, 968, 2001.

62. Fang, Z. et al., estrogen depletion induces NaCl-sensitive hypertension in female spontaneously hypertensive rats, *Am. J. Physiol. Regul. Integr. Comp. Physiol.*, 281, R1934, 2001.

63. Clarkson, T.B., Soy, soy phytoestrogens and cardiovascular disease, *J. Nutr.*, 132, 566S, 2002.

64. Adams, M.R. et al., The inhibitory effect of soy protein isolate on atherosclerosis in mice does not require the presence of LDL receptors or alteration of plasma lipoproteins, *J. Nutr.*, 132, 43, 2002.

65. Kirk, E.A. et al., Dietary isoflavones reduce plasma cholesterol and atherosclerosis in C57BL/6 mice but not LDL receptor-deficient mice, *J. Nutr.*, 128, 954, 1998.

66. Ni, W. et al., Dietary soy protein isolate compared with casein reduces atherosclerotic lesion area in apolipoprotein E-deficient mice, *J. Nutr.*, 128, 1884, 1998.

67. Wagner, J.D. et al., Dietary soy protein and estrogen replacement therapy improve cardiovascular risk factors and decrease aortic cholesteryl ester content in ovariectomized cynomolgus monkeys, *Metab. Clin. Exp.*, 46, 698, 1997.

68. Duncan, A.M. et al., Modest hormonal effects of soy isoflavones in postmenopausal women, *J. Clin. Endocrinol. Metab.*, 84, 3479, 1999.

69. Appt, S.E., Clarkson, T.B., and Anthony, M.S., Soy attenuates the high density lipoprotein cholesterol lowering effects of tibolone in atherogenic diet-fed cynomologus monkeys, *FASEB J.*, in press.

14 Malnutrition and the Heart: A Pediatric Perspective

Poothirikovil Venugopalan

CONTENTS

0-8493-1674-X/04/$0.00+$1.50

14.1 INTRODUCTION

Every year millions of children are subjected to the effects of malnutrition — long-standing deleterious effects on growth and development. Statistics published by the United Nations Educational Scientific and Cultural Organization (UNESCO) place the incidence of low birth weight (less than 2500 grams) at 18% among developing countries.[1] Thirty-one percent of children under the age of 5 years in these countries suffer from moderate to severe malnutrition (weight more than two standard deviations from median weight for age of reference population) that correlates to poor dietary intake of calories and/or proteins.[2,3]

Supplementation studies such as those carried out in Guatemala and Colombia have shown significant improvement in weight and linear growth in children with the addition of calories and proteins to the diet.[4,5] The dietary requirements of children of different ages have also been computed.[6,7] However, poverty and illiteracy among other factors have rendered difficult the realization of these recommended allowances to a significant proportion of the population. Table 14.1 lists various factors that contribute to the development of protein energy malnutrition (PEM).

Although PEM is a disease of poorer countries, it has also been observed in the U.S. in children with unusual or deficient diets, especially in children with organic disorders such as enteropathies and malignancies and with anorexia nervosa.[8,9] Chase et al. of Denver[10] reported a series of 14 infants with severe malnutrition and attributed the condition to vegetarian dietary habits, alleged refusal of food, food deprivation as part of diarrhea treatment, and excessive dilution of infant formula.

TABLE 14.1
Factors Contributing to Protein Energy Malnutrition

Factor	Possible Cause
Inadequate food availability	Poverty, ignorance, unusual dietary habits, parental neglect, quiet baby, depressed mother, substance abuse
Inadequate food intake	Anorexia, swallowing dysfunction, cerebral palsy, mental retardation, cleft palate, obstructing tonsils or adenoids, dental caries, oral cavity infections
Increased loss of nutrients	Persistent vomiting, gastroesophageal reflux, chronic diarrhea
Inadequate absorption	Cystic fibrosis, biliary atresia, cirrhosis of liver, celiac disease, dietary protein intolerance, giardiasis, short bowel syndrome, chronic pancreatitis, Shwachman–Diamond syndrome, tropical sprue
Increased requirement	Hyperthyroidism, thermal stress, chronic illness, malignancy, renal failure, chronic heart failure, acquired immune deficiency syndrome
Decreased growth potential	Down syndrome, other chromosomal anomalies, Russell Silver syndrome, intrauterine infection

It is more disturbing to note that these children were younger compared to those seen in the developing countries and possibly face greater long-term consequences.

14.2 CLINICAL SYNDROMES ASSOCIATED WITH PROTEIN ENERGY MALNUTRITION

PEM is a state of undernutrition that can manifest as marasmus, kwashiorkor, or marasmic kwashiorkor[11] (Table 14.2).

14.2.1 MARASMUS

Marasmus is general malnutrition with a proportionate deficiency of proteins and energy. Marasmic patients have less than 60% of expected weight for age and do not exhibit edema. They demonstrate loss of subcutaneous fat, muscle wasting, and

TABLE 14.2
Clinical Classification of Protein Energy Malnutrition

Undernutrition:	*Kwashiorkor:*
Weight 60 to 80%	Weight 60 to 80%
Edema absent	Edema present
Marasmus:	*Marasmic Kwashiorkor:*
Weight <60%	Weight <60%
Edema absent	Edema present

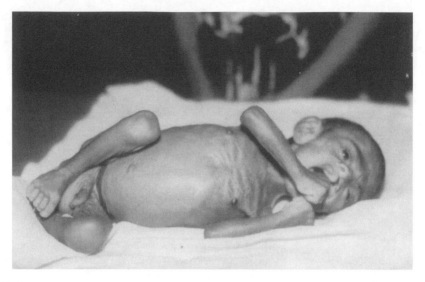

FIGURE 14.1 Eight-month-old infant with marasmus. Note severe wasting and loss of subcutaneous fat and muscle. This infant also had a cleft palate that contributed to the feeding difficulty and consequent marasmus.

atrophy of most organs (Figure 14.1). Endocrine changes that result from marasmus lead to mobilization of fatty acids from adipose tissue and amino acids from muscles.[12] Hepatic gluconeogenesis is enhanced and plasma proteins maintained at normal levels.[13] No edema occurs as long as cardiac output is sufficient to maintain renal perfusion.

Marasmus is more common in infants, presents initially as failure to gain weight, and later is characterized by loss of weight leading to severe emaciation. The skin becomes wrinkled and loses turgor. Buccal pads of fat are retained until late in the illness, when the infant develops sunken cheeks and a wizened appearance. Initially the infant is fretful and later becomes listless. The abdomen becomes distended due to prominent bowel loops secondary to bowel wall hypotonia. Constipation is common, and occasionally frequent small stools from a starvation type of diarrhea may appear.

14.2.2 KWASHIORKOR

Kwashiorkor means *deposed child*, i.e., a child who is no longer breast-fed. The condition manifests after weaning and hence presents itself at a slightly later age compared to marasmus, usually between 1 and 5 years. A disproportionate deficiency of protein and general undernourishment are present. Kwashiorkor patients have edema; their weights are between only 60 and 80% of expected weight (Figure 14.2). Edema dominates the clinical picture and loss of subcutaneous tissue is less pronounced. Mobilization of fatty acids and amino acids occurs, but not to the same extent as in marasmus. Presence of proteinase inhibitors may also contribute to the derangement of homeostasis.[14]

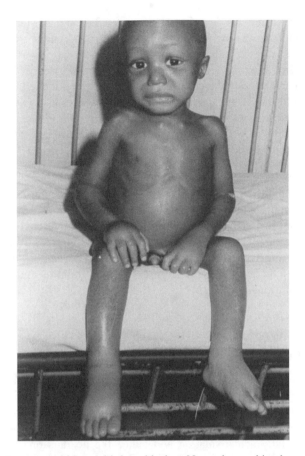

FIGURE 14.2 Two-year-old boy with kwashiorkor. Note edema, skin changes, and apathy.

Low plasma oncotic pressure leads to edema formation, and the resultant reduction in effective circulating blood volume leads to reduced renal perfusion and activation of the renin angiotensin system. Retention of salt and water then exacerbates edema accumulation. Since the disease results from a predominant protein deficiency, the adaptive endocrine mechanisms are not activated to the extent seen in marasmus. The clinical features thus result from both the reduced cardiac output and accumulation of extravascular fluid. The edema is initially evident on the feet and it then spreads to involve the whole body. The resultant rounded "moon face" gives kwashiorkor patients a characteristic appearance. Ascites and pleural effusion may also develop.

Hepatomegaly secondary to fatty infiltration is common in African and West Indian children but less frequently reported for Asian and Ugandan children. Skin and hair changes are common in kwashiorkor. Hyperpigmentation at sites of irritation, followed by desquamation gives the picture of "crazy pavement" dermatitis. Other skin changes include flexural ulcers, hypopigmented patches, and punched-out ulcers. Hair is sparse, thin, dry, brittle, and dyspigmented. A band of hypopigmented hair next to the scalp in an otherwise dark-haired child associated at times with kwashiorkor is referred to as a "flag sign." Mental changes are common and include apathy and irritability. Stupor and coma are late manifestations. Acute and chronic infections and parasitic infestations are common. Secondary to acquired immunodeficiency, relatively benign diseases like measles can have fulminant and devastating courses in kwashiorkor patients. Intercurrent infections associated with HIV infection are also more common and severe in HIV patients who develop kwashiorkor.

14.2.3 MARASMIC KWASHIORKOR

Marasmic kwashiorkor is characterized by edema and weight below 60% of expected weight.[15] The manifestations are a combination of wasting and fluid retention, and bear a worse prognosis than either marasmus or kwashiorkor alone.

Clinical features in patients with PEM are also influenced by coexisting factors like anemia, infections, thiamine deficiency, and electrolyte disturbances. These complicating factors are more frequent with kwashiorkor. Local dietary practices favor deficiencies of certain minerals and vitamins and may dictate the mode of presentation.

14.3 CARDIOVASCULAR CHANGES IN PROTEIN ENERGY MALNUTRITION

This section examines the clinical and pathologic changes in the cardiovascular system that result from PEM — marasmus, kwashiorkor, and deficiencies of essential vitamins and other nutrients.[16,17] Because cardiac muscle contracts actively throughout life, it requires constant supplies of energy to sustain health. Most of this energy is derived from fatty acid oxidation and hence the heart is one of the important organs to be affected by PEM.

14.3.1 CLINICAL FEATURES

The major cardiovascular manifestations are the results of impaired cardiac output and sluggish peripheral perfusion (Table 14.3). Bradycardia, weak peripheral pulses, low blood pressure, narrow pulse pressure, hypothermia, and even circulatory collapse may ensue.[18] Innocent cardiac murmurs secondary to anemia are common both in marasmus and in kwashiorkor. Cardiac output is low[19] and cardiac failure is unusual at presentation.[20] An infant or child with kwashiorkor is frequently pale or dusky and may exhibit hypotension and hypothermia.[20] The precordial cardiac impulse is hardly palpable, the heart sounds are distant and muffled, and pericardial effusion and cardiac arrhythmias occasionally occur.

Sudden deaths have been reported both in marasmus and in kwashiorkor during or following therapy and apparent recovery.[16,20] These may be attributed to fatal cardiac arrhythmias, either secondary to coexisting electrolyte disturbances (particularly sodium, potassium, calcium, and magnesium) or as a result of degenerative changes in the conducting tissues, but these hypotheses are not well established or substantiated.

TABLE 14.3
Clinical Manifestations of
Cardiovascular Involvement
in Malnutrition

Bradycardia
Weak peripheral pulse
Narrow pulse pressure
Hypotension
Hypothermia
Circulatory collapse
Cardiac failure
Weak apical impulse
Muffled heart sounds
Innocent cardiac murmurs
Pericardial effusion
Cardiac arrhythmia
Sudden death

14.3.2 INVESTIGATIONS

Table 14.4 shows cardiac investigation abnormalities in children with malnutrition. Chest radiographs reveal small cardiac silhouettes attributable to both muscle atrophy and decreases in systolic and diastolic blood volume secondary to reduced whole body blood volume and diminished venous return.[20–22] Coexisting pericardial effusion may cast a large cardiac shadow and complicating pneumonia and pleural effusion may also be evident in the lung fields.[21,23]

Electrocardiograms reflect the malnutrition and coexisting electrolyte disturbances. Sinus bradycardia, diminished QRS voltage, shortened P waves and PR intervals, flattened or inverted T waves over left precordial leads and U waves are the usual changes.[20,21,24] Based on the types of ST-T wave changes, different ECG patterns were reported by Smythe et al.[20] but their clinical or prognostic significance has not been established by subsequent reports. Prolonged QT intervals and normal QT intervals have been reported[21,25] and may simply depend on electrolyte status. Sinus tachycardia was prominent in the series of Smythe et al.[20] and is usual at presentation, especially when associated with hypomagnesemia,[24] anemia, and underlying infectious diseases.[22] Cardiac arrhythmias like ventricular ectopics, junctional rhythm, escape beats, and atrial fibrillation have been described. Lethal ventricular arrhythmia remains a possibility although not documented conclusively.

Echocardiographic studies of left ventricular ejection fraction, shortening fraction, and fiber shortening rate have not revealed any significant abnormality. Heymsfield et al.[22] noted that these indices of cardiac function were normal or above normal when adjusted for body weight, although the absolute values were depressed. Moreover, during therapy, these remained steady even in patients who

TABLE 14.4
Abnormalities in Cardiac Investigations of Children with Malnutrition

Investigation	Abnormality
Chest radiograph	Small cardiac silhouette
	Cardiomegaly
	Pneumonia
	Pleural effusion
Electrocardiogram	Sinus bradycardia
	Sinus tachycardia
	Diminished QRS voltage
	Shortened P wave and PR interval
	Flattened or inverted T waves
	Prolonged QT interval
	U waves
	Atrial arrhythmias
	Ventricular arrhythmias
Echocardiogram	Normal LV ejection fraction
	Normal LV shortening fraction
	Reduced LV muscle mass
	Reduced cardiac chamber volumes
	Reduced stroke volume
	Reduced cardiac output
	Pericardial effusion
Cardiac catheterization	Low cardiac output
	Low systemic and pulmonary pressures
	High vascular resistance
	Bradycardia
	Low myocardial compliance (late stages)
	Low plasma volume
	Reduced body oxygen consumption
	Reduced oxygen transport
	Reduced tissue delivery of oxygen

showed symptoms resembling heart failure. However, Shoukry et al.[26] reported slightly different findings in infants with severe PEM. They performed echocardiography before and after therapy and demonstrated slight reduction in baseline left ventricular muscle mass and shortening fraction when compared with healthy controls matched for age and body length. During therapy, these measurements returned toward normal, except for a slight increase in left ventricular end diastolic dimension.

Cardiac catheter studies revealed decrease in cardiac output, lowered pressures in systemic and pulmonary circulations with high vascular resistances,[19,27] and bradycardia, reflecting the low output state.[28] Thus the myocardial mechanics were intact and contractility normal. Toward terminal stages of the illness, with superadded infection and associated anemia, myocardial compliance would be expected to decrease, contractility to reduce, and heart failure to ensue. Studies have also shown reduction in plasma volume, total body oxygen consumption, oxygen transport, and tissue oxygen delivery in patients with severe malnutrition, consistent with the reported reduction in thyroid and adrenal activity.[29-31]

14.3.3 PATHOLOGIC CHANGES

Our knowledge of the pathologic changes in PEM comes partly from reports on autopsy studies and partly from animal models. The heart is almost always abnormal; the changes are related to the malnutrition per se along with associated anemia and the terminal infection (Table 14.5). In autopsy analysis of 93 malnourished children in Costa Rica, 14 (15%) were considered to have primary congestive heart failure resulting from either marasmus or kwashiorkor.[23] The heart appears small and the loss of cardiac mass[23,29,32] reflects the hypometabolic state with reduced thyroid and adrenal activity.[29,30] In the presence of severe anemia or volume overload, heart size may increase instead. This is often the case as death occurs during the course of acute therapy.

Gross examination revealed a pale flabby heart with a thin wall. The cardiac muscle was wasted, consistent with generalized wasting of other muscles. Subepicardial fat was absent,[20,21,33] and pericardial effusion was common with kwashiorkor. The coronary arteries, valves, and endocardium were normal. Histological findings included thinning and shrinkage of myofibers in marasmic patients; interstitial edema was prominent with kwashiorkor.[20,21,23,33,34] Connective tissue increased and apparent disorganization of myofibrillar structure was also frequent. Studies of kwashiorkor

TABLE 14.5
Pathology of the Heart in Malnutrition

Study Type	Pathology
Macroscopy	Small cardiac size
	Pale, thin, and flabby muscle
	Wasting of cardiac muscle
	Loss of subpericardial fat
	Pericardial effusion
Light microscopy	Thinning and shrinkage of myofibers in marasmus
	Interstitial edema in kwashiorkor
	Increase in fibrous tissue
	Myofibrillar disorganization
	Loss of fiber striations
	Vacuolization of fibers
	Patchy muscle necrosis
	Atrophy of atrioventricular conducting system
Electron microscopy	Muscle atrophy
	Loss of myofibrils
	Loss of muscle glycogen
	Mitochondrial degeneration

patients also revealed small myocardial fibers with poorly staining areas of the myocardium and indistinct striations, vacuolations in many, and deformed nuclei in others, reflecting fragmentation of myofibrils, loss of striations, and patchy necrosis.[21] Small muscle fibers were separated by edematous stroma.[8]

Pathologic changes in the conduction system that could explain sudden deaths have also been reported.[35] These changes include atrophy of the atrioventricular conducting system and myocytolysis in the absence of any cellular reaction or fibrosis.[23] Patchy myofiber necrosis and fibrosis have also been described.[21,34] Electron microscopic changes include foci of atrophy, loss of myofibrils and glycogen, decreased mitochondria, and swelling of matrix with disruption of cristae.

14.3.4 Animal Models

Experimentally produced PEM has been most extensively studied in rat models (Table 14.6). The animals were fed special low-protein formulae and the cardiovascular changes were studied by comparing them with well-fed cohort animals.

Rossi et al. studied the effects of 6 weeks of protein depletion in rats and demonstrated myocardial damage associated with electrocardiographic abnormalities and increased myocardial catecholamine levels.[36–41] They postulated that the stress of PEM enhanced levels of catecholamines. However, this could be associated with a down-regulation of beta-adrenergic receptors of the heart, thus explaining the cardiovascular changes observed. Later in the course of food deprivation, the catecholamine levels reduced, consistent with the cardiac changes. Grossly, the heart was small and its weight was reduced. Myocardial changes included myofiber atrophy with hyalinization and vacuolization, and occasional small foci of necrosis, interstitial fibrosis, and mononuclear cell infiltrates. Electron microscopy revealed myofibrillar degeneration, contraction band formation, dilatation of sarcoplasmic reticulum, mitochondrial swelling, dehiscence of intercalated discs,

---

TABLE 14.6
Summary of Cardiac Effects of Malnutrition in Rat Models

Study	Findings
Rossi et al.[36–39]	Myocardial damage
	Electrocardiographic abnormalities
	Elevated myocardial catecholamine levels
Benfey et al.[42]	Normal response to isoproterenol, phenylephrine, or calcium infusion
	Normal alpha and beta receptors in ventricular membranes
Freund et al.[43]	Low myocardial force and force-velocity that returned to control levels on therapy
	Bradycardia, hypotension, and low cardiac output
Nutter et al.[44]	Increase in left ventricular DNA
	Low cardiac protein/DNA ratio
	Increase in ventricular collagen
Gold et al.[45]	Elevated myocardial adenosine triphosphate
	Increased oxidation of amino acids for energy
Zahringer et al.[46]	Low microsomal RNA and messenger RNA

and widened interstitial spaces around blood vessels secondary to fluid and mono-nuclear cell infiltrates.

Benfey et al. studied the inotropic effects of isoproterenol, phenylephrine, and calcium on the left atria of 5-week-old rats with PEM induced by 3 weeks of low-protein formula.[42] Heart weights adjusted for body weights were slightly increased when compared to weights in normal rats. However, no difference was noted in the atrial resting tension and peak developed tension in response to isoproterenol, phenylephrine, or calcium. The number of alpha and beta receptors and receptor affinities in ventricular membranes were also normal.

Freund and Holroyde studied cardiac function in the isolated rat heart using a Langendorff isolated heart perfusion apparatus.[43] Myocardial-developed force and force-velocity were lower in PEM cases than in controls and returned to control levels on therapy. Even in the absence of myocardial edema, the rat heart evidenced bradycardia, systemic hypotension, and diminished cardiac output.[44] When output was adjusted for total body mass, the cardiac output index was normal. No evidence of loss of myocardial reserve in ventricular function curves was noted. This study did not uncover any myocardial stiffness, although ventricular contractility was enhanced and the duration of contraction prolonged.[44]

Nutter et al.[44] in their study of marasmic rats showed normal myocardial structure and function. However the left ventricular concentration of DNA, an index of cell number, was found to be greater by 45%, consistent with a higher cell density in the atrophic myocardium. The total cardiac protein/DNA ratio was lower by 30% as was the reduction in myofiber diameter. There was a 95% increase in ventricular collagen, with normal actomyosin levels. These findings supported the fibrotic changes in the myocardium, with reduction in the contractile protein per unit of tissue.

Significant metabolic changes have also been recorded in the myocardia of malnourished rats. It appears that cardiac muscle plays a role in energy metabolism similar to that observed in liver and skeletal muscle by undergoing glycogenolysis and proteolysis. Fasting leads to increased fatty acid oxidation and the by-product citrate accumulates in the intracellular compartment. Rising citrate inhibits the key regulatory enzyme, phosphofructokinase. Also, despite fasting, myocardial levels of adenosine triphosphate (ATP) were high, indicating an ample supply of ATP to satisfy myocardial demands.[45]

These studies have also given evidence of a shift in amino acid metabolism from anabolic to oxidative pathways, consistent with the increasing role of amino acids as myocardial energy sources late in starvation.[45] Myocardial levels of alanine were low and the alanine/pyruvate equilibrium ratios fell. Alanine yielded pyruvate on transamination with alpha-ketoglutarate, and pyruvate was then converted to glucose or oxidized in the citric acid cycle. Glutamate also entered the citric acid cycle and a similar fall in glutamate/alpha-ketoglutarate ratio occurred.

Myocardial messenger RNA in malnourished rats was studied at the molecular level. Significant reductions in extractable amounts of both microsomal RNA and messenger RNA have been reported.[46] When a normal energy but protein-deficient diet was fed, the decreases in extractable microsomal RNA and mRNA were quantitatively similar but slightly less severe. Analysis of the intracellular distribution of cardiac microsomal RNA and mRNA indicated that mRNA did not accumulate in the cytoplasm but was rapidly degraded. During refeeding, mRNA was transported from the nucleus to the cytoplasm and engaged in polyribosome formation. The specific mRNA species coding for the myofibrillar proteins was affected to a similar extent by starvation, protein deprivation, and refeeding.

Other animal models studied include dogs, rabbits, and monkeys. A PEM syndrome in young monkeys showed early as well as late changes. The early changes included swelling and hydropic changes in the myofibers, together with eosinophilic coagulation and fragmentation of the sarcoplasm, hazy striations, small foci of necrosis, and infiltration with lymphocytes.[47] As the deficiency syndrome progressed, atrophy of muscle fibers dominated, with reduced heart size resulting from diminished muscle fiber size, without diminution in the number of fibers present. The sarcoplasmic reticulum and sarcolemmal membrane were normal.

Abel et al. in their study of dogs with PEM reported similar findings — atrophy of myofibers, interstitial edema,[48] and decreased left ventricular compliance and contractility.[48] They also documented significant depression of left ventricular systolic function at high filling pressures and decrease in left ventricular compliance and contractility.[48]

A rabbit model of PEM produced a reduction in total cardiac mass due to decreased nitrogen and glycogen content and an increase in fat content. Myocardial performance has also been shown to be depressed in rabbit models subjected to 6 weeks of protein depletion.[49]

Thus we find that animal studies have documented serially the myocardial changes of malnutrition similar to those observed in human autopsy findings. However, the functional significance of the degree of myocardial atrophy described has not been directly investigated. A critical degree of atrophy may affect cardiac function and sudden death may result from the predisposition of an atrophic heart to sudden cardiac arrest or ventricular fibrillation.

14.3.5 VITAMIN DEFICIENCIES

Vitamin A has been shown to be essential for normal fetal development in rats.[50] Maternal vitamin A deficiency in these animal models is associated in the offspring with defects in the aortic arch and dysmorphic hypoplastic ventricles.[51] No human counterpart has been described.

Thiamine (vitamin B_1) is essential for myocardial energy production; it is a coenzyme in the decarboxylation of alpha-keto acids and in the utilization of pentose in the hexose monophosphate shunt pathway. Deficiency leads to beriberi characterized by a high cardiac output state associated with arteriolar vasodilatation. Cardiac symptoms are common in infants breast-fed by thiamine-deficient mothers and mainly consist of right ventricular failures (systemic venous congestion). Clinical features include marked edema, warm extremities, wide pulse pressure, a third heart sound, and apical systolic murmur. Left ventricular failure including frank pulmonary edema is less frequent, although studies have documented elevated left ventricular end diastolic and pulmonary capillary wedge pressures[52,32] in affected patients.

Chest radiographs showed cardiomegaly, and ECG changes included low voltage QRS complexes, prolonged QT intervals, and inverted T waves. The abnormalities were reversible with thiamine therapy. Blood examination revealed elevated pyruvate and lactate and low red blood cell transketolase levels. Confirmation was by assay of thiamine in blood and other biological fluids. Although serum pyruvate levels were elevated in kwashiorkor patients, thiamine deficiency has not been identified to play a role in the pathogenesis of cardiac changes in this disease.

Vitamin C deficiency (scurvy) has been associated with sudden death from cardiac hypertrophy, especially of the right ventricle.[54] Chest pain and shortness of breath have been reported by human volunteers on a vitamin C-deficient diet. ECG changes included prolongation of PR intervals and abnormalities of the ST segments. These changes reversed rapidly with parenteral vitamin C administration. Degenerative changes of the myocardium have also been reported in the presence of deficiency.[55]

Pyridoxine (vitamin B$_6$)-deficient rats showed cardiomyopathic changes at postmortem examination; similar changes have not been described in humans. Vitamin D deficiency leads to hypocalcemia with associated cardiac changes (see calcium section below). Vitamin E deficiency in association with selenium deficiency has been shown to produce cardiomyopathy in young swine (see selenium section below).[56,57] Chronic vitamin E deficiency alone can produce cardiomyopathy in rats, zoo animals, and birds.[58,59]

14.3.6 ELECTROLYTE AND OTHER MINERAL DISTURBANCES

Electrolyte changes frequently complicate and influence the cardiac manifestations of PEM. Potassium, sodium, calcium, magnesium, and phosphorus are the most frequently implicated elements.[60]

14.3.6.1 Potassium

Potassium is the principal intracellular cation and helps regulate muscle contractions and cardiac rhythm. Deficiency associated with excess loss and poor oral intake accompanying gastroenteritis affects myocardial function profoundly.[61] Muffled heart sounds, poor myocardial systolic function, cardiac arrhythmias, and potentiation of digitalis effects are the manifestations. ECG changes include diminished voltages, prolongation of QT intervals, prominent U waves, and broadening and lowering of T waves. Histopathologic changes attributed to hypokalemia are myocyte necrosis with infiltration by neutrophils, lymphocytes, and macrophages.[54]

Hyperkalemia can complicate PEM, especially when associated with renal failure or severe metabolic acidosis. Cardiac arrhythmias and cardiac standstill are the manifestations. ECG changes parallel the degree of hyperkalemia. Tall (tented) T waves are early changes, followed progressively by prolongation of PR interval and QRS duration, and finally disappearance of P waves and formation of a sine-wave pattern.[62]

14.3.6.2 Sodium

Sodium is the principal cation in the extracellular compartment and plays an important role in the maintenance of osmotic equilibrium and systemic blood pressure. Hyponatremia, a frequent accompaniment of PEM, is the result of decreased intake and increased loss. Inappropriate antidiuretic hormone secretion associated with intercurrent infections also contributes. The major clinical manifestation are hypotension and cerebral edema.[63]

14.3.6.3 Calcium

Calcium ions are concerned in the linking of electrical stimulation to the contractile process in all muscle cells including cardiac muscles.[64] Coagulation of blood and maintenance of nerve irritability are also dependent on adequate calcium levels. Vitamin D deficiency is the major underlying factor leading to calcium deficiency in PEM. Acute heart failure and dilated cardiomyopathy responding to calcium infusion have been described in association with hypocalcemia.[65,66] Chest radiographs show cardiomegaly and pulmonary congestion. ECG changes include prolonged QT intervals.

Echocardiographic studies in patients with vitamin D deficiency (rickets) revealed left ventricular dilatation and dysfunction even in the absence of overt heart failure.[64] The most striking echocardiographic finding was an increase in the ratio of interventricular septal thickness to left ventricular posterior wall thickness that returned to normal after treatment. The heart failure of hypocalcemia is refractory to digitalis and diuretics, but responds to specific therapy that restores serum calcium to normal.[67]

14.3.6.4 Magnesium

Magnesium is a cofactor in all transphosphorylation reactions involving ATP and is therefore essential for energy metabolism. Prolonged losses of body fluids can result in magnesium deficiency[68] which in infants and children can manifest with hypotension, hypothermia, weak pulse, and shallow respiration. ECG studies showed unstable rate and rhythm, atrial dysrrhythmmias, low amplitude complexes, and inversion of left precordial T waves. These changes reversed with normalization of serum magnesium levels.[69] Hypomagnesemia also predisposed patients to digoxin toxicity. Animal models showed mitochondrial degeneration, focal myocardial hemorrhage, and myocardial necrosis and fibrosis.[70] Hypocalcemia and hypomagnesemia often coexisted.

14.3.6.5 Phosphate

Phosphorus forms an essential component of cells and plays a key role in energy transfer mechanisms. Deficiency can predispose individuals to cardiac arrhythmias[71] and myocardial dysfunction.[72] Replacement therapy helps restore these effects.

14.3.6.6 Selenium

Selenium is an essential component of the glutathione peroxidase enzyme that protects cells against oxidative damage by maintaining stability of mitochondrial membranes. Deficiency of selenium leads to defective cell membranes and disturbances of intracellular electrolytes and water composition as well as energy production. Experimental selenium deficiency in monkeys produced degeneration and necrosis of cardiac muscle.[73]

A combined deprivation of selenium and vitamin E produced patchy necrosis of the myocardium in young swine. Keshan disease, a form of necrotizing cardiomyopathy described in infants and children from China, is believed due to chronic selenium deficiency.[56] The disease is characterized by focal myocardial necrosis, fibrosis, and hypercontraction bands. Children with this disease develop heart failure and mortality is high. Provision of selenium resolves the cardiomyopathy. ECG changes include cardiac arrhythmias, varying forms of heart block, abnormal Q waves, and ST-T depression. Echocardiography reveals dilatation of cardiac chambers, especially the left ventricle, with hypokinesia.[56] Replacement therapy with selenium is known to reverse these changes.[74] In heart failure accompanying PEM, selenium deficiency has not been shown to have any etiologic role.

14.3.6.7 Iron

Iron is essential for blood formation and for the functioning of several enzymes.[75] Iron deficiency is the most common nutritional deficiency in developing and developed countries.[76,77] Cardiac effects are secondary to the increased blood volume and the effects of hypoxemia and iron deficiency on myocardial function. Tachycardia, cardiomegaly, and systolic murmurs are common manifestations.[78] Impaired ventricular performance observed in patients with iron deficiency anemia has been shown to improve following total dose infusion of iron, suggesting that the impairment was due to electrophysiological abnormalities of the heart induced by iron deficiency,[79] but these findings are not consistent.[78]

14.3.6.8 Copper

Copper is essential for red blood cell production, cytochrome C oxidase activity, and collagen formation. Deficiency occurs in preterm babies who have low copper reserves when fed modified cow's milk that is poor in copper. Impaired cardiac function, cardiac arrhythmias, and nonspecific ECG changes disappear on copper supplementation.[76]

14.3.7 MANAGEMENT OF PROTEIN ENERGY MALNUTRITION

Nutritional assessment forms an essential part of pediatric history taking and physical examination. Failure to thrive evokes a nutritional history and the need for a careful evaluation for features of PEM such as inappropriately low body weight and length and loss of muscle and subcutaneous fat with or without overt edema. The hair is thin, with bald patches on the occiput. Skin is hyperpigmented or hypopigmented, with areas of peeling and maculopapular eruptions. Other features include hepatomegaly, moon face, apathy, and hypotonia.

Laboratory studies show an early fall in blood urea and serum proteins, with later decreases of transferrin and hemoglobin.[80,81] Hypomagnesemia, hyponatremia, and hypokalemia should always be evaluated.[60] To achieve the best results in the treatment of PEM, it is recommended that a definitive and rational plan be followed, that common and serious complications be investigated and promptly treated, and intensive monitoring be undertaken. At the onset of therapy, fluid and electrolyte alterations should be treated slowly because of the risk of cardiac failure.[82,83] The same caution applies to restoring serum protein levels and to blood transfusions. Initial feeding should consist of an easily digestible lactose-free formula such as Pregestimil®, Nutramigen® or Vivonex®. The formula should be given in a diluted form initially, and then gradually increased to minimize the risk of diarrhea or syndromes of nutrition recovery.[84] Total parenteral nutrition should be used very sparingly and restricted to infants with persisting diarrhea in view of the high risk for serious infections. Antibiotics are administered only when specifically indicated. Finally, other specific nutrients such as iron, vitamins A, B complex, C, D, and K, zinc, and magnesium may also be needed. Magnesium is poorly absorbed from the gastrointestinal tract and must be included in parenteral fluids in cases where deficiency exists. Finally, prevention and early rehabilitation of PEM should focus on (1) special care and close follow-up of infants with high risk factors, (2) parent education concerning nutritional needs of children, especially those on vegetarian diets and those who do not consume adequate amounts of whole milk, and (3) better utilization of growth charts to screen children for malnutrition to facilitate early diagnosis and intervention.

14.3.8 Cardiac Complications during Recovery

During recovery, cardiac abnormalities are common[16,20,21,83] (Table 14.7). In one test series of Smythe et al.,[20] 13 of 98 infants with PEM died during therapy. Hypervolemia associated with the mobilization of edema fluid and severe anemia imposed excessive loads on the atrophic myocardium.[85] A hypermetabolic state accompanied by an increase in heart rate, blood pressure, and cardiac output ensued.[19,86] Large blood transfusions and high-sodium diets may also have contributed to the heart failure.[82] Wharton et al. also reported heart failure in malnourished children during recovery.[21,82]

TABLE 14.7
Cardiac Changes during Recovery from Malnutrition

Hypervolemia
Fluid and electrolyte disturbances
Ventricular arrhythmias
Cardiac failure
Cardiomegaly on chest radiograph
Normalization of electrocardiographic changes
Dilated cardiac chambers on echocardiography
Short circulation time
Low vascular resistance
Narrow arteriovenous oxygen difference

Congestive cardiac failure is common during the first week of therapy.[10,21,22,82] Fluid and electrolyte disturbances, infections, and anemia contribute to the pathogenesis.[87] High protein and salt intakes also contribute,[20,88] and vigorous diuretic use only worsens the outcome. Sudden death attributed to malignant ventricular arrhythmias can also occur during the first week. During therapy, chest radiographs initially show an increase in heart size in the first week attributable to increased chamber filling and subsequent slower increases that may be due to an increase in muscle bulk.

Signs of pulmonary venous congestion become evident occasionally during recovery, but cardiac size ultimately returns to normal. Cardiomegaly on a chest radiograph without overt heart failure is not uncommon.[20] The T wave and QRS voltage changes normalize. Echocardiography shows an enlarging cardiac mass, normal systolic function, and an increase in cardiac output.[22,26] Exercise testing or ambulatory ECG recording may reveal ventricular irritability during refeeding, and digitalis should be used with caution in such situations.[89] Failure to provide magnesium and potassium supplements may lead to progressive ECG abnormalities and arrhythmias that are potentially dangerous.[24,90] With refeeding and gain in weight, the cardiac output rises, and the T wave and QRS voltage changes normalize.[21,90] On echocardiography, left ventricular diameter enlarges with weight gain, but increases in wall thickness are more delayed.[22,89,91] Resting and maximal heart rates with exercise normalize, as do peak oxygen consumption and exercise duration.

Indicator dilution techniques show cardiac output in excess of age-matched controls,[18] but this may be only a reflection of the general increase in body metabolism as catch-up growth takes place. This is further supported by the short circulation time, low vascular resistance, and narrow arteriovenous oxygen differences in recovering patients.[28,92]

14.3.9 STUDIES OF ADULTS WITH SEVERE MALNUTRITION

Malnutrition is a feature of several adult diseases like anorexia nervosa, chronic illnesses including malignancy, and acquired immune deficiency disease, and also inflicts postoperative patients placed on prolonged periods of nutritional deprivation.[27,93–95] In human adult volunteers on a semistarvation regimen, significant reductions of heart rate, stroke volume, cardiac output, and heart size were observed. The fall in cardiac output, as in children, was only proportionate to the diminished metabolic requirements or reduction in body weight. The reduced cardiac output was associated with echocardiographically measured reductions in left ventricular end diastolic diameter and mass.[27]

Shortening fraction and radionuclide left ventricular ejection fraction were generally normal.[89,96,97] Hypotension and bradycardia were attributed to reduced levels of norepinephrine neurotransmitter during starvation.[98]

Cardiac changes are pronounced also in anorexia nervosa.[99] Responses of heart rate and blood pressure to exercise are reduced substantially, although resting bradycardia and hypotension are less common. Patients may develop arrhythmias including tachycardia, sinus arrest, and ectopic rhythms. Myocardial damage leading to nutritional cardiomyopathy has also been reported. ECG results are generally normal, but some patients exhibit nonspecific ST and T wave changes.[100] Some studies have found prolonged QT intervals, while others have not supported these findings.[27] A prolonged QT interval is an independent marker for arrhythmias and sudden death, and necessitates urgent attention especially when associated with bradycardia.[99]

Echocardiography revealed a reduced left ventricular mass and left ventricular afterload. Significant decreases in interventricular septal thickness and left ventricular posterior wall thickness have also been reported.[89,91] The systolic ejection phase indices of left ventricular function were normal and responded normally to exercise. With decrease in skeletal muscle mass, the response to exercise became restricted, with lower peak oxygen consumption. Reduced increments in heart rate and systolic pressure were also noted. Mitral valve prolapse (MVP) that resolved with weight gain was reported in as many as a third of patients.[101] It was attributed to enhanced ability to detect MVP in starving patients based on their intravascular volume depletion.[99]

Exercise testing was abnormal in patients with anorexia nervosa.[89,91,96,102] Other findings included decreased working capacity, maximal heart rate, increment in systolic blood pressure, and maximal VO_2. Norepinephrine and dopamine levels were significantly lower at peak exercise, but epinephrine levels were not significantly different from those of control patients.[102] Electrophysiologic changes included prolonged sinus node recovery time and AV nodal block at 70 beats/minute. Both conditions reversed with refeeding.

Experimental studies of food deprivation in rats showed biphasic responses in plasma catecholamine levels, with an initial increase followed 14 days later by a fall. Greater release of norepinephrine secondary to the stress of food deprivation explains the initial rise; the later fall is attributed to chronically reduced calorie intake.[103]

Patients who recover from anorexia show improvement in heart rate, posterior wall dimension, systolic wall stress, and left ventricular internal dimension.[104] A significant risk of heart failure exists in the first two weeks of recovery.[95] This has been attributed to reduced cardiac contractility and refeeding edema. Electrolyte disturbances also may be a factor.[105]

14.3.10 CONCLUSION

The major cardiovascular manifestations of malnutrition are related to the atrophy of the cardiac muscle, loss of energy sources, and complicating factors like infection, fluid retention, and electrolyte mineral disturbances. Cardiac failure and arrhythmias can lead to death especially during therapy. The paucity of recent human studies in relation to the cardiovascular manifestations of PEM is worth noting. Echocardiographic investigations of cardiac dimensions and systolic and diastolic function incorporating larger volumes of case material should be pursued. The feasibility of using other non-invasive techniques like magnetic resonance imaging should be explored during active disease process and recovery.

Animal studies should involve growing mammals and include ultrastructural studies of the disease process, myocardial metabolism, cardiac mechanics, responses to volume loading, afterloading, heart rate and changes in the inotropic state, and the assessment of effects of therapeutic interventions on contractile and electrophysiologic status. Although sudden death in PEM patients has been attributed to cardiac arrhythmias, more solid proof is required to support this hypothesis. At the molecular level, studies should be carried out to assess possible alterations in the contractile proteins, e.g., myosin heavy chains, as PEM develops. Molecular genetic studies should also be encouraged in order to determine the feasibility of genetic intervention in the prevention and therapy of cardiac complications of PEM.

14.4 MALNUTRITION IN CHILDREN WITH HEART DISEASES

This next section deals with the prevalence and pathogenesis of malnutrition in children with congenital and acquired heart diseases.

14.4.1 Nutritional Requirements in Children

Normal growth in infants and children depends on adequate nutrient deposit in two tissue compartments: lean body mass and fat mass. Lean body mass consists of proteins, minerals, water, and carbohydrates. Nutritional needs change as a child's body composition is altered by growth, age, gender, hormonal status, and genetic potential. Growth requires adequate intake of macronutrients (proteins, carbohydrates, and fats), as well as water, vitamins, minerals, and trace elements defined as per the recommended dietary allowances (RDAs) by the National Research Council.[6,7] These recommendations are based on studies of controlled diets, nutrient balance data, biochemical measurements, intake data of breast-fed infants, epidemiological studies, and in some instances, animal experimentation.

Several factors, including chronic illness, nutrient intolerance, and high nutrient losses, influence these recommendations. The route of delivery of nutrition (enteral versus parenteral) also alters the requirements. In addition, psychological factors within the family and society influence nutrient intake and eating behavior. Infants are at high risk of malnutrition because of their relatively high requirements for proteins, calories, and other nutrients when expressed per kilogram of body weight. Energy needs are supplied by carbohydrates and fat. When energy needs exceed intake and available stores, protein is used for energy. To promote nitrogen retention and growth, adequate energy calories must be available.

The identification and classification of malnutrition were discussed in a previous section of this chapter. Acute malnutrition causes a decrease in subcutaneous fat and muscle mass and is identified by more pronounced loss of weight rather than height. In chronic malnutrition, height and weight are affected proportionately. The severity of the deficit and whether it is acute or chronic affect a child's ability to return to previous growth potential with nutritional therapy.

14.4.2 Prevalence of Malnutrition in Children with Heart Disease

Malnutrition remains a major problem among children with CHD, especially those who are symptomatic with cardiac failure or cyanosis (Table 14.8). In 1962,

TABLE 14.8
Studies on Prevalence of Malnutrition in Children with Congenital Heart Diseases

Study	Year	Prevalence of Acute Malnutrition	Prevalence of Chronic Malnutrition
Mehzivi et al.[106]	1962	55%	52%
Cameron et al.[107]	1995	33%	64%
Thompson-Chagoyan et al.[109]	1998	Not reported	76%
Varan et al.[108]	1999	65%	42%
Venugopalan et al.[110]	2001	23%	24%

Mehzivi and Drash[106] reported 55 and 52% prevalence of acute and chronic malnutrition, respectively, in children with CHD. Cameron et al.[107] later found that both types of malnutrition still occurred in 33 and 64%, respectively, of hospitalized children with CHD even in the U.S. In Turkey, the frequency rates of acute and chronic malnutrition were reported as 65 and 42%, respectively,[108] while chronic malnutrition was documented in 76% of patients in a hospital-based study from Spain.[109]

Recent reports also have placed the prevalence of acute and chronic malnutrition among children with CHD attending a pediatric cardiology outpatient clinic at more than 20%.[110] The reports also noted that symptomatic infants are more severely affected, namely those with heart failure or cyanosis.[106,108,110] This is understandable because symptomatic infants have severe forms of CHD that can interfere with growth to a greater extent. Also infants were more severely affected than older children, as the symptomatic infants either underwent surgical intervention for their heart disease or had subsidence of symptoms secondary to the natural history of the CHD (e.g., reduction in size of ventricular septal defect).

Autopsy studies confirmed the frequent occurrence of malnutrition in CHD. Naeye[111] evaluated 220 individuals with congenital heart disease aged 1 month to 44 years and found that their body and organ weights were significantly reduced when compared to those of controls without CHD. Children aged 1 month to 8 years dying from congenital heart disease exhibited growth retardation and organ and cellular abnormalities seen in chronic malnutrition. Brain weights on autopsy showed growth retardation related to the degree of undernutrition. Measurements of brain weight, cell number, and cell size correlated with head circumference in infants. Winick et al.[112] showed that a reduction in head circumference was proportional to losses of brain weight, protein, and DNA content.

14.4.3 MECHANISMS AND CONSEQUENCES OF MALNUTRITION IN CHILDREN WITH HEART DISEASE

Several possible explanations for the poor growth of children with CHD exist.[113] See Table 14.9.

TABLE 14.9
Mechanisms Underlying Malnutrition in Congenital Heart Diseases

Mechanism	Cause
Inadequate intake	Poor appetite
	Feeding difficulty
	Respiratory infection
	Fluid restriction
	Side effects of medications
Poor absorption	Venous congestion
	Decreased lymphatic flow
Increased loss	Excessive vomiting
	Diarrhea
	Gastroesophageal reflux
Increased demand	Increased energy expenditure
	Greater proportion of lean body mass
	Catabolic state
Decreased growth potential	Decreased levels of IGF-I
	Chronic hypoxemia
	Poor glucose tolerance
	Low serum insulin levels
Extracardiac factors	Chromosomal anomalies
	Genetic syndromes
	Chronic systemic diseases
	Psychosocial problems

14.4.3.1 Poor Intake and Absorption

Inadequate calorie intake or absorption remains the predominant cause in most patients, especially for those who are symptomatic from congestive heart failure.[114] Several investigators documented low calorie intakes in patients with CHD compared with intakes of age-matched controls.[115] In their study of 22 children with CHD, Hansen and Dorup noted that the children consumed only 88% of RDAs and that most did not meet the recommendations for iron, zinc, calcium, and vitamins D, E, C, B_1, and B_6.[116] The energy intakes correlated with weight standard deviation (SD) scores. Thommessen et al. reported poor appetite and feeding problems among children with CHD, and the problems related well with the degree of malnutrition.[117]

Children with feeding problems also tended to eat less than children without feeding problems. Unger et al. found that underweight children with CHD consumed only 89% of RDAs whereas the figure was 108% in those with normal weights.[118] For most parents, feeding of infants and children with CHD involves difficulties, time, and anxiety. The feeding problems are related to anorexia, tachypnea, fatigue, excessive vomiting, and respiratory infections. The importance of poor intake is emphasized by studies that have shown significant improvement in growth with nutrient supplementation.[118,119] Rigorous fluid restriction before the advent of powerful diuretics also led to calorie restriction. However, the metabolic alkalosis and hypokalemia associated with diuretic use can also lead to anorexia and may inhibit effective protein anabolism by interfering with the maintenance of adequate sodium balance. Digitalis intoxication is another recognized cause of anorexia, but the symptom can occur even as a side effect of a standard dose.

Edema of the intestinal wall and mucosal surfaces may lead to impaired nutrient absorption and lymphatic drainage. Sondheimer and Hamilton[120] reported calorie losses in stools as both proteins and fats, but Menon and Poskitt[114] found no significant difference between stool losses of infants with heart disease and control patients. This factor is of importance when aggressive nutritional therapy with supplemental enteral feedings is attempted in these children. Excessive vomiting caused partly by gastroesophageal reflux may reduce the net intake of food.[121]

14.4.3.2   Energy Expenditure

Earlier studies by Krauss et al.[122] and Stocker et al.[123] revealed relative hypermetabolism in neonates and infants with CHD. More recently, Barton et al.[124] demonstrated significant elevation of total daily expenditures of energy in underweight infants with severe cardiac failure (CCF). In their study of 14 infants with CHD and severe failure to thrive, Yahav et al.[115] showed that an intake as high as 170 cal/kg was necessary for significant growth.

Clinical features that suggest increased metabolic rate in children with CHD include tachycardia, tachypnea, increased work of breathing, profuse sweating, early fatigue, and prolonged feedings. One of the reasons for this excess metabolic rate is the greater proportion of lean body mass, which expends greater energy compared to adipose tissue. Increased concentrations of tumor necrosis factor recorded in patients with cardiac cachexia may contribute by enhancing tissue catabolism.[125] It is also possible that increased energy expenditures in malnourished children with CHD are related to the malnutrition per se, as suggested by Krieger et al.[126] who found no significant differences in oxygen consumption in underweight infants with and without CHD.

14.4.3.3   Potential for Growth

Cyanotic heart disease is associated with proportionate retardation of weight and height, the severity depending on the degree of cyanosis.[127] Some studies suggest lower oxygen consumptions in cyanotic patients compared to those in heart failure,[122,128] although low calorie intake and high metabolic rate may still play roles in growth retardation in these children. Endocrine factors have also been implicated. Cyanotic newborn lambs have decreased levels of serum insulin-like growth factor I (IGF-I) without corresponding decreases in growth hormone and hepatic growth factor receptors.

Weintraub et al.[129] report that while IGF-I levels were linearly related to height and weight in patients with acyanotic CHD, no such correlation was found in their cyanotic patients. However, in their study of 29 children with cyanotic CHD Dundar et al.[130] found a positive correlation between serum IGF-I and degree of oxygen saturation. Thus, chronic hypoxemia may exert a direct or indirect effect to reduce serum IGF-I concentrations, thereby contributing to growth failure. Kanazawa found that children with left-to-right shunt lesions had poorer glucose tolerance and lower levels of serum insulin that improved after surgical correction of the heart disease.[131]

14.4.3.4 Extracardiac factors

Several factors like chromosomal anomalies, genetic syndromes, low birth weights, chronic systemic diseases affecting other organs, and psychosocial problems play major roles in significant numbers children with CHD and failure to thrive.[132–135] A population-based study reports that among children with CHD, 12.9% had chromosomal abnormalities and 13.9% had a recognizable or suspect syndrome, heritable disorder, or nonsyndromic malformation.[134] A significant number of patients had other extracardiac anomalies involving the musculoskeletal, neurologic, renal, and gastrointestinal systems. It is also worth noting that the birth weights of infants with major CHDs regardless of the presence or absence of extracardiac anomalies were reported to be low.[136]

14.4.3.5 Consequences of Malnutrition

Both short-term and long-term consequences of malnutrition associated with CHD have been described. Leite et al.[137] in their follow-up of surgically corrected CHD noted that malnourished children tended to have higher risks of postoperative complications including infections. Correction of a defect in early infancy will usually alleviate or prevent malnutrition and result in catch-up growth.[137] Sholler and Celermajer[138] analyzed 47 infants with CHD who underwent surgical correction in infancy and noted overall preoperative decreases in growth velocity that were reversed after surgery. At follow-up, 12 to 18 months later, most infants had regained at least their birth weight percentiles, while the subgroup with ventricular septal defects exceeded them.

Levy et al.[139] reported their results on the effect of surgical intervention on growth in 45 infants with simple D-transposition of the great arteries (DTGA) and found that growth failure was present in 8 of 45 patients 1 year postoperatively compared to preoperative presence in 25 patients. They also noted that all 8 patients with postoperative growth failure had one or more major residual hemodynamic abnormalities. The effect of surgical intervention on asymptomatic children with CHD has also been evaluated. Rhee et al. studied asymptomatic children with atrial septal defect (ASD) and failure to thrive of no obvious extracardiac etiology and found significant catch-up growth after surgical closure of ASD. This improvement was greater in children who were younger at the time of the repair.[140] This improvement may not occur in patients in whom a noncardiac factor is responsible for the failure to thrive, as was reported by Mainwaring et al.[141] in 1996. Poor growth without any other obvious contributing factor should be considered a relative indication for early ASD repair. This should be feasible with the widespread use of device (nonsurgical) closure ASDs and patent ductus arteriosus (PDAs), although the technique has still to catch up in the developing world.

Children with CHD are also at significant risk for long-term consequences of malnutrition, including continued growth failure, delayed development, and delayed cognitive skills, especially if intervention is delayed.[142,143] Compromised immune function has also been associated with cardiac cachexia.[144,145] Prolonged inadequate nutritional supplementation in a postcardiac surgery state worsens the deleterious effects of cardiac cachexia.[146]

14.4.4 MANAGEMENT

Children with CHD have been referred to as *nutritional challenges*. Most treatment strategies aim to facilitate catch-up growth by providing extra calories (as many as 220 cal/kg) and protein (as much as 4 gm/kg) that exceed the RDAs.[147] However, no single generally accepted set of guidelines defines appropriate caloric intake for catch-up growth. Even simple nutritional counseling has been shown to improve dietary intake and consequent catch-up growth in CHD patients.[118]

Follow-up evaluation in underweight patients showed improvement in mean dietary intakes (from 90 to 104% of the RDA of calories) and in mean percentage of ideal body weight for length after intervention (from 83.1 to 88.3%). Marin et al.[119] studied the effect of supervised administration of a hypercaloric whole cow's milk formula with sucrose, butter oil, and corn starch (1.29 kcal/ml) on nutritional recovery in malnourished infants with CHD and documented a mean weight gain of 2.7 g/kg/day.

When oral intake is insufficient to sustain growth, continuous feeding through nasogastric tube or gastrostomy is often helpful. Santini et al.[148] tried home enteral nutrition and found it effective and well-tolerated in a group of malnourished infants who included CHD patients. Percutaneous endoscopic gastrostomy provides a major improvement for children requiring long-term tube feeding, with high efficacy and low rates of complication,[149] even in infants with CHD. Despite all attempts, corrective intervention for the CHD where feasible provides the most gratifying results in terms of catch-up growth and development, and this should be possible with improvements in the surgical and nonsurgical management of CHD in the current decade.

14.4.5 CONCLUSION

Despite advances in the management of children with CHD, associated malnutrition continues to be a problem. For several decades, investigators have tried to identify the factors affecting growth in children with CHD. Cardiac malformations are undoubtedly responsible for malnutrition, but other associated diseases should not escape attention. Malnutrition per se can undermine the outcome of corrective surgical operations and postoperative recovery. Mechanisms linking CHD to malnutrition may be related to decreased energy intake and/or increased energy requirements.

Most treatment strategies aim to facilitate catch-up growth by providing extra calories and protein that exceed the RDAs for age. Early attention to the correction of the cardiac defect supplemented by a balanced nutritional care will help children with CHD thrive better.

14.5 FETAL ORIGIN OF ADULT HEART DISEASE

Fetal and infant nutrition have been postulated to influence adult onset cardiovascular and metabolic diseases, namely coronary heart disease, hypertension, and maturity onset diabetes mellitus. Scattered reports as early as 1934 made the observation that early environment in which a child grows may exert long-lasting effects on health.[150,151]

The hypothesis was formally suggested and substantiated first by David Barker and his team from the Medical Research Council's Environmental Epidemiology Unit at Southampton, U.K. They observed that the impact of the 20th century epidemic of coronary heart disease in Western countries paradoxically coincided with improved standards of living and nutrition, while prevalence was greatest in the most deprived areas.[152] These areas in the early 20th century had high rates of neonatal mortality and possibly of low birth weight. This led to the postulate that impaired fetal growth may have predisposed the survivors to heart disease in later life. The epidemiologic study that followed, although criticized by several sources, served to establish the need for further research. Several studies subsequently supported the association, but a few cast doubts on the validity of the concept. This section attempts to examine relevant studies in this regard and explain the basis of the suggested association.

14.5.1 EPIDEMIOLOGIC STUDIES

14.5.1.1 Fetal Growth and Coronary Heart Disease

14.5.1.1.1 Cross-Sectional Studies
These studies depend heavily on availability of accurate anthropometric measurements at birth and during infancy. Barker's group originally examined cardiovascular mortality in men born in Hertfordshire, England, in the early decades of the 20th century, for whom reliable records of weight at birth and at 1 year were available. They studied 5654 men born between 1911 and 1930 and found a progressive fall in future deaths from coronary heart disease between birth weights of 2500 and 4310 g.[153]

In a similar study involving 1586 men at Sheffield, standardized mortality ratios for cardiovascular disease fell from 119 in men with birth weights of 2495 g or less to 74 in those who weighed more than 3856 g.[154] Records of head circumference and length were also available for these patients, and the association of increased cardiovascular mortality also held true with decreasing head circumference and decreasing ponderal index (weight/length^2).

Periods of famine during the siege of Leningrad and later in the Netherlands provided opportunities to test the hypothesis. Stanner et al. investigated the development of risk factors for coronary heart disease in subjects exposed to starvation during the siege of Leningrad from 1941 through 1944.[155] They found no association between intrauterine exposure to maternal malnutrition and glucose intolerance, dyslipidemia, hypertension, and cardiovascular disease in adulthood. The intrauterine group showed higher concentrations of von Willebrand factor, a marker of endothelial damage, compared to the infant group; female subjects in the intrauterine group had stronger interactions between obesity and systolic and diastolic blood pressures than those in the infant group.

In contrast, studies of the Dutch famine in 1944 and 1945 revealed that among 736 subjects evaluated, the prevalence of coronary heart disease was higher in those exposed in early gestation than in nonexposed people (odds ratio = 3).[156] The prevalence was not increased in those exposed in mid- or late gestation. People with coronary heart disease tended to have lower birth weights and smaller head circumferences at birth, but the effect of exposure to famine in early gestation was independent of birth weight.

The lack of association noted in the seige of Leningrad study has been attributed to the longer duration of the famine and scarcity of food in the postfamine period that did not permit catch-up growth[157] (see Section 14.15.2 covering the "thrifty" phenotype hypothesis). Sampling bias, loss of patients during follow-up, and lack of reliable data on birth weight may explain the lack of association. Other possible explanations for the negative findings include the possibility that the effect of protein deprivation on fetal development is more marked in offspring of women with high carbohydrate intakes during pregnancy — a situation likely to prevail in malnourished populations of developing countries. This explanation follows the observations from human studies by Godfrey et al.[158] and in sheep by Barker et al.[159] Studies have also shown maternally transmitted intergenerational effects on birth weight.[160] It is possible that malnutrition for more than one generation is necessary before the relations between growth retardation and adult disease are seen.[161]

14.5.1.1.2 Longitudinal Studies

Forsen et al.[162] followed up 3447 women whose body sizes at birth were known and for whom an average of 10 measurements of height and weight were made during childhood. The researchers noted that the hazard ratio for women developing coronary heart disease increased by 10.2% for each centimeter decrease in length at birth. They also showed that the effect of short length at birth was greatest in women who achieved catch-up growth in height after birth. In contrast, men in the same cohort who developed the disease were thin at birth and showed catch-up growth in weight.

Thus, coronary heart disease in both men and women reflected poor prenatal nutrition and consequent catch-up growth in childhood. Martyn et al. commented that stunting and thinness at birth may represent two different responses to fetal undernutrition. Both have been associated with adult hypertension,[163] but stunting is associated with persistent changes in liver function (raised serum cholesterol[164] and plasma fibrinogen levels[165]), while thinness is associated with features of insulin resistance syndrome (impaired glucose tolerance and dyslipidemia).[166]

In another longitudinal study of 4630 men born in Helsinki, Erickson et al.[167] showed that regardless of size at birth, low weight gain during infancy was associated with increased risk of coronary heart disease. However after the age of 1 year, rapid weight gain was associated with further increase in risk, but only among boys who were thin at birth. The adverse effects of this association were evident even by the age of 3 years. They found two paths of growth associated with coronary heart disease. In one, thinness at birth was followed by rapid weight gain in childhood.

In the other, failure of infant growth was followed by persistent thinness during childhood. Both were associated with short stature in childhood.

Subsequent studies published by Barker et al.[168] attempted to evaluate the effects of poor living conditions in later life on the risk of coronary heart disease in the presence of small birth size. They studied 3676 men born in Helsinki, who were small at birth, or who grew slowly in infancy. They noted their social class and household income and evaluated their risk of death from coronary heart disease. The highest risk was in men who were thin at birth, but had accelerated weight gain after the age of 1 year followed by poor living standards in adult life. Low rates of fetal and infant growth, poor educational attainment, and low adult social class had independent effects on coronary heart disease. Low social class in childhood and low adult income did not give any additional prediction of disease. The psychosocial consequences of a low position in the social hierarchy as indicated by low income may lead to changes in the neuroendocrine pathways,[169] abnormal response to stress,[170] and earlier cardiovascular disease. This effect was more pronounced in those who had poor intrauterine and infantile growth.[171]

This study did not analyze the influences of diet, smoking, alcoholism, and other factors that have established associations with coronary heart disease. Of interest in this context is a study from Aberdeen, Scotland,[172] reporting that those who had lower scores in a mental ability test at the age of 12 years died younger. The authors suggested that performance in intelligence tests might also reflect general aspects of childhood fitness related to long-term health. Better intelligence may also act by modifying diet and social behavior in adult life.

14.5.1.2 Fetal Growth and Hypertension

The evidence for the association of adverse adult outcomes with lower birth weights is strongest for blood pressure and impaired glucose tolerance. In a 1988 study of a hospital-based Swedish population, Gennser et al. reported a higher risk of increased diastolic blood pressure in early adult life among men who were growth-retarded at birth than among those whose birth weights were appropriate for gestational age.[173]

Barker et al. published in 1989 an inverse relation independent of gestational age between systolic blood pressure and birth weight among a British sample of 9921 10-year-olds and 3259 adults aged 36 years.[174] They also showed that 10-year-olds living in areas with high cardiovascular mortality in England and Wales were shorter and had higher resting pulse rates than those living in other areas. Their mothers were also shorter and had higher diastolic blood pressures. The authors suggested that besides intrauterine environment, persisting geographical differences in childhood environment may contribute to the observed risk from hypertension. Another report from Barker's team in 1992 showed a strong trend of higher blood pressure in adult life with lower birth weight, lower ponderal index, and greater placental weight.[175]

Law et al. reported in 1993 that people of all ages beyond infancy who had lower birth weights also had higher systolic blood pressures. The systolic blood pressure was not related to growth during infancy independently of birth weight. The relation between systolic pressure and birth weight became larger with increasing age. Thus, after allowing for current body mass, systolic pressure at ages 64 through 71 years decreased by 5.2 mmHg for every kilogram increase in birth weight. They concluded that essential hypertension was initiated in fetal life, and elevated blood pressure was amplified from infancy to old age.[176]

Martyn et al., in a study of 337 adults reported in 1995, documented raised blood pressure in adult life in association with impaired fetal growth and showed that it was associated with decreased compliance in the conduit arteries of the trunk and legs.[163] Leon et al. suggested in 1996 that adult blood pressure is more markedly affected by obesity in individuals with intrauterine growth retardation than in those without growth retardation.[177]

A systematic review by Law et al. of all studies available in 1996 revealed that cross-sectional studies of prepubertal children and adults showed a negative relationship between blood pressure and birth weight that was independent of size at the time of the study.[178] The magnitude of the change in blood pressure tended to increase with age during childhood and adult life. However, the relationship in adolescents was inconsistent.

A subsequent study of Leningrad siege victims published in 1997 by Stanner et al. also showed that blood pressure was positively related to obesity.[155] However, the relationship between body mass index (BMI) and blood pressure (systolic and diastolic) was significantly stronger in the intrauterine group than in the infant group. This suggests that siege exposure and adult obesity may act synergistically to increase susceptibility to hypertension.

The latest publication of Barker's team[179] notes that children with low birth weights and thinness at birth followed by rapid compensatory growth (high BMIs at age 12), living in poor social conditions during childhood (low social class, few rooms in homes, poor educational achievements) had added risks of developing hypertension. However, the team's finding that living conditions in adult life did not present this influence is not well explained. One suggested explanation is that the influence of small birth weight on adult hypertension is related to the reduced number of nephrons in the kidneys of these children secondary to intrauterine malnutrition.[180] This reduction led to hyperperfusion of existing nephrons and early nephrosclerosis.[181] Rapid growth in childhood may exacerbate this process by increasing hyperperfusion and may explain the lack of influence of factors in adult life.

14.5.1.3 Fetal Growth and Other Risk Factors for Ischemic Heart Disease

Almost half the mass of beta cells present in the adult pancreas is formed during fetal life and early infancy.[182] In this context, adult onset diabetes mellitus and insulin deficiency and resistance have been studied in relation to fetal underweight. Hales et al. performed glucose tolerance tests in 64-year-old men from Hertfordshire, England, in 1991 and found that the odds ratios for development of glucose intolerance in those with birth weights <2500 g were 7 times those of men whose birth weights were above 4300 g.[183]

Similar risk was also associated with weight at 1 year of age after adjusting for current BMI and social class. Low birth weight was also shown in another study to be associated (odds ratio = 18) with a metabolic syndrome (postprandial hyperglycemia, systolic hypertension, and fasting hypertriglyceridemia) that has a well-known association with ischemic heart disease.[184] McCance et al. reported in 1994 a higher rate of diabetes in adults with birth weights < 2500 g compared to those with weights between 2500 and 4499 g (odds ratio = 3.8) when age, sex, BMI, maternal diabetes during pregnancy, and birth year were controlled.[185]

Increased serum cholesterol and fibrinogen and factor VII concentrations in adult life have also been linked to restricted fetal growth.[164,165] Phillips et al. reported that men and women who were thin at birth as measured by low ponderal indices were more prone to develop insulin resistance in adulthood.[186] Insulin resistance has also been documented in otherwise well prepubertal children born with intrauterine growth retardation (IUER), suggesting that insulin resistance may be one of the earliest metabolic abnormalities of such children.[187]

A study published in 2002[188] evaluated the influence of size at birth, during infancy, and throughout childhood growth (from ages 3 to 11 years) on the occurrence of coronary heart disease, type II diabetes mellitus, and hypertension. This longitudinal study by Barker et al. involved 13,517 men and women born from 1924 through 1944. Men and women who had birth weights above 4 kg and whose prepubertal BMIs at age 11 were in the lowest fourth had half the risk of coronary heart disease when compared with people whose birth weights were below 3 kg and BMIs were in the highest fourth. Similar strong associations were also recorded for hypertension and type II diabetes mellitus.

14.5.2 MECHANISMS PROPOSED TO EXPLAIN REPORTED ASSOCIATIONS

14.5.2.1 Fetal Origins Hypothesis

Fetal growth mainly occurs in the second and third trimesters of pregnancy. This growth is associated with cell division and depends on adequate supplies of nutrients and oxygen. Nutritional deficiency slows cell division directly or indirectly, acting through changes in growth factors or hormones, especially insulin and growth hormone. The timing of the malnutrition results in varying involvement of different organ systems, depending on their "critical periods" of growth. The size of the organ, distribution of cell types, patterns of hormonal secretion, metabolic activity, and structure may all be affected in such situations. The changes may persist and produce further alterations in function later in life.

In other words, fetal malnutrition may permanently change or "program" the body (fetal programming). For example, the critical period for muscle growth is around 30 weeks of gestation and little cell replication occurs after birth.[189] Babies who are thin at birth have thin muscles and this deficiency will persist. If these babies develop rapidly after birth, the development is often due to deposit of fat — a known cardiovascular and metabolic risk factor in adult life. Similarly, impaired liver development *in utero* may permanently impair liver function in later life, leading to high concentrations of low density lipoprotein cholesterol and fibrinogen.[190]

The epidemiologic association between low birth weight and increased risk of developing coronary heart disease, hypertension, and type II diabetes mellitus has been consistent.[184,191] The evidence led to the concept of fetal programming and the fetal origins hypothesis.[192–194] The hypothesis proposes that an adverse intrauterine environment alters the fetal metabolic and hormonal milieu, resulting in developmental adaptations to ensure fetal survival. If these adaptive responses designed for survival in a substrate-limited fetal environment persist into postnatal life, it is proposed that they lead to metabolic, cardiovascular, and endocrine disorders. Growth retardation that affects the development and vascularization of particular organs at different stages of fetal development will predispose an individual to impaired organ function, with consequent disease in later life.[192]

14.5.2.2 "Thrifty" Phenotype Hypothesis

This hypothesis has been invoked to explain why people with similar intrauterine exposures to malnutrition behave differently later, depending on the degree of catch-up growth after birth. Animal studies show that this "compensatory growth" shortens survival.[195] The consequent rapid rates of cell division may lead to changes in genetic material and earlier cell death.[196] Rapid childhood weight gain also has been shown to increase the risk of disease associated with small body size at birth and during infancy.

The structural and metabolic alternations induced *in utero* by adverse environment entrain both selective preservation of key organs and metabolic adaptations that are of advantage in a restricted postnatal life. If nutrition becomes plentiful postnatally, these changes predispose to obesity and impaired glucose tolerance. This has been substantiated by the Dutch Famine study in which poor nutrition in the first trimester was associated with increased obesity in 19-year-old males.[197] This obesity and the consequent metabolic syndrome predispose an individual to coronary heart disease later in life.

These studies led to the "thrifty" phenotype hypothesis that attributes these suggested associations to the programming of metabolism and function of a tissue or organ as a result of diminished supplies of certain nutrients during critical stages of development.[184,198] The effects of impaired fetal growth are modified by subsequent growth; the highest risks of heart disease, type II diabetes, insulin resistance syndrome, and impaired glucose tolerance (all but heart disease are collectively referred to below as *impaired glucose tolerance*) appear in those who were small at birth and became overweight adults.[199]

14.5.2.3 Genetic Explanations

Three genetic mechanisms have been postulated to explain the fetal origin of adult heart disease, but none has been confirmed by strong evidence. The thrifty genotype hypothesis[200] suggests that in the early stages of evolution, a series of genes that adapted the individual to the intermittent availability of food may have been selected. This survival advantage may be detrimental to health when food availability is in abundance — leading to cardiovascular and metabolic diseases.

The surviving small baby genotype hypothesis states that babies with low birth weights also have an enrichment of genes that initially confers a survival advantage but becomes detrimental to health in later life.[186] The fetal insulin hypothesis proposes that genetically determined insulin resistance causes growth retardation *in utero* and cardiovascular and metabolic diseases in later life.[201] Experimental support for all these hypotheses is·lacking, and no single hypothesis can explain fully the reported strong epidemiologic association between fetal and infant nutrition and adult onset cardiovascular and metabolic diseases.

14.5.3 ANIMAL STUDIES

Animal models have shown that even brief periods of undernutrition can reduce the sizes of organs[202] and also lead to persisting changes in blood pressure, cholesterol metabolism, insulin response to glucose, and other metabolic, endocrine, and immune functions.[203] Animals also exhibit "phenotypic plasticity" and express a range of different phenotypes dependent on environmental conditions during development.[204] The size of an offspring is dependent on the size of the mother and on the availability of food.[205] Size at birth for gestational age serves as a marker of fetal nutrition.[206]

Studies have confirmed the association of intrauterine protein deficiency in pregnant animals with impaired pancreatic function[207–209] and increased blood pressure in later life.[210] These conditions may be explained by permanent alterations in the expressions of glucocorticoid receptors in specific tissues of the offspring and hyperactivity of the hypothalamic–pituitary–adrenal axis documented in animal studies.[211] Exposure of the fetus to excess glucocorticoids has been shown to result in both reduced weight at birth and permanent hypertension and hyperglycemia in adult life.[212,213]

Postnatal environmental factors are important in the etiology of adult onset disease, and studies on the effect of hypercaloric nutrition in growth-retarded animals have supported this observation. Hyperphagia in rats subjected to fetal food deprivation led to hyperinsulinism and hyperleptinemia.[214] Although increased plasma insulin levels are normally associated with reduced appetite,[215] the hyperinsulinism seen in experimentally programmed rats likely reflects insulin resistance and reduced insulin action, as seen in children born with IUGR.[187] This secondary hyperinsulinism can have stimulating and undesirable effects such as chronic renal sodium retention and increased sympathetic nervous system activity, whereas resistance in other tissues such as endothelium can result in impaired vasodilatation.[216,217] In addition, the kidneys in the growth-retarded animals were smaller, suggesting a renal component of the hypertension.[218]

Vitamin A deficiency *in utero* in animal models has been shown to result in a decrease in elastin and increase in growth arrest-specific gene-6 expression in both lungs and heart of the offspring. The consequent changes in lung function led to higher neonatal mortality in the offspring. Those who did not succumb to lung failure may have been affected by later-appearing heart defects.[219] Studies with cell culture systems have shown that the active forms of vitamin A, retinal and retinoic acid, serve as signals to regulate the expression of genes during vertebrate development.[220]

14.5.4 CONCLUSION

Epidemiologic evidence supports the association between poor growth *in utero* and higher prevalence of adult onset ischemic heart disease, hypertension, and diabetes

---

TABLE 14.10
Influence of Fetal and Infant Nutrition on Adult Onset Cardiovascular and Metabolic Diseases

What We Know

Low birth weight is associated with increased risk of coronary heart disease, hypertension, and adult onset diabetes mellitus.

Thinness and shortness at birth have been specifically associated with a metabolic syndrome, while both large and small placenta may lead to hypertension.

The increased risk is independent of confounding variables like smoking, diet, exercise, etc.

Influences that act in postnatal life such as low socioeconomic status, accelerated weight gain in childhood, and adult onset obesity can add to the effects of low birth weight.

What We Do Not Know

Retrospective studies establish only an association and do not necessarily mean a cause-and-effect relationship.

Smallness or thinness at birth need not always imply maternal malnutrition.

Explanations offered for the observed association are not fully evidence based.

Further prospective clinical studies and basic research on pathophysiology are needed.

---

mellitus (Table 14.10). The most unfavorable growth pattern seems to be smallness and thinness at birth, continued slow growth in early childhood, and then accelerated growth secondary to dietary excesses. In the case of hypertension, the risk has been shown to be increased by low social class, few rooms in the home, and poor educational achievement. Improving maternal and infant health may be the key to effective prevention of cardiovascular disease in adult life.

However, prospective controlled studies are lacking and the economic, political, and social contexts of life have not been taken into account in most of the available studies. The explanations for the observed associations must be understood better, and closer awareness and cooperation between epidemiological investigators and those studying mechanistic biological issues will hopefully solve these issues.

Most studies have assumed that early growth retardation is synonymous with fetal malnutrition, and this in turn is related to maternal supplies of nutrients during pregnancy. Finally, the question remains whether improving a mother's growth and nutrition before and during pregnancy will translate into decreasing prevalence of these adult onset cardiovascular and metabolic diseases.

REFERENCES

1. Bellamy C., *The State of the World's Children 2000*, United Nations Children's Fund, Geneva, 2000, 3.
2. Allen, L.H., Nutritional influences on linear growth: a general review, *Eur. J. Clin. Nutrition*, 48 (Suppl. 1), S75, 1994.
3. Neumann, C.G. and Harrison, G.G., Onset and evolution of stunting in infants and children: examples from the Human Collaborative Research Support Programme Kenya and Egypt studies, *Eur. J. Clin. Nutr.*, 48 (Suppl. 1), S90, 1994.

4. Martorell, R., Results and implications of the INCAP follow-up study, *J. Nutr.*, 125, 1127S, 1995.

5. Super, C.M., Herrera, M.G., and Mora, J.O., Long-term effects of food supplementation and psychosocial intervention on the physical growth of Colombian infants at risk of malnutrition, *Child Dev.*, 61, 29, 1990.

6. Food and Nutrition Board, *Recommended Dietary Allowances*, 10th ed., National Academy of Sciences, Washington, D.C., 1989, 3.

7. World Health Organization Study Group, *Diet, Nutrition, and the Prevention of Chronic Diseases*, WHO Technical Report Series 797, Geneva, 1990, 1.

8. John, T.J. et al., Kwashiorkor not associated with poverty, *J. Pediatr.*, 90, 730, 1977.

9. Committee on Nutrition, *Pediatric Nutrition Handbook*, American Academy of Pediatrics, Elk Grove Village, IL, 1979, 59.

10. Chase, H.P. et al., Kwashiorkor in the United States, *Pediatrics*, 66, 972, 1980.

11. Waterlow, J.C., Classification and definition of protein-calorie malnutrition, *Br. Med. J.*, 3, 566, 1972.

12. Oslon, R.E., Introductory remarks: nutrient, hormone, enzyme interactions, *Am. J. Clin. Nutr.*, 28, 626, 1975.

13. Jaya-Rao, K.S., Evolution of kwashiorkor and marasmus, *Lancet*, I, 709, 1974.

14. Schelp, F.P. et al., Are proteinase inhibitors a factor for the derangement of homeostasis in protein-energy malnutrition? *Am. J. Clin. Nutr.*, 31, 451, 1978.

15. Classification of infantile malnutrition (editorial), *Lancet*, 1, 302, 1970.

16. Heymsfield, S.B. and Nutter, D.O., The heart in protein-calorie undernutrition, in *The Heart Update*, Hurst, J.W., Ed., McGraw-Hill, New York, 1979, 191.

17. Chaithiraphan, S., The heart in protein-energy malnutrition, *J. Med. Assoc. Thailand*, 69, 170, 1986.

18. Alleyne, G.A., Cardiac function in severely malnourished Jamaican children, *Clin. Sci.*, 30, 553, 1966.

19. Viart, P., Hemodynamic findings during treatment of protein-calorie malnutrition, *Am. J. Clin. Nutr.*, 31, 911, 1978.

20. Symthe, P.M., Swanepoel. A., and Campbell, J.A.H., The heart in kwashiorkor, *Br. Med. J.*, 1, 67, 1962.

21. Wharton, B.A. et al., The myocardium in kwashiorkor, *Q. J. Med.*, 38, 106, 1969.

22. Heymsfield, S.B. et al., Cardiac abnormalities in cachectic patients before and during nutritional repletion, *Am. Heart J.*, 95, 584, 1978.

23. Piza, J. et al., Myocardial lesions and heart failure in infantile malnutrition, *Am. J. Trop. Med. Hyg.*, 20, 343, 1971.

24. Caddell, J.L. and Goddard, D.R., Studies in protein-calorie malnutrition, *New Engl. J. Med.*, 276, 533, 1967.

25. Thurston, J. and Marks, P., Electrocardiographic abnormalities in patients with anorexia nervosa, *Br. Heart J.*, 36, 719, 1974.

26. Shoukry, I. et al., Cardiac atrophy and ventricular function in infants with severe protein-calorie malnutrition (kwashiorkor disease), in *Pediatric Cardiology*, Doyle, E.E. et al., Eds., Springer-Verlag, New York, 1986, 1169.

27. Moodie, D.S., Anorexia and the heart: results of studies to assess effects, *Postgrad. Med.*, 81, 46, 1987.

28. Viart, P., Hemodynamic findings in severe protein-calorie malnutrition, *Am. J. Clin. Nutr.* 30, 334, 1977.

29. Schimmel, M. and Utiger, R.D., Thyroidal and peripheral production of thyroid hormones, *Ann. Intern. Med.*, 87, 760, 1977.

30. Landsberg, L. and Young, J.B., Fasting, feeding and regulation of the sympathetic nervous system, *New Engl. J. Med.*, 298, 12951, 1978.
31. Alleyne, G.A.O., Plasma and blood volume in severely malnourished Jamaican children, *Arch. Dis. Child.*, 41, 313, 1960.
32. Mukherjee, A., Dey, T.K., and Battacharya, A.K., Cardiac pathology in classical and marasmic kwashiorkor, *Indian J. Pathol. Microbiol.*, 25, 207, 1982.
33. Ramalingaswami, V., Nutrition and the heart, *Cardiologia*, 52, 57, 1968.
34. Isner, J.M. et al., Anorexia nervosa and sudden death, *Ann. Intern. Med.* 102, 49, 1985.
35. Sims, B.A., Conducting tissue of the heart in kwashiorkor, *Br. Heart J.*, 34, 828, 1972.
36. Rossi, M.A. et al., Effect of protein-calorie malnutrition on catecholamine levels and weight of heart in rats, *J. Neural. Transm.*, 48, 85, 1980.
37. Rossi, M.A. et al., Noradrenaline levels and morphological alterations of myocardium in experimental protein-calorie malnutrition, *J. Pathol.* 131, 83, 1980.
38. Pissaia, O., Rossi, M.A., and Oliveira, J.S., The heart in protein-calorie malnutrition in rats: morphological, electrophysiological and biochemical changes, *J. Nutr.*, 110, 2035, 1980.
39. Rossi, M.A. and Zucoloto, S., Ultrastructural changes in nutritional cardiomyopathy of protein-calorie malnourished rats, *Br. J. Exp. Pathol.*, 63, 242, 1982.
40. Alden, P.B. et al., Left ventricular function in malnutrition, *Am. J. Physiol.*, 253, H380, 1987.
41. Balasubramanian, V. and Dhalla, N.S., Biochemical basis of heart function: effect of starvation on storage, transport and synthesis of cardiac norepinephrine in rats, *Can. J. Physiol. Pharmacol.*, 50, 238, 1972.
42. Benfey, B.G., Varma, D.R., and Yue, T.L., Myocardial inotropic responses and adrenoreceptors in protein-deficient rats, *Br. J. Pharmacol.*, 80, 527, 1983.
43. Freund, H.R. and Holroyde, J., Cardiac function during protein malnutrition and refeeding in the isolated rat heart, *J. Parenter. Enteral Nutr.*, 10, 470, 1986.
44. Nutter, D.O. et al., The effect of chronic protein-calorie undernutrition in the rat on myocardial function and cardiac function, *Circ. Res.*, 45, 144, 1979.
45. Gold, A.M. and Yaffe, S.R., Effect of prolonged starvation on cardiac energy metabolism in the rat, *J. Nutr.*, 108, 410, 1978.
46. Zahringer, J. et al., Influence of starvation and total protein deprivation on cardiac mRNA levels, *Basic Res. Cardiol.*, 80, 1, 1985.
47. Chauhan, S., Nayak, N.C., and Ramalingaswami, V., The heart and skeletal muscle in experimental protein-calorie malnutrition in rhesus monkeys, *J. Pathol. Bacteriol.*, 90, 301, 1965.
48. Abel, R.M. et al., Adverse hemodynamic and ultrastructural changes in dog hearts subjected to protein-calorie malnutrition, *Am. Heart J.*, 97, 733, 1979.
49. Kuykendall, R.C. et al., Biochemical consequences of protein depletion in the rabbit heart, *J. Surg. Res.* 43, 62, 1987.
50. Antipatis, C., Grant, G., and Ashworth, C.J., Moderate maternal vitamin A deficiency affects perinatal organ growth and development in rats, *Br. J. Nutr.*, 84, 125, 2000.
51. Wilson, J.G. and Warkany, J., Aortic arch and cardiac anomalies in the offspring of vitamin A deficient rats, *Am. J. Anat.*, 85, 113, 1949.
52. Akbarian, M., Yankopoulos, N.A., and Abelmann, W.H., Hemodynamic studies in beriberi heart disease, *Am. J. Med.*, 41, 197, 1966.
53. Ayzenberg, O., Silber, M.H., and Bortz, D., Beriberi heart disease: a case report describing the hemodynamic features, *S. Afr. Med. J.*, 68, 263, 1985.
54. Scotti, T.M., Heart, in *Pathology*, 7th ed., Anderson, W.A.D. and Kissane, J.M., Eds., Mosby–Year Book, St. Louis, 1977, 737.

55. Levine, M., New concepts in the biology and biochemistry of ascorbic acid, *New Engl. J. Med.*, 314, 892, 1986.

56. Xu, G.L. et al., Further investigation on the role of selenium deficiency in the aetiology and pathogenesis of Keshan disease, *Biomed. Environ. Sci.*, 10, 316, 1997.

57. Van Vleet, J.F., Ferrans, V.J., and Ruth, G.R., Ultrastructural alterations in nutritional cardiomyopathy of selenium-vitamin E deficient swine I: fiber lesions, *Lab. Invest.*, 37, 188, 1977.

58. Lin, C.T. and Chen, L.H., Ultrastructural and lysosomal enzyme studies of skeletal muscle and myocardium in rats with long-term vitamin E deficiency, *Pathology*, 14, 375, 1982.

59. Liu, S.K., Dolensek, E.P., and Tappe, J.P., Cardiomyopathy and vitamin E deficiency in zoo animals and birds, *Heart Vessels* 1 (Suppl.), 288, 1985.

60. Leier, C.V., Dei-Cas, L., and Metra, M., Clinical relevance and management of the major electrolyte abnormalities in congestive heart failure: hyponatremia, hypokalemia, and hypomagnesemia, *Am. Heart J.* 128, 564, 1994.

61. Dietz, T., Bissett, J.K., and Talley, J.D., The effects of hypokalemia on the heart, *J. Ark. Med. Soc.*, 94, 79, 1997.

62. Mattu, A., Brady, W.J., and Robinson, D.A., Electrocardiographic manifestations of hyperkalemia, *Am. J. Emerg. Med.*, 18, 721, 2000.

63. Gross, P., Wehrle, R., and Bussemaker, E., Hyponatremia: pathophysiology, differential diagnosis and new aspects of treatment, *Clin. Nephrol.* 46, 273, 1996.

64. Uysal, S., Kalayci, A.G., and Baysal, K., Cardiac functions in children with vitamin D deficiency rickets, *Pediatr. Cardiol.*, 20, 283, 1999.

65. Abdullah, M. et al., Dilated cardiomyopathy as a first sign of nutritional vitamin D deficiency rickets in infancy, *Can. J. Cardiol.*, 15, 699, 1999.

66. Gulati, S. et al., Hypocalcemic heart failure masquerading as dilated cardiomyopathy, *Indian J. Pediatr.*, 68, 287, 2001.

67. Bashour, T., Basha, H.S., and Cheng, T.O., Hypocalcemic cardiomyopathy, *Chest*, 78, 663, 1980.

68. Al-Ghamdi, S.M., Cameron, E.C., and Sutton, R.A., Magnesium deficiency: pathophysiologic and clinical overview, *Am. J. Kidney Dis.*, 24, 737, 1994.

69. Agus, M.S. and Agus, Z.S., Cardiovascular actions of magnesium, *Crit. Care Clin.*, 17, 175, 2001.

70. Freedman, A.M. et al., Magnesium deficiency-induced cardiomyopathy: protection by vitamin E, *Biochem. Biophys. Res. Commun.*, 170, 1102, 1990.

71. Venditti, F. et al., Hypophosphatemia and cardiac arrythmias, *Min. Electrolyte Metab.*, 13, 19, 1987.

72. Zazzo, J.F. et al., High incidence of hypophosphatemia in surgical intensive care patients: efficacy of phosphorus therapy on myocardial function, *Intensive Care Med.*, 21, 826, 1995.

73. Burke, R.F., Selenium in man, in *Trace Elements in Human Health and Disease*, Prasad, A.S., Ed., Academic Press, New York, 1976, 105.

74. Saito, Y. et al., Effect of selenium deficiency on cardiac function of individuals with severe disabilities under long-term tube feeding, *Dev. Med. Child Neurol.*, 40, 743, 1998.

75. Uchida, T., Overview of iron metabolism, *Int. J. Hematol.*, 62, 193, 1995.

76. National Research Council, *Diet and Health: Implications for Reducing Chronic Disease Risk (Report of Committee on Diet and Health, Food and Nutrition Board)*, National Academy Press, Washington, D.C., 1989, 750.

77. Cook, J.D., Skikne, B.S., and Baynes, R.D., Iron deficiency: the global perspective, *Adv. Exp. Med. Biol.*, 356, 219, 1994.
78. Hayashi, R. et al., Cardiovascular function before and after iron therapy by echocardiography in patients with iron deficiency anemia, *Pediatr. Int.* 41, 13, 1999.
79. Alvares, J.F., Oak, J.L., and Pathare, A.V., Evaluation of cardiac function in iron deficiency anemia before and after total dose iron therapy, *J. Assoc. Physicians India*, 48, 204, 2000.
80. Kumar, V. et al., Alterations in blood biochemical tests in progressive protein malnutrition, *Pediatrics*, 49, 736, 1972.
81. Kumar, V., Chandrasekran, R., and Belavalgidad, M.S., Blood biochemical tests in the diagnosis of malnutrition in children, *Indian Pediatr.*, 12, 955, 1975.
82. Wharton, B.A., Howels, G.R., and McCance, R.A., Cardiac failure in kwashiorkor, *Lancet*, 2, 384, 1967.
83. Foxx-Orenstein, A., Jensen, G.L., and McMahon, M.M., Overzealous resuscitation of an extremely malnourished patient with nutritional cardiomyopathy, *Nutr. Rev.*, 48, 406, 1990.
84. Wharton, B.A., Syndromes of treatment in infantile malnutrition, *East Afr. Med. J.*, 43, 570, 1966.
85. Webb, J.G., Kiess, M.C., and Chan-Yan, C.C., Malnutrition and the heart, *Can. Med. Assoc. J.*, 135, 753, 1986.
86. Montgomery, R.D., Changes in the basal metabolic rates of the malnourished infant and their relation to body composition, *J. Clin. Invest.*, 41, 1653, 1962.
87. Viart, P., Blood volume changes during treatment of protein-calorie malnutrition, *Am. J. Clin. Nutr.*, 30, 349, 1977.
88. Edozien, J.C. and Rahim-Khan, M.A., Anemia in protein malnutrition, *Clin. Sci.*, 34, 315, 1968.
89. Gottdiener, J.S. et al., Effects of self-induced starvation on cardiac size and function in anorexia nervosa, *Circulation*, 58, 425, 1978.
90. Caddell, J.L. and Olson, R.E., An evaluation of the electrolyte status of malnourished Thai children, *J. Pediatr.*, 83, 124, 1973.
91. St. John Sutton, M.G. et al., Effects of reduced cross-ventricular mass on chamber architecture, load, and function: a study of anorexia nervosa, *Circulation*, 72, 991, 1985.
92. Viart, P., Blood volume changes during treatment of protein-calorie malnutrition, *Am. J. Clin. Nutr.*, 30, 349, 1977.
93. Bistrian, B.R. et al., Prevalence of malnutrition in general medical patients, *JAMA*, 235, 1567, 1976.
94, Abel, R.M. et al., Malnutrition in cardiac surgical patients: results of a prospective randomized evaluation of early post-operative parenteral nutrition, *Arch. Surg.*, 111, 45, 1976.
95. Fisler, J.S., Cardiac effects of starvation and semi-starvation diets: safety and mechanisms of action, *Am. J. Clin. Nutr.*, 56 (Suppl.), 230S, 1992.
96. Moodie, D.S. and Salcedo, E., Cardiac function in adolescents and young adults with anorexia nervosa, *J. Adol. Health Care*, 4, 9, 1983.
97. Kothari, S.S. et al., Left ventricular mass and function in children with severe protein energy malnutrition, *Int. J. Cardiol.*, 35, 19, 1992.
98. Pirke, K.M., Central and peripheral noradrenaline regulation in eating disorders, *Psychiatr. Res.*, 62, 43, 1996.
99. Cooke, R.A. and Chambers, J.B., Anorexia nervosa and the heart, *Br. J. Hosp. Med.* 54, 313, 1995.

100. Palossy, B. and Oo, M., ECG alterations in anorexia nervosa, *Adv. Cardiol.*, 19, 280, 1977.
101. Meyers, D.G. et al., Mitral valve prolapse in anorexia nervosa, *Ann. Intern. Med.*, 105, 384, 1986.
102. Nudel, D.B. et al., Altered exercise performance and abnormal sympathetic responses to exercise in patients with anorexia nervosa, *J. Pediatr.*, 105, 34, 1984.
103. Hilderman, T. et al., Effects of long-term dietary restriction on cardiovascular function and plasma catecholamines in the rat, *Cardiovasc. Drugs Ther.*, 10, 247, 1996.
104. Gould, L. et al., Evaluation of cardiac conduction in anorexia nervosa, *Pacing Clin. Electrophysiol.*, 3, 660, 1980.
105. Veverbrants, E. and Arky, R.A., Effects of fasting and refeeding I: studies on sodium, potassium and water excretion on a constant electrolyte and fluid intake, *J. Clin. Endocrinol. Metab.*, 29, 55, 1969.
106. Mehziri, A. and Drash, A., Growth disturbance in congenital heart disease, *J. Pediatr.*, 61, 418, 1962.
107. Cameron, J.W., Rosenthal, A., and Olson, A.D., Malnutrition in hospitalized children with congenital heart disease, *Arch. Pediatr. Adolesc. Med.*, 149, 1098, 1995.
108. Varan, B., Tokel, K., and Yilmaz, G., Malnutrition and growth failure in cyanotic and acyanotic congenital heart disease with and without pulmonary hypertension, *Arch. Dis. Child.*, 81, 49, 1999.
109. Thompson-Chagoyan, O.C. et al., The nutritional status of the child with congenital cardiopathy, *Arch. Inst. Cardiol. Mex.*, 68, 119, 1998.
110. Venugopalan, P. et al., Malnutrition in children with congenital heart defects, *Saudi Med. J.*, 22, 964, 2001.
111. Naeye, R.L., Anatomic features of growth failure in congenital heart disease, *Pediatrics*, 39, 433, 1967.
112. Winick, M. and Rosso, P., Head circumference and cellular growth of the brain in normal and marasmic children, *J. Pediatr.*, 74, 774, 1969.
113. World Heath Organization, *Management of Severe Malnutrition: A Manual for Physicians and Senior Health Workers*, Geneva, 1999, 41.
114. Menon, G. and Poskitt, E., Why does congenital heart disease cause failure to thrive? *Arch. Dis. Child.*, 60, 1134, 1985.
115. Yahav, J. et al., Assessment of intestinal and cardiorespiratory function in children with congenital heart disease on high caloric formulas, *J. Pediatr. Gastroenterol. Nutr.*, 4, 778, 1985.
116. Hansen, S.R. and Drup, I., Energy and nutrition intakes in congenital heart disease, *Acta Paediatr.*, 82, 166, 1993.
117. Thommessen, M., Heiberg, A., and Kase, B.F., Feeding problems in children with congenital heart disease: the impact on energy intake and growth outcome, *Eur. J. Clin. Nutr.*, 46, 457, 1992.
118. Unger, R. et al., Calories count: improved weight gain with dietary intervention in congenital heart disease, *Am. J. Dis. Child.*, 146, 1078, 1992.
119. Marin, V. et al., Nutritional recovery in infants with congenital heart disease and severe malnutrition using a hypercaloric diet, *Rev. Child Pediatr.*, 61, 303, 1990.
120. Sondheimer, J.M. and Hamilton, J.R., Intestinal function in infants with severe congenital heart disease, *J. Pediatr.*, 92, 572, 1978.
121. Weesner, K.M. and Rosenthal, A., Gastroesophageal reflux in association with congenital heart disease, *Clin. Pediatr.*, 22, 424, 1983.
122. Krauss, A.N. and Auld, P.A.M., Metabolic rate of neonates with congenital heart disease, *Arch. Dis. Child.*, 50, 539, 1975.

123. Stocker, F.P. et al., Oxygen consumption in infants with heart disease: relationship to severity of congestive failure, relative weight and caloric intake, *J. Paediatr.*, 80, 43, 1972.

124. Barton, J.S. et al., Energy expenditure in congenital heart disease, *Arch. Dis. Child.*, 70, 5, 1994.

125. McMurray, J. et al., Increased concentrations of tumor necrosis factor in cachectic patients with severe chronic heart failure, *Br. Heart J.*, 66, 356, 1991.

126. Krieger, I., Growth failure in congenital heart disease: energy and nitrogen balance in infants, *Am. J. Dis. Child.*, 120, 497, 1970.

127. Baum, D., Beck, R.Q., and Haskell, W.L., Growth and tissue abnormalities in young people with cyanotic congenital heart disease receiving systemic pulmonary shunts, *Am. J. Cardiol.*, 52, 349, 1983.

128. Kennaird, D.L., Oxygen consumption and evaporative water loss in infants with congenital heart disease, *Arch. Dis. Child.*, 51, 34, 1976.

129. Weintraub, R.G., Menahem, S., and Werther, G., Serum Insulin-like growth factor I levels in patients with congenital heart disease, *Aust. Paediatr. J.*, 25, 324, 1989.

130. Dundar, B. et al., Chronic hypoxemia leads to reduced serum IGF-I levels in cyanotic congenital heart disease, *J. Pediatr. Endocrinol. Metab.*, 13, 431, 2000.

131. Kanazawa, H., Glucose tolerance and insulin secretion in infants with the left-to-right shunt congenital heart disease, *Nippon Kyobu. Geka. Gakkai. Zasshi.*, 40, 1675, 1992.

132. Levy, R.J. et al., Birthweight of infants with congenital heart disease, *Am. J. Dis. Child.*, 132, 249, 1978.

133. Rosenthal, G.L. et al., Birthweight and cardiovascular malformations: a population-based study, *Am. J. Epidemiol.*, 133, 1273, 1991.

134. Ferencz, C. et al., Congenital cardiovascular malformations associated with chromosome abnormalities: an epidemiologic study, *J. Pediatr.*, 114, 79, 1989.

135. Lavigne, J.V. and Burns, W.J., The impact of a chronic illness on the family, in *Pediatric Psychology: An Introduction for Pediatricians and Psychologists*, Grune & Stratton, New York, 1981, 331.

136. Levy, R.J. et al., Birthweight of infants with congenital heart disease, *Am. J. Dis. Child.*, 132, 249, 1978.

137. Leite, H.P. et al., Nutritional assessment and surgical risk markers in children submitted to cardiac surgery, *Rev. Paul Med.*, 113, 706, 1995.

138. Sholler, G.F. and Celermajer, J.M., Cardiac surgery in the first year of life: the effect on weight gains of infants with congenital heart disease, *Aust. Paediatr. J.*, 22, 305, 1986.

139. Levy, R.J. et al., Growth after surgical repair of simple D-transposition of the great arteries, *Ann. Thorac. Surg.*, 25, 225, 1978.

140. Rhee, E.K. et al., Impact of anatomic closure on somatic growth among small, asymptomatic children with secundum atrial septal defect, *Am. J. Cardiol.*, 85, 1472, 2000.

141. Mainwaring, R.D. et al., Secundum-type atrial septal defects with failure to thrive in the first year of life, *J. Card. Surg.*, 11, 116, 1996.

142. Loeffel, M., Developmental considerations of infants and children with congenital heart disease, *Heart Lung*, 14, 214, 1985.

143. Rudolph, A.M., Developmental considerations in neonatal failure, *Hosp. Pract.*, 20, 53, 1985.

144. Freeman, L.M. and Roubenoff, R., The nutrition implications of cardiac cachexia, *Nutr. Rev.*, 52, 340, 1994.

145. Morrison, W.L. and Edwards, R.H.T., Cardiac cachexia, *Br. Med. J.*, 302, 301, 1991.

146. Rosenthal, A., Nutritional considerations in the prognosis and treatment of children with congenital heart disease, in *Textbook of Pediatric Nutrition*, 2nd ed., Suskind, R.M. and Lewinter-Suskind, I., Eds., Raven Press, New York, 1993, 383.

147. Forchielli, M.L. et al., Children with congenital heart disease: a nutrition challenge, *Nutr. Rev.*, 52, 348, 1994.

148. Santini, B. et al., Home enteral nutrition in pediatric age based on the Torino experience, *Minerva Pediatr.*, 48, 429, 1996.

149. Behrens, R. et al., Percutaneous endoscopic gastrostomy in children and adolescents, *J. Pediatr. Gastroenterol. Nutr.*, 25, 487, 1997.

150. Kermack, W.O., McKendrick, A.G., and McKinlay, P.L., Death rates in Great Britain and Sweden, *Lancet*, 1, 698, 1934.

151. Forsdahl, A., Are poor living conditions in childhood and adolescence an important risk factor for arteriosclerotic heart disease? *Br. J. Prev. Soc. Med.*, 31, 91, 1977.

152. Barker, D.J. and Osmond, C., Infant mortality, childhood nutrition, and ischaemic heart disease in England and Wales, *Lancet*, 1, 1077, 1986.

153. Barker, D.J. et al., Weight in infancy and death from ischaemic heart disease, *Lancet*, 2, 577, 1989.

154. Barker, D.J. et al., The relation of small head circumference and thinness at birth to death from cardiovascular disease in adult life, *Br. Med. J.*, 306, 422, 1993.

155. Stanner, S.A. et al., Does malnutrition *in utero* determine diabetes and coronary heart disease in adulthood? Results from the Leningrad siege study, a cross sectional study, *Br. Med. J.*, 315, 1342, 1997.

156. Roseboom, T.J. et al., Coronary heart disease after prenatal exposure to the Dutch famine, 1944–45, *Heart*, 84, 595, 2000.

157. Stanner, S. and Yudkin, J.S., Fetal programming and the Leningrad Siege Study, *Twin Research*, 4, 287, 2001.

158. Godfrey, K. et al., Maternal nutrition in early and late pregnancy in relation to placental and fetal growth, *Br. Med. J.*, 312, 410, 1996.

159. Barker, D.J., Gluckman, P.D., and Robinson, J.S., Conference report: fetal origins of adult disease, report of the First International Study Group, Sydney, 29–30 October 1994, *Placenta*, 16, 317, 1995.

160. Emanuel, J.I. et al., Intergenerational studies of human birthweight from the 1958 birth cohort 1: evidence for a multigenerational effect, *Br. J. Obstet. Gynaecol.*, 99, 67, 1992.

161. Martyn, C.N., Barker, D.J., and Osmond, C., Mothers' pelvic size, fetal growth, and death from stroke and coronary heart disease in men in the U.K., *Lancet*, 348, 1264, 1996.

162. Forsen, T. et al., Growth *in utero* and during childhood among women who develop coronary heart disease: longitudinal study, *Br. Med. J.*, 319, 1403, 1999.

163. Martyn, C.N. et al., Growth *in utero*, adult blood pressure, and arterial compliance, *Br. Heart J.*, 73, 116, 1995.

164. Barker, D.J. et al., Growth *in utero* and serum cholesterol concentrations in adult life, *Br. Med. J.*, 307, 1524, 1993.

165. Martyn, C.N. et al., Plasma concentrations of fibrinogen and factor VII in adult life and their relation to intra-uterine growth, *Br. J. Haematol.*, 89, 142, 1995.

166. Lithell, H.O. et al., Relation of size at birth to non-insulin dependent diabetes and insulin concentration in men aged 50–60 years, *Br. Med. J.*, 312, 406, 1996.

167. Eriksson, J.G. et al., Early growth and coronary heart disease in later life: longitudinal study, *Br. Med. J.*, 322, 949, 2001.

168. Barker, D.J. et al., Size at birth and resilience to effects of poor living conditions in adult life: longitudinal study, *Br. Med. J.*, 323, 1, 2001.

169. Marmot, M. and Wilkinson, R.G., Psychosocial and material pathways in the relation between income and health: a response to Lynch et al., *Br. Med. J.*, 322, 1233, 2001.

170. Phillips, D.I.W. et al., Low birth weight predicts elevated plasma cortisol concentrations in adults from three populations, *Hypertension*, 35, 1301, 2000.

171. Forsen, T. et al. The fetal and childhood growth of persons who develop type 2 diabetes, *Ann. Intern. Med.*, 133, 176, 2000.

172. Whalley, L.J. and Deary, I.J., Longitudinal cohort study of childhood IQ and survival up to age 76, *Br. Med. J.*, 322, 819, 2001.

173. Gennser, G., Rymark, P., and Isberg, P.E., Low birth weight and risk of high blood pressure in adulthood, *Br. Med. J.*, 296, 1498, 1988.

174. Barker, D.J. et al. Growth *in utero*, blood pressure in childhood and adult life, and mortality from cardiovascular disease, *Br. Med. J.*, 298, 564, 1989.

175. Barker, D.J. et al. The relation of fetal length, ponderal index and head circumference to blood pressure and the risk of hypertension in adult life, *Paediatr. Perinat. Epidemiol.*, 6, 35, 1992.

176. Law, C.M. et al. Initiation of hypertension *in utero* and its amplification throughout life, *Br. Med. J.*, 306, 24, 1993.

177. Leon, D.A. et al. Failure to realise growth potential *in utero* and adult obesity in relation to blood pressure in 50-year old Swedish men, *Br. Med. J.*, 312, 401, 1996.

178. Law, C.M. and Shiell, A.W., Is blood pressure inversely related to birth weight? The strength of evidence from a systematic review of the literature, *J. Hypertens.*, 14, 935, 1996.

179. Barker, D.J. et al., Growth and living conditions in childhood and hypertension in adult life: a longitudinal study, *J. Hypertens.*, 20, 1951, 2002.

180. Merlet-Benichou, C. et al., Intrauterine growth retardation leads to a permanent nephron deficit in the rat, *Pediatr. Nephrol.*, 8, 175, 1994.

181. Brenner, E. and Chertow, G.M., Congenital oligonephropathy and the etiology of adult hypertension and progressive renal injury, *Am. J. Kidney Dis.*, 23, 171, 1994.

182. Rahier, J., Wallon, J., and Henquin, J.C., Cell populations of the endocrine pancreas of human neonates and infants, *Diabetologia*, 20, 540, 1981.

183. Hales, C.N. et al., Fetal and infant growth and impaired glucose tolerance at age 64, *Br. Med. J.*, 303, 1019, 1991.

184. Barker, D.J. et al., Type 2 (non-insulin dependent) diabetes mellitus, hypertension and hyperlipidemia (syndrome X): relation to reduced fetal growth, *Diabetologia*, 36, 62, 1993.

185. McCance, D.R. et al., Birth weight and non-insulin dependent diabetes: thrifty genotype, thrifty phenotype, or surviving small baby genogype? *Br. Med. J.,* 308, 942, 1994.

186. Phillips, D.I.W. et al., Thinness at birth and insulin resistance in adult life, *Diabetologia*, 37, 150, 1994.

187. Hofman, P.L. et al., Insulin resistance in short children with intrauterine growth retardation, *J. Clin. Endocrinol. Metab.*, 82, 402, 1997.

188. Barker, D.J. et al., Fetal origins of adult disease: strength of effects and biological basis, *Int. J. Epidemiol.*, 31, 1235, 2002.

189. Widdowson, E.M., Crabb, D.E., and Milner, R.D.G., Cellular development of some human organs before birth, *Arch. Dis. Child.*, 47, 652, 1972.

190. Gebhardt, R., Metabolic zonation of the liver: regulation and implications for liver function, *Pharmacol. Therapeut.*, 53, 275, 1992.

191. Martyn, C.N. and Barker, D.J., Reduced fetal growth increases risk of cardiovascular disease, *Health Rep.*, 6, 45, 1994.
192. Barker, D.J., The fetal and infant origins of disease, *Eur. J. Clin. Invest.*, 25, 457, 1995.
193. Lucas, A., Role of nutritional programming in determining adult morbidity, *Arch. Dis. Child.*, 71, 288, 1994.
194. Reynolds, R.M. and Phillips, D.I., Long-term consequences of intrauterine growth retardation, *Horm. Res.* 49 (Suppl. 2), 28, 1998.
195. Metcalfe, N.B. and Monaghan, P., Compensation for a bad start: grow now, pay later, *Trends Ecol. Evol.*, 16, 254, 2001.
196. Hales, C.N., Suicide of the nephron, *Lancet,* 357, 136, 2001.
197. Ravelli, G.P., Stein, Z.A., and Susser, M.W., Obesity in young men after famine exposure *in utero* and early infancy, *New Engl. J. Med.*, 295, 349, 1976.
198. Barker, D.J., The intrauterine origins of cardiovascular disease and obstructive lung disease in adult life, *J. R. Coll. Physicians Lond.*, 25, 129, 1991.
199. Hales, C.N. and Barker, D.J., Type 2 (non-insulin-dependent) diabetes mellitus: the thrifty phenotype hypothesis, *Diabetologia*, 35, 595, 1992.
200. Neel, J.V., Diabetes mellitus: a 'thrifty' genotype rendered detrimental by 'progress'? *Am. J. Hum. Genet.*, 14, 353, 1962.
201. Hattersley, A.T. and Tooke, J.E., The fetal insulin hypothesis: an alternative explanation of the association of low birthweight with diabetes and vascular disease, *Lancet*, 353, 1789, 1999.
202. Widdowson, E.M. and McCance, R.A., The determinants of growth and form, *Proc. R. Soc. Lond.*, 185, 1, 1974.
203. Widdowson, E.M. and McCance, R.A., A review: new thoughts on growth, *Pediatr. Res.*, 9, 154, 1975.
204. West-Eberhard, M.J., Phenotypic plasticity and the origins of diversity, *Ann. Rev. Ecol. Syst.*, 20, 249, 1989.
205. McCance, R.A., Food, growth and time, *Lancet*, 2, 621, 1962.
206. Harding, J.E., The nutritional basis of fetal origins of adult disease, *Int. J. Epidemiol.*, 30, 15, 2001.
207. Weinkove, C., Weinkove, E.A., and Pimstone, B.L., Insulin release and pancreatic islet volume in malnourished rats, *S. Afr. Med. J.*, 48, 1888, 1974.
208. Swenne, I., Crace, C.J., and Milner, R.D.G., Persistent impairment of insulin secretory response to glucose in adult rats after limited period of protein-calorie malnutrition early in life, *Diabetes*, 36, 454, 1987.
209. Snoeck, A. et al., Effect of a low protein diet during pregnancy on the fetal rat endocrine pancreas, *Biol. Neonate*, 5, 107, 1990.
210. Langley, S.C. and Jackson, A.A., Increased systolic blood pressure in adult rats induced by fetal exposure to maternal low protein diets, *Clin. Sci.*, 86, 217, 1994.
211. Levitt, N. et al., Dexamethasone in the last week of pregnancy attenuates hippocampal glucocorticoid receptor gene expression and elevates blood pressure in the adult offspring in the rat, *Neuroendocrinology*, 64, 412, 1996.
212. Benediktsson, R. et al., Glucocorticoid exposure *in utero*: a new model for adult hypertension, *Lancet*, 341, 339, 1993.
213. Lindsay, R.S. et al., Programming of glucose tolerance in the rat: role of placental 11β-hydroxysteroid dehydrogenase, *Diabetologia*, 39, 1299, 1996.
214. Vickers, M.H. et al., Fetal origins of hyperphagia, obesity, and hypertension and postnatal amplification by hypercaloric nutrition, *Am. J. Physiol. Endocrinol. Metab.*, 279, E83, 2000.

215. Schwartz, M.W. et al., Insulin in the brain: a hormonal regulator of energy balance, *Endocr. Rev.*, 13, 387, 1992.

216. Anderson, E.A. and Mark, A.L., The vasodilator action of insulin: implications for the insulin hypothesis of hypertension, *Hypertension*, 21, 136, 1993.

217. Steinberg, H.O. et al., Obesity/insulin resistance is associated with endothelial dysfunction. Implications for the syndrome of insulin resistance, *J. Clin. Invest.*, 97, 2601, 1996.

218. Kingdom, J.C. et al., Intrauterine growth restriction is associated with persistent juxtamedullary expression of renin in the fetal kidney, *Kidney Int.*, 55, 424, 1999.

219. Antipatis, C. et al., Effects of maternal vitamin A status on fetal heart and lung: changes in expression of key developmental genes, *Am. J. Physiol.* 275, L1184, 1998.

220. Chambon, P., A decade of molecular biology of retinoic acid receptors, *FASEB J.*, 10, 940, 1991.

15 Plant Sterols and Stanols, Lipoprotein Metabolism, and Cardiovascular Disease

Elke Naumann, Jogchum Plat, and Ronald P. Mensink

CONTENTS

15.1 INTRODUCTION

Several risk factors for cardiovascular disease — still the most important cause of death in the Western world — are known. Certain factors such as age, gender, and family history of coronary heart disease cannot be modified, but other factors like high blood pressure, diabetes mellitus, and smoking can be changed. This chapter will focus on another important modifiable risk factor: high serum concentration of cholesterol.

It is well established that the mortality of coronary heart disease increases continuously and progressively with increasing serum cholesterol concentrations.[1] From this finding, we can predict that lowering serum cholesterol concentrations is especially beneficial for mildly cholesterolemic and hypercholesterolemic subjects. In addition to drugs, serum cholesterol concentrations can be lowered by diet. A decrease in intakes of saturated and *trans* fatty acids and cholesterol and an increase in intakes of unsaturated fatty acids and fiber have been advocated.[2] Another successful way to lower serum cholesterol concentrations is through the consumption of plant sterols and stanols. Their cholesterol lowering effects are widely accepted and functional foods enriched with plant sterols and stanols are currently on the market to help people lower their cholesterol levels.

15.2 WHAT ARE PLANT STEROLS AND STANOLS?

Plant sterols are structurally related to cholesterol, but differ by having a methyl group (campesterol) or ethyl group (sitosterol) at position 24 or an additional double bond at position 22 (stigmasterol). The structures of plant stanols resemble those of plant sterols, but lack the double bonds (Figure 15.1). Since humans cannot synthesize these compounds, all plant sterols and stanols in the body originate from diet.

Western diets provide 160 to 437 mg plant sterols a day, which is approximately similar to the amount of cholesterol in the diet.[3] A recent survey from the Netherlands found that important sources of plant sterol and stanol intake are brown bread,

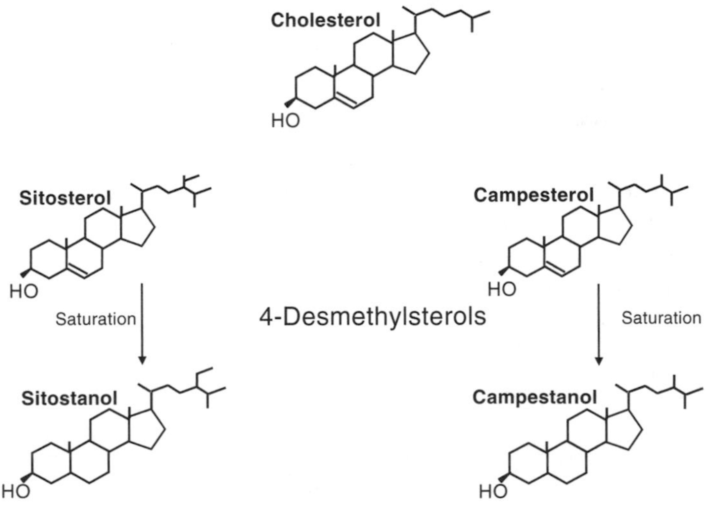

FIGURE 15.1 Molecular structures of cholesterol and two 4-desmethylsterols (sitosterol and campesterol). Saturation of the double bonds in sitosterol and campesterol results in the formation of sitostanol and campestanol, respectively.

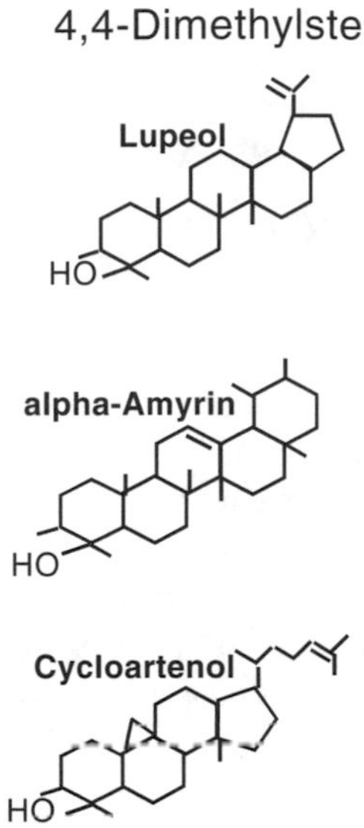

4,4-Dimethylsterols

FIGURE 15.2 Molecular structures of three 4,4-dimethylsterols.

vegetable fats and oils, vegetables, and fruits. Plant stanols are present in these products in only very small amounts and estimated daily intake is less than 30 mg.[4] It should be noted that it is difficult to estimate plant sterol and stanol intake accurately due to wide variations in the compositions of comparable products, differences in harvesting periods, and geographic locations.[5]

The most common plant sterol in the Western diet is sitosterol, which contributes about 65% to total daily plant sterol and stanol intake. For campesterol and stigmasterol, these values are about 20 and 10%, respectively. Sitostanol and campestanol contribute about 5% to daily plant sterol and stanol intake.[4]

Sitosterol, campesterol, and stigmasterol are 4-desmethylsterols. Their cholesterol lowering effects and the effects of plant stanols have been proven in many trials.[3] In contrast, 4,4-dimethylsterols like lupeol, alpha-amyrin, and cycloartenol (Figure 15.2) present in rice bran and shea nut oil hardly lower serum cholesterol.[6] The structures of 4-desmethylsterols resemble the structure of cholesterol more than they resemble the structures of 4,4-dimethylsterols. This may be the reason for the difference in cholesterol lowering effect.

Plant sterols and stanols are added to a wide variety of products such as margarines, yogurts, cream cheese, milk, and snack bars. The plant stanols present in these products are mainly produced by hydrogenation of plant sterols. Hydrogenation of sitosterol and campesterol results in the formation of sitostanol and campestanol, respectively. Stigmasterol is then converted to sitostanol.

As mentioned, plant sterols and stanols effectively lower serum cholesterol concentrations. To understand (1) why these effects are beneficial with respect to the development of cardiovascular disease and (2) the mechanisms of actions of plant sterols and stanols, it is necessary to be familiar with some basic principles of cholesterol metabolism and the relation between cholesterol concentrations and cardiovascular disease. These issues will be discussed in Section 15.3 and Section 15.4 before the discussion of the effects of plant sterols and stanols on lipid and lipoprotein metabolism.

15.3 CHOLESTEROL METABOLISM

Cholesterol is an essential component for the human body. It is one of the building blocks for cell membranes and serves as a precursor for a number of compounds such as steroid hormones and bile acids. Because of the low solubility of cholesterol in the hydrophilic environment of the circulation, it is transported through the blood stream in lipoproteins. A lipoprotein consists of a hydrophilic coat that contains free cholesterol, phospholipids, and apolipoproteins, as well as a hydrophobic core consisting of cholesterol esters and triacylglycerols. Lipoproteins differ in their amounts of cholesterol and triacylglycerol (Table 15.1). The cholesterol the lipoproteins contain is derived from two pathways: dietary cholesterol (exogenous route) and endogenous synthesis.

15.3.1 EXOGENOUS ROUTE

Cholesterol esters and triacylglycerol from the diet are first hydrolyzed within the small intestine. This results in the formation of free cholesterol, fatty acids, monoglycerides, diglycerides, and glycerol. These components along with phospholipids and bile acids are incorporated into mixed micelles. The individual components of the micelles can be taken up by the enterocytes. Within the intestinal cells, the free cholesterol is re-esterified by an enzyme called ACAT (acyl-coenzyme A: cholesterol acyltransferase). Monoglycerides and diglycerides, however, are first hydrolyzed into free fatty acids and glycerol and then used for the formation of new triacylglycerols. These triacylglycerols and the cholesterol esters are, together with apolipoproteins and phopholipids, used for the synthesis of chylomicrons.

The lipoproteins are secreted into the lymph and reach the circulation in the vena subclavia. The triacylglycerols from the chylomicrons are taken up by various peripheral tissues (for example, adipose tissue and muscle cells) after hydrolysis into free fatty acids and glycerol through the action of lipoprotein lipase, an enzyme.

TABLE 15.1
Mean Compositions of Lipoproteins (Percent of Total Mass)

	Chylomicron	VLDL	IDL	LDL	HDL
Triacylglycerol	87	52	26	6	6
Cholesterol ester	3	9	28	40	21
Free cholesterol	2	6	7	9	3
Phospholipids	6	23	22	22	24
Apolipoprotein	2	10	14	23	46

VLDL = very low density lipoprotein; IDL = intermediate density lipoprotein; LDL = low density lipoprotein; HDL = high density lipoprotein.

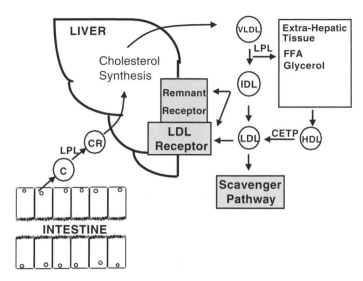

FIGURE 15.3 Metabolism of cholesterol. Dietary cholesterol enters the circulation in chylomicrons (C). After removal of triacylglycerols from the chylomicrons through the action of the lipoprotein lipase (LPL) enzyme, chylomicron remnants (CR) are taken up by the liver. The liver can resecrete cholesterol, together with endogenously synthesized cholesterol, into the circulation in very low density lipoproteins (VLDL). As for chylomicrons, most of the triacylglycerol is hydrolyzed into free fatty acids (FFA) and glycerol and taken up by peripheral tissues. The remaining particles are intermediate density lipoproteins (IDL) that can be taken up by the liver. IDL particles that are not taken up are converted into cholesterol-rich low density lipoproteins (LDL). LDL particles are also cleared from the circulation by LDL receptors. Part of the LDL is also removed by the scavanger pathway. Cholesterol from extrahepatic tissues can be removed via high density lipoproteins (HDL) that transfer it to the liver or with the help of cholesterol ester transfer protein (CETP) to LDL and VLDL particles.

The particles formed by the gradual delipidation are relatively rich in cholesterol and are now called chylomicron remnants. They are taken up by the liver, which can store the cholesterol as cholesterol esters through the action of ACAT or resecrete it along with endogenously synthesized cholesterol into the circulation in very low density lipoprotein (VLDL) particles (Figure 15.3).

15.3.2 ENDOGENOUS ROUTE

The liver produces and secretes VLDL particles that contain mainly triacylglycerol and cholesterol. As described for chylomicrons, most of the triacylglycerol is taken up by peripheral tissues. The remaining particle, now called an intermediate density lipoprotein (IDL), can be taken up through hepatic low density lipoprotein (LDL) receptors. IDL particles not taken up are converted into cholesterol-rich LDL particles that are also cleared from the circulation by LDL receptors. Some of the LDL, however, is also removed by the scavenger pathway (Figure 15.3). The higher the LDL cholesterol concentration in the blood, the more LDL cholesterol is removed from the circulation via this pathway. The scavenger pathway is mainly involved in the development of atherosclerosis.

15.4 LIPOPROTEINS AND RISK OF CORONARY HEART DISEASE

15.4.1 LDL CHOLESTEROL

High serum concentrations of LDL cholesterol are positively and causally related to the risk of coronary heart disease.[7] Reducing serum LDL cholesterol concentrations will decrease the risk of coronary heart disease. Serum LDL cholesterol concentrations can be lowered by drugs that inhibit HMG-CoA-reductase, the rate limiting enzyme for endogenous cholesterol synthesis. These drugs are called statins and they reduce serum concentrations of total cholesterol by approximately 20% and LDL cholesterol by approximately 30%.[8-11] The decreases are associated with reductions in the relative risk of death from coronary heart disease of 24 to 42%.[8-11]

One reason LDL cholesterol is atherogenic is the presence of several components in the LDL that are easily oxidized like the unsaturated fatty acids from phospholipids. The formation of oxidized LDL is an important step in the development of atherosclerosis. Oxidized LDL is not recognized by LDL receptors, but is instead efficiently cleared by scavenger receptors on macrophages found in the arterial walls. The macrophages then develop into foam cells. Many of these foam cells form a fatty streak that may ultimately turn into an atherosclerotic plaque. As a consequence, the diameter and elasticity of the vessel wall diminish and endothelial function is impaired. If a plaque ruptures, a part may loosen from the vessel wall. This embolus enters the circulation and may obstruct an artery, and this can lead to a myocardial infarction or cerebrovascular accident.

15.4.2 HDL CHOLESTEROL

In contrast to high serum LDL cholesterol concentrations, high HDL cholesterol levels are negatively associated with the risk for cardiovascular disease. The reason for this protective effect of HDL is its role in reverse cholesterol transport. Cholesterol from extrahepatic tissues, including vessel walls, is taken up by an HDL particle that transfers cholesterol directly or via LDL and VLDL particles to the liver for secretion (Figure 15.3).

15.5 PLANT STEROLS AND STANOLS AND THEIR EFFECTS ON CHOLESTEROL METABOLISM

15.5.1 EFFECTS OF PLANT STEROLS AND STANOLS ON SERUM LIPID AND LIPOPROTEIN CONCENTRATIONS

The fact that plant sterols from soybeans lowered serum cholesterol concentrations in chickens,[12,13] rabbits,[14] and humans[15] was known in the 1950s. However, plant sterols could not easily be incorporated into food products and intakes of large amounts in the forms of capsules and syrups were necessary to achieve substantial reductions in plasma cholesterol concentrations. Interest in the cholesterol lowering properties of plant sterols decreased until the discovery in the 1970s that esterification of plant sterols facilitated their incorporation into various food products.

Since then, many studies have shown that both plant sterol and stanol esters lower serum LDL cholesterol concentrations without effects on serum HDL cholesterol concentrations. In one study of patients with type II diabetes, consumption of plant stanol esters even increased serum HDL cholesterol concentrations by 11%,[16] but this could not be confirmed in another study.[17] In recent years, free plant sterols and stanols have been incorporated into food products by improved techniques. Their effects on serum lipoprotein concentrations are the same as those of esterified plant sterols and stanols.

Heinemann et al.[18] studied the effects of plant sterols and stanols on cholesterol absorption over a 40-cm segment of the small intestine during passage of a liquid diet containing sitosterol or sitostanol. Cholesterol absorption decreased by 50% after sitosterol infusion and by almost 85% after sitostanol infusion. This suggested that plant stanols might be more effective than plant sterols. However, recent studies demonstrated that plant sterols and stanols, either free or esterified, are equally effective in reducing serum LDL cholesterol concentrations.[19–23]

Daily intakes of 2 to 3 g of plant sterols and stanols result in decreases in LDL cholesterol concentrations of 10 to 15% (Figure 15.4).[24] Increasing the daily intake to more than 3 g hardly reduces LDL cholesterol any further. Plant sterols as present naturally in vegetable oils also reduce LDL cholesterol concentrations. This has been known for more than 40 years[25] and was confirmed recently in an elegant study. Cholesterol absorption was measured after consumption of a commercial corn oil containing 270 mg of plant sterols per treatment, purified corn oil from which the

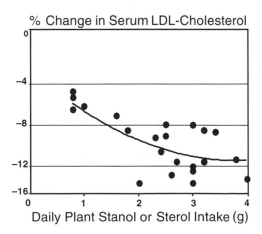

FIGURE 15.4 Relative changes in serum LDL cholesterol during different intakes of plant sterols or stanols. Daily intakes of 2 to 3 g of plant sterols and stanols decrease serum LDL cholesterol concentrations by 10 to 15%.[24]

plant sterols were removed, or purified corn oil to which the plant sterols were added back at two different amounts (150 and 300 mg per treatment). Compared with corn oil without plant sterols, cholesterol absorption was decreased by 27.5% after consumption of the commercial corn oil. A similar decrease was observed when plant sterols were added to the sterol-free corn oil to a nearly equal amount as that in the commercial oil. The decrease was 12% when only 150 mg of plant sterols were added back to the purified corn oil.[26]

Plant sterols and stanols lower LDL cholesterol in people with elevated and normal serum cholesterol concentrations, in people with diabetes mellitus, and in children. Furthermore, effects of plant sterols and stanols do not depend on the amount of fat or cholesterol in the diet, which means they are also effective when consumed as part of a recommended diet.[27] In subjects receiving statin therapy, the LDL cholesterol lowering effects of plant sterols and stanols is still present and is additive to the LDL cholesterol lowering effect of statins alone.[28] Although plant sterols and stanols are often esterified to improve their fat solubility, they need not be incorporated into high-fat food products. Plant stanol esters incorporated into low-fat yogurt also effectively decreased serum LDL concentrations.[29]

15.5.2 EFFECTS OF PLANT STEROLS AND STANOLS ON DEVELOPMENT OF ATHEROSCLEROSIS

Although plant sterols and stanols lower serum LDL cholesterol levels, this does not mean that consumption of plant sterols and stanols lowers the risk for atherosclerosis. Theoretically, it is possible that plant sterols and stanols have unfavorable effects on other risk factors for atherosclerosis. Effects of diet on atherosclerosis are not easy to study in humans. Biomarkers for atherosclerosis such as flow-mediated vasodilation or ultrasound techniques can be used to examine effects of plant sterols and stanols on the condition of vessel walls, but such studies have not yet been carried out. Several animal studies have evaluated effects of plant sterols and stanols on plaque formation. Transgenic and knock-out mouse models such as the apoE knock-out and apoE3-Leiden, which are validated models for studying the effects of diet on plaque formation, have been used.

In studies of Moghadasian et al.,[30–32] a diet enriched with a mixture of plant sterols and stanols resulted in smaller lesions in the aortic roots and sinuses of male apoE knock-out mice as compared to those in control animals that received a diet without added plant sterols and stanols. Plant stanol esters reduced atherosclerotic lesion area in female apoE*3-Leiden transgenic mice.[33] *In vitro* studies suggest anti-atherogenic effects of plant sterols not directly related to effects on LDL cholesterol. Plant sterols, especially sitosterol, inhibited vascular smooth muscle cell growth and proliferation without cytotoxic effects or reduction in cell viability. Sitosterol increased prostacyclin release, which may improve endothelial function. Taken together, these animal and cell studies indicate that plant sterols and stanols exert favorable effects on the development and progression of atherosclerosis.[34] Only long-term human intervention studies can actually prove whether consumption of plant sterols and stanols truly affects atherosclerotic risk.

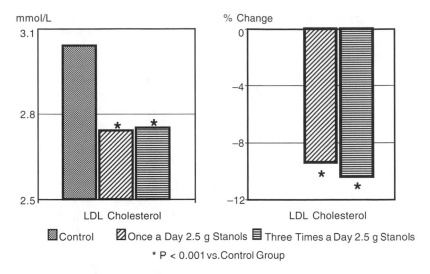

FIGURE 15.5 Effect of consumption frequency of plant stanols on their serum LDL cholesterol lowering properties. Consumption of 2.5 g of plant stanols once a day is as effective as consumption of 2.5 g of plant stanols three times a day.[35]

15.5.3 MECHANISM OF ACTION

Plant sterols and stanols have a higher affinity for incorporation into micelles and occupy more space in micelles than cholesterol. These effects will result in decreased incorporation of cholesterol into micelles, a consequent reduced availability of cholesterol for absorption, and lower serum LDL cholesterol concentrations. However, if effect on micellar composition is the only mechanism, plant sterols and stanols should be most effective when consumed with cholesterol. A study reported in 2000 that a daily intake of 2.5 g of plant stanols once a day is as effective as consumption of the same amount of plant stanols divided over three meals (Figure 15.5).[35] This indicates that replacement of plant sterols and stanols for cholesterol in micelles is not the only mechanism causing a reduction in serum LDL cholesterol.

It was suggested that plant sterols and stanols produce effects in the lumen of the small intestine and also inside the enterocytes. In a caco-2 cell line — an accepted model to study human intestinal lipoprotein metabolism — sitostanol increased the expression of ABCA1. ABCA1 transfers cholesterol from the enterocytes back into the intestinal lumen. This suggests that plant sterols and stanols also lower the absorption of cholesterol by transporting cholesterol out of enterocytes (Figure 15.6).

The cholesterol lowering properties of plant sterols and stanols can be explained by reduced incorporation of cholesterol into mixed micelles along with increased transport of cholesterol from enterocytes back into the intestinal lumen. As a result of decreased cholesterol absorption, endogenous cholesterol synthesis increases. Despite this increase, the net result will be reduced LDL cholesterol concentration after plant sterol or stanol consumption.

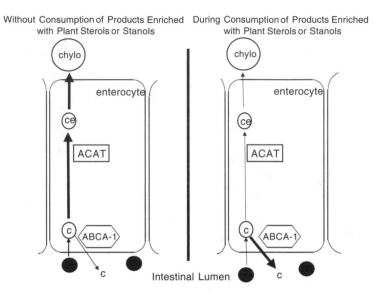

FIGURE 15.6 Suggested effects of plant sterols and stanols on cholesterol metabolism. In addition to reduced incorporation of cholesterol into mixed micelles (●) in the intestinal lumen, plant sterols and stanols may also affect intestinal walls. Cholesterol can be esterified into cholesterol esters (ce) by acyl-coenzyme A: cholesterol acyltransferase (ACAT) and then incorporated into chylomicrons (chylo) inside enterocytes. Part of the cholesterol can also be resecreted back into the intestinal lumen through ABCA-1. It is suggested that plant sterols and stanols increase expression of ABCA-1, which shuttles cholesterol from enterocytes back into the intestinal lumen, and thus decreases cholesterol absorption.

15.5.4 METABOLISM OF PLANT STEROLS AND STANOLS

After consumption, about 80% of campesterol and 50 to 60% of the sitosterol, campestanol, and sitostanol esters are hydrolyzed in the upper part of the small intestine by intestinal sterol ester hydrolase.[36] As 90% of plant sterols and stanols are in the unesterified form in feces,[37] further hydrolysis should occur in other parts of the intestine. The free plant sterols and stanols are incorporated into mixed micelles and taken up by enterocytes. As compared to cholesterol, of which approximately 30 to 80% is absorbed, plant sterols and stanols are poorly absorbed. Estimated uptake of campesterol (1.89%) is higher than that of sitosterol (0.51%), while campestanol absorption (0.16%) is higher than sitostanol absorption (0.04%).[38]

Saturation of the plant sterol lowers absorption. Absorption efficiency decreases when the length of the side chain at position 24 of the molecule increases. Absorption of sitosterol, with an ethyl group at position 24, is lower than that of campesterol, which contains a methyl group. Similarly, absorption of sitostanol is lower than that of campestanol. Cholesterol only contains a hydrogen atom at position 24 and has the highest absorption (Figure 15.1).

Plant sterols and stanols are poor substrates for ACAT and after absorption only a very small part of the plant sterols and stanols is esterified. Since free plant sterols and stanols are poorly incorporated into chylomicrons, their absorption is very low as compared to cholesterol. In analogy with cholesterol, which is resecreted from enterocytes into the intestinal lumen via ABCA1, other ABC-transporters (ABCG5 and ABCG8) may be involved in the resecretion of free plant sterols and stanols from the enterocytes back into the intestinal lumen.[39,40]

Once taken up by the liver through lipoproteins, plant sterols and stanols are incorporated into VLDL or secreted via bile. ABCG5 and ABCG8 are involved in secretion of free plant sterols and stanols from the liver into the bile.[37,41] Due to a lower affinity of ACAT for sitosterol in the liver, biliary excretion is faster for sitosterol than for campesterol.[42] This, along with higher absorption of campesterol from the gut, explains the higher serum concentrations of campesterol than of sitosterol. Serum concentrations of plant stanols are lower as compared with plant sterol concentrations, which can at least partly be explained by lower absorption of plant stanols than of plant sterols from the gut. Consumption of products enriched with plant sterols or stanols increases their respective serum concentrations but they are still less than 1% of serum cholesterol concentrations.

15.5.5 SITOSTEROLEMIA

Sitosterolemia is a rare inherited disease characterized by xanthomas in skin, tendons, and coronary arteries and early development of atherosclerosis. It often results in an early myocardial infarction, sometimes before the age of 20.[43,44] These patients have extremely high serum concentrations of plant sterols and stanols. Sitosterol in particular is extremely elevated and plasma concentrations in these patients are about 0.48 mmol/L. In nonsitosterolemic people, concentrations are more than 40 times lower. The high serum plant sterol and stanol concentrations are due to increased absorption of plant sterols and stanols in combination with slow elimination.

Patients with sitosterolemia have mutations in ABCG5 and ABCG8 that may result in reduced transport from plant sterols and stanols from enterocytes back into the intestinal lumen and in reduced secretion into bile.[45–47] Mice overexpressing ABCG5 and ABCG8 showed clear reductions in plasma sitosterol and campesterol concentrations as compared with wild-type mice,[40] while an increase in plasma plant sterol concentrations was found in ABCG5 and ABCG8 knock-out mice.[39] Whether the high plant sterol concentrations cause the high risk of coronary heart disease in sitosterolemic patients is not known.

15.5.6 SIDE EFFECTS

Safety studies have shown that consumption of plant sterols and stanols is nontoxic and does not cause adverse effects on liver, kidney, and gastrointestinal function or on hematological, coagulation, and fibrinolytic parameters.[48–52] One aspect related to plant sterol and stanol consumption that may need attention is the lowered serum concentrations of fat-soluble antioxidants.

Since plant sterols and stanols interfere with the absorption of cholesterol, they may also influence the absorption of other lipophilic substances. Most studies have found decreases in plasma concentrations of alpha-carotene, beta-carotene, lycopene, lutein/zeaxanthin, beta-cryptoxanthin, and tocopherols after plant sterol or stanol

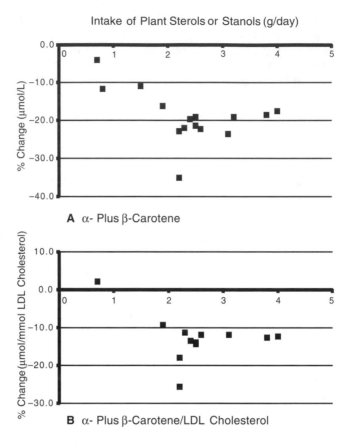

FIGURE 15.7 Percent changes in absolute (A) and LDL cholesterol-standardized (B) plasma concentrations of alpha- plus beta-carotene at different intakes of plant sterols or stanols.

consumption.[53] These lipophilic substances are transported in lipoproteins and the observed decrease may be simply due to a decrease in serum LDL cholesterol. Therefore, plasma concentrations are usually standardized for plasma LDL cholesterol concentrations. In general, LDL cholesterol standardized changes were negative for the hydrocarbon carotenoids (alpha-carotene, beta-carotene, and lycopene), about zero for oxygenated carotenoids (lutein/zeaxanthin and beta-cryptoxanthin), and positive for tocopherols.[54] Results of several studies of alpha-carotene, beta-carotene, and alpha-tocopherol are shown in Figure 15.7 and Figure 15.8. For LDL cholesterol, standardized concentration effects are most pronounced at daily intakes above 2 g; effects are hardly evident below this level. Whether the lowered serum hydrocarbon carotenoid concentrations at higher intakes have any functional consequences is unknown. However, all plasma concentrations remained within normal ranges. Plasma concentrations of fat-soluble vitamin A, vitamin D, and vitamin K are not affected by plant sterols and stanols.

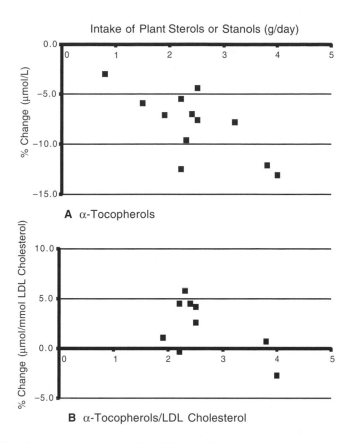

FIGURE 15.8 Percent changes in absolute (A) and LDL cholesterol-standardized (B) plasma concentrations of alpha-tocopherol at different intakes of plant sterols or stanols.

15.6 CONCLUSION

Many studies have shown that a wide variety of functional foods enriched with plant sterols and stanols reduce absorption of cholesterol. Daily intakes of 2 to 3 g of these components reduce serum LDL cholesterol concentrations by 10 to 15%. As high serum LDL cholesterol concentrations increase the risk for coronary heart disease, decreases in serum LDL cholesterol through consumption of plant sterols and stanols may be beneficial with regard to the development of atherosclerosis. Reductions in atherosclerotic lesion sizes were found in animals after plant sterol and stanol consumption and *in vitro* plant sterols reduced smooth muscle cell growth and proliferation.

Consumption of plant sterols and stanols is considered safe. The only possible relevant side effect reported is a reduction in serum cholesterol-standardized hydrocarbon carotenoid concentrations, although they remained within normal ranges. Thus, functional foods enriched with plant sterols and stanols as components of a prudent diet are helpful for lowering serum LDL cholesterol concentrations.

REFERENCES

1. Martin, M.J. et al., Serum cholesterol, blood pressure, and mortality: implications from a cohort of 361,662 men, *Lancet*, 2, 932, 1986.
2. National Cholesterol Education Program, Third Report of the National Cholesterol Education Program (NCEP) Expert Panel on Detection, Evaluation, and Treatment of High Blood Cholesterol in Adults (Adult Treatment Panel III). Final Report, National Heart, Lung, and Blood Institute, National Institutes of Health, Bethesda, MD, 2002.
3. Ostlund, R.E., Jr., Phytosterols in human nutrition, *Annu. Rev. Nutr.*, 22, 533, 2002.
4. Normen, A.L. et al., Plant sterol intakes and colorectal cancer risk in the Netherlands Cohort Study on Diet and Cancer, *Am. J. Clin. Nutr.*, 74, 141, 2001.
5. Weihrauch, J.L. and Gardner, J.M., Sterol content of foods of plant origin, *JADA*, 73, 39, 1978.
6. Sierksma, A., Weststrate, J.A., and Meijer, G.W., Spreads enriched with plant sterols, either esterified 4,4-dimethylsterols or free 4-desmethylsterols, and plasma total and LDL cholesterol concentrations, *Br. J. Nutr.*, 82, 273, 1999.
7. Pekkanen, J. et al., Ten-year mortality from cardiovascular disease in relation to cholesterol level among men with and without preexisting cardiovascular disease, *New Engl. J. Med.*, 322, 1700, 1990.
8. Sacks, F.M. et al., The effect of pravastatin on coronary events after myocardial infarction in patients with average cholesterol levels, *New Engl. J. Med.*, 335, 1001, 1996.
9. Shepherd, J. et al., Prevention of coronary heart disease with pravastatin in men with hypercholesterolemia, *New Engl. J. Med.*, 333, 1301, 1995.
10. Long-Term Intervention with Pravastatin in Ischaemic Disease (LIPID) Study Group, Prevention of cardiovascular events and death with pravastatin in patients with coronary heart disease and a broad range of initial cholesterol levels, *New Engl. J. Med.*, 339, 1349, 1998.
11. Scandinavian Simvastatin Survival Study Group, Randomised trial of cholesterol lowering in 4444 patients with coronary heart disease: the Scandinavian Simvastatin Survival Study (4S), *Lancet*, 344, 1383, 1994.
12. Peterson, D.W. et al., Dietary constituents affecting plasma and liver cholesterol in cholesterol-fed chicks, *J. Nutr.*, 50, 191, 1952.
13. Peterson, D., Effect of soybean sterols in the diet on plasma and liver cholesterol in chicks, *Proc. Exp. Biol. Med.*, 78, 143, 1951.
14. Pollak, O., Successful prevention of experimental hypercholesterolemia and cholesterol atherosclerosis in the rabbit, *Circulation*, 7, 696, 1953.
15. Peterson, D., Nichols, L., and Peck, N., Depression of plasma cholesterol in human subjects consuming butter containing soy sterols, *Fed. Proc.*, 65, 569, 1956.
16. Gylling, H. and Miettinen, T.A., Serum cholesterol and cholesterol and lipoprotein metabolism in hypercholesterolaemic NIDDM patients before and during sitostanol ester-margarine treatment, *Diabetologia*, 37, 773, 1994.
17. Gylling, H. and Miettinen, T.A., Effects of inhibiting cholesterol absorption and synthesis on cholesterol and lipoprotein metabolism in hypercholesterolemic noninsulin-dependent diabetic men, *J. Lipid Res.*, 37, 1776, 1996.
18. Heinemann, T. et al., Comparison of sitosterol and sitostanol on inhibition of intestinal cholesterol absorption, *Agents Actions Suppl.*, 26, 117, 1988.

19. Weststrate, J.A. and Meijer, G.W., Plant sterol-enriched margarines and reduction of plasma total and LDL cholesterol concentrations in normocholesterolaemic and mildly hypercholesterolaemic subjects, *Eur. J. Clin. Nutr.*, 52, 334, 1998.
20. Hallikainen, M.A. et al., Comparison of the effects of plant sterol ester and plant stanol esters-enriched margarines in lowering serum cholesterol concentrations in hypercholesterolaemic subjects on a low-fat diet, *Eur. J. Clin. Nutr.*, 54, 715, 2000.
21. Normen, L. et al., Soy sterol esters and beta-sitostanol ester as inhibitors of cholesterol absorption in human small bowel, *Am. J. Clin. Nutr.*, 71, 908, 2000.
22. Noakes, M. et al., An increase in dietary carotenoids when consuming plant sterols or stanols is effective in maintaining plasma carotenoid concentrations, *Am. J. Clin. Nutr.*, 75, 79, 2002.
23. Vanstone, C. et al., Unesterified plant sterols and stanols lower LDL-cholesterol concentrations equivalently in hypercholesterolemic persons, *Am. J. Clin. Nutr.*, 76, 1272, 2002.
24. Law, M.R., Plant sterol and stanol margarines and health, *West. J. Med.*, 173, 43, 2000.
25. Keys, A., Anderson, J.T., and Grande, F., Serum cholesterol response to change in the diet I: Iodine value of dietary fat versus 2S-P, *Metabolism*, 14, 747, 1965.
26. Ostlund, R.E., Jr. et al., Phytosterols that are naturally present in commercial corn oil significantly reduce cholesterol absorption in humans, *Am. J. Clin. Nutr.*, 75, 1000, 2002.
27. Hallikainen, M.A. and Uusitupa, M.I., Effects of 2 low-fat stanol ester-containing margarines on serum cholesterol concentrations as part of a low-fat diet in hypercholesterolemic subjects, *Am. J. Clin. Nutr.*, 69, 403, 1999.
28. Simons, L.A., Additive effect of plant sterol-ester margarine and cerivastatin in lowering low-density lipoprotein cholesterol in primary hypercholesterolemia, *Am. J. Cardiol.*, 90, 737, 2002.
29. Mensink, R.P. et al., Effects of plant stanol esters supplied in low-fat yoghurt on serum lipids and lipoproteins, non-cholesterol sterols and fat soluble antioxidant concentrations, *Atherosclerosis*, 160, 205, 2002.
30. Moghadasian, M.H. et al., Lack of regression of atherosclerotic lesions in phytosterol-treated apo E-deficient mice, *Life Sci.*, 64, 1029, 1999.
31. Moghadasian, M.H. et al., Proatherogenic and antiatherogenic effects of probucol and phytosterols in apolipoprotein E-deficient mice: possible mechanisms of action, *Circulation*, 99, 1733, 1999.
32. Moghadasian, M.H. et al., "Tall oil"-derived phytosterols reduce atherosclerosis in ApoE-deficient mice, *Arterioscler. Thromb. Vasc. Biol.*, 17, 119, 1997.
33. Volger, O.L. et al., Dietary vegetable oil and wood derived plant stanol esters reduce atherosclerotic lesion size and severity in apoE*3-Leiden transgenic mice, *Atherosclerosis*, 157, 375, 2001.
34. Awad, A.B., Smith, A.J., and Fink, C.S., Plant sterols regulate rat vascular smooth muscle cell growth and prostacyclin release in culture, *Prostaglandins Leukot. Essent. Fatty Acids*, 64, 323, 2001.
35. Plat, J. et al., Effects on serum lipids, lipoproteins and fat soluble antioxidant concentrations of consumption frequency of margarines and shortenings enriched with plant stanol esters, *Eur. J. Clin. Nutr.*, 54, 671, 2000.
36. Nissinen, M. et al., Micellar distribution of cholesterol and phytosterols after duodenal plant stanol ester infusion, *Am. J. Physiol. Gastrointest. Liver Physiol.*, 282, G1009, 2002.

37. Miettinen, T.A. et al., Serum, biliary, and fecal cholesterol and plant sterols in colectomized patients before and during consumption of stanol ester margarine, *Am. J. Clin. Nutr.*, 71, 1095, 2000.

38. Ostlund, R.E., Jr. et al., Gastrointestinal absorption and plasma kinetics of soy δ(5)-phytosterols and phytostanols in humans, *Am. J. Physiol. Endocrinol. Metab.*, 282, E911, 2002.

39. Yu, L. et al., Disruption of ABCG5 and ABCG8 in mice reveals their crucial role in biliary cholesterol secretion, *Proc. Natl. Acad. Sci. USA*, 99, 16237, 2002.

40. Yu, L. et al., Overexpression of ABCG5 and ABCG8 promotes biliary cholesterol secretion and reduces fractional absorption of dietary cholesterol, *J. Clin. Invest.*, 110, 671, 2002.

41. Salen, G., Ahrens, E.H., and Grundy, S.M., Metabolism of beta-sitosterol in man, *J. Clin. Invest.*, 49, 952, 1970.

42. Tavani, D.M., Nes, W.R., and Billheimer, J.T., The sterol substrate specificity of acyl CoA cholesterol acyltransferase from rat liver, *J. Lipid Res.*, 23, 774, 1982.

43. Salen, G. et al., Sitosterolemia, *J. Lipid Res.*, 33, 945, 1992.

44. Salen, G. et al., Lethal atherosclerosis associated with abnormal plasma and tissue sterol composition in sitosterolemia with xanthomatosis, *J. Lipid Res.*, 26, 1126, 1985.

45. Berge, K.E. et al., Accumulation of dietary cholesterol in sitosterolemia caused by mutations in adjacent ABC transporters, *Science*, 290, 1771, 2000.

46. Chen, H.C., Molecular mechanisms of sterol absorption, *J. Nutr.*, 31, 2603, 2001.

47. Hubacek, J.A. et al., Mutations in ATP-cassette binding proteins G5 (ABCG5) and G8 (ABCG8) causing sitosterolemia, *Hum. Mutat.*, 18, 359, 2001.

48. Plat, J., van Onselen, E.N.M., and Mensink, R.P., Dietary plant stanol ester mixtures: effects on safety parameters and erythrocyte membrane fatty acid composition in non-hypercholesterolemic subjects, *Eur. Heart J.*, 1 (suppl.), S58, 1999.

49. Hepburn, P.A., Horner, S.A., and Smith, M., Safety evaluation of phytosterol esters 2: subchronic 90-day oral toxicity study on phytosterol esters — a novel functional food, *Food Chem. Toxicol.*, 37, 521, 1999.

50. Sanders, D.J. et al., The safety evaluation of phytosterol esters 6: comparative absorption and tissue distribution of phytosterols in the rat, *Food Chem. Toxicol.*, 38, 485, 2000.

51. Davidson, M.H. et al., Safety and tolerability of esterified phytosterols administered in reduced-fat spread and salad dressing to healthy adult men and women, *J. Am. Coll. Nutr.*, 20, 307, 2001.

52. Turnbull, D. et al., 13-week oral toxicity study with stanol esters in rats, *Regul. Toxicol. Pharmacol.*, 29, 216, 1999.

53. Plat, J., Kerckhoffs, D.A., and Mensink, R.P., Therapeutic potential of plant sterols and stanols, *Curr. Opin. Lipidol.*, 11, 571, 2000.

54. Plat, J. and Mensink, R.P., Effects of diets enriched with two different plant stanol ester mixtures on plasma ubiquinol-10 and fat-soluble antioxidant concentrations, *Metabolism*, 50, 520, 2001.

16 Non-Nutrient Food Factors and Cardiovascular Diseases

Simin Bolourchi-Vaghefi

CONTENTS

16.1 PROTECTIVE EFFECTS OF FLAVONOIDS ON CARDIOVASCULAR DISEASES: INTRODUCTION

Atherosclerosis and its related complications, coronary heart disease (CHD), myocardial infarction and stroke, have been identified as the major causes of mortality and morbidity in the Western world. Atherosclerosis is a progressive build-up of fatty streaks on the interior arterial walls that prevents adequate blood supply to the myocardium. Although many factors are involved in atherosclerosis, oxidation of low-density lipoprotein (LDL) by free radicals may initiate the lesions and lead to the development and progression of cardiovascular disease (CVD).

Development of atherosclerotic plaques in arteries involves accumulations of oxidized LDL cholesterol and lipids in macrophages and smooth muscle cells that lead to foam cell formation. Enzymes from injured endothelia, macrophages, and smooth muscle cells can produce oxidized free radicals — molecules with unpaired electrons that damage cells and tissues. Various reactive oxygen species are generated daily during normal aerobic metabolic processes and exposure to smog, chemicals, drugs, radiation, and high oxygen intake. Free radicals propagate more radicals, taking electrons from cell constituents including cell membranes, nucleic acids, and amino acids. Damage due to free radicals results in DNA mutations, protein structural disruption, and lipid degradation —processes implicated in the etiology of athero-sclerosis, cancer, and many other degenerative diseases.

Antioxidants provide the electrons that neutralize free radicals and protect LDL from oxidation to reduce the risk of CVD. Low dietary intakes of food sources of antioxidants (vitamins A, C, E, and beta-carotene and flavonoids) increase the prob-ability of oxidized LDL production in the body. Individuals with high dietary cho-lesterol and fat intakes who develop hypercholesterolemia are at a greater risk of developing cardiovascular disease due to increased LDL oxidation.[1] Dietary factors play a major role in the development or prevention of chronic diseases such as CVD and foods that enhance health and prevent diseases have gained interest and directed attention to naturally occurring non-nutrients such as polyphenolic compounds found in plants (flavonoids). Many different non-nutrient factors contained in foods of plant origin produce antioxidant activity or other important health effects for humans. These compounds are widely distributed among foods and beverages and include fruits, vegetables, whole grains, legumes, tea, wine, and cocoa. Epidemiological studies have shown that populations with high dietary intakes of fruits and vegetables have lower rates of heart disease, cancer, and other ailments of aging.[2] The roles that factors other than nutrients (vitamins, minerals, amino acids, and fatty acids) play in preven-tion or treatment of cardiovascular diseases will be discussed in this chapter.

16.2 ANTIOXIDANT ACTIVITIES OF FLAVONOIDS*

Oxidative stress and reactive oxygen species are major factors in the pathophysiology of CVD. The protective mechanism of flavonoids associated with reducing CVD is believed to be due to the potent antioxidant and free radical scavenging abilities that prevent oxidation of LDL.[1,2] Cao et al. studied the serum antioxidant capacities of eight elderly women after intake of strawberries, spinach, red wine, and vitamin C to determine which antioxidant nutrients provided the best protection. The study indicated that the potentially important antioxidants other than vitamin C contained in the foods consumed produced over 80% of the total antioxidant capacity. Cao et al. concluded that the consumption of the rich antioxidant phenolic compounds contained in strawberries, spinach, and red wine are able to increase serum antiox-idant capacities in humans.[3]

High flavonoid intake is directly correlated with decreased risk of CVD. The potent antioxidant abilities of flavonoids have been demonstrated in various studies. Noroozi et al. compared the antioxidant abilities of vitamin C with flavonoids and concluded that flavonoids were more protective than vitamin C in reducing oxidative

---

* The assistance of Carlie Abersold in preparation of this section is greatly appreciated.

DNA damage.[4] The unpaired electrons formed *in vivo* during regular aerobic metabolism damage DNA, proteins, and lipids without adequate antioxidant protection.

Flavonoids are the largest class and the most common group of plant polyphenols with over 5000 subclasses identified, and are responsible for giving most of the flavor and color to fruits and vegetables. Sunlight is required for synthesis of polyphenols in plants. That means higher concentrations appear in areas with the most exposure to the sun — the skins of fruits and outer layers of vegetables. The basic flavonoid is low in molecular weight, is often bound to a sugar molecule (glycoside), and tends to be water-soluble, thus enhancing absorption from the gut into the blood. The flavonoid molecular structure consists of two aromatic rings linked through three carbons. The six major subclasses of flavonoids based upon heterocyclic C-ring variations are anthocyanidins found in berries, grapes, fruit, and juices; catechins found in black, green, and oolong teas; flavonones found in citrus fruits; flavones found in grains and herbs; flavonols found in fruits, onions, and botanicals; and isoflavones found in legumes.[2]

Flavonoids have received considerable attention for their specific properties and health benefits although conflicting data have been reported. Intakes of flavonoids and their effects on CVD were the focus of the Zutphen study conducted with 805 men aged 65 to 84 in 1985. Food intake was recorded using diet histories. Flavonoid consumption averaged 26 mg/day. Data from health records including morbidity and mortality rates after 5 years were examined. The intake of flavonoids, specifically quercetin, was found to be inversely associated with CHD mortality. The subjects of this study were followed up 10 years later, when the results showed that the group of men with highest flavonoid intakes had decreased risk of all-cause mortality compared to those with lowest flavonoid intakes.[5]

The prevalence of CVD is different among various populations. The U.S., Finland, and the Netherlands have higher heart disease mortality rates compared to southern European countries and Japan, which have the lowest rates of cardiac-related mortality. It is interesting that in the diets of people in the U.S., Finland, and the Netherlands intakes of saturated fats, meats, and sugars are very high and intakes of fruits, vegetables, whole grains, and legumes are low, thus indicating low intakes of all types of antioxidants and phytochemicals.

The Seven Countries Study followed 12,763 men aged 40 to 59 at the onset and continued for 25 years to test the hypothesis that a diet similar to the Mediterranean diet is correlated with decreased risk of all-cause and CVD-related deaths. Flavonoid intake was estimated by using an equivalent food composite of the participants' average reported diets. The study reported flavonoid intakes of 2.6 mg/day in Finland, 68.2 mg/day in Japan, and 12.9 mg/day consumed by U.S. railroad workers. Study data convincingly found protective roles for fruits and vegetables in CVD and showed that average flavonoid intakes were inversely associated with CHD.[6]

According to the Second Joint Task Force of European and Other Societies on Coronary Prevention **at least** 400 g/day of fruits and vegetables is recommended to provide protective cardiac benefits.[7] Many studies have fallen short of this recommendation and may be responsible for some of the conflicting results. The U.S. government endorses and promotes increased intakes of fruits and vegetables for improved health. The combined benefits of antioxidants, fiber, potassium, magnesium, and other phytochemicals in fruits, berries, and vegetables may be the key to reducing CVD.[8] However, a U.S. study of health professional males aged 40 to 75 did not find a significant relationship of CHD and flavonoid intake.[9]

The Kuopio Ischaemic Heart Disease (KIHD) Risk Factor Study investigated the risk factors for CVD, atherosclerosis, and related outcomes associated with dietary intake of food groups including fruits, berries, and vegetables. Participants included 2641 Finnish men aged 42 to 60 at baseline with no previous CVD history. Daily intake of fruits, berries, and vegetables was 284 g (mean SD +/− 182 g). Subjects were divided into five groups according to their mean daily intakes (below 133, 133 to 214, 215 to 293, 294 to 408, and above 408 g/day). Participants' dietary intakes were assessed using their 4-day food intake records during the baseline phase of the study and blood samples were obtained for analysis. Men in the highest fruit-and-vegetable intake group had healthier lifestyle behaviors — not smoking and drinking less alcohol than those of the lower intake groups. These men also had lower blood pressure, plasma fibrinogen levels, and total and LDL cholesterol levels compared with the others. Of the men who died of CVD in the first 5 years of follow-up, intakes of fruits, berries, and vegetables were 41% lower. Men in the lowest fifth of intake level had the highest rates of CVD death, non-CVD death, and total mortality during a mean follow-up of 12.8 years. A significant inverse relationship was observed between intakes of fruits, berries, and vegetables and all-cause CVD- and non-CVD-related mortality.[10]

Bazzano et al., in an epidemiologic survey follow-up of data from the National Health and Nutrition Examination, showed an inverse relationship of fruit and vegetable intake with CVD risk and all-cause mortality in the general U.S. population. This study followed 9,600 participants representing over 160,000 person-years. Findings indicated that multiple mechanisms might be involved in the protective effects of fruits, berries, and vegetables against CHD. The beneficial components proposed in this study included antioxidant compounds and polyphenols such as vitamin C, carotenoids, and flavonoids in fruits and vegetables.[11]

The benefits of a high-grain, fruit-and-vegetable, low-fat diet were evaluated by Singh et al.[12] in a study including 1066 sedentary middle-age participants in a randomized, single-blind study. Over a 2-year period, a diet high in fruits, vegetables, legumes, and whole grains, including plant oils high in linolenic acid consumed as mustard or soybean oil and walnuts, reduced serum total cholesterol, LDL cholesterol, and tryglycerides significantly. Singh et al. noted a significant reduction in nonfetal myocardial infarction, sudden cardiac death, and total cardiac endpoints. They concluded that in the south Asian population, increased susceptibility to CVD is due to decreased consumption of fruits and vegetables that causes a deficiency of antioxidants, vitamins A and C, and n-3 fatty acids and overproduction of free radicals.

Liu et al. reported a prospective cohort of 75,521 U.S. women 38 to 63 years old with no previous diagnoses of diabetes mellitus or CVD who participated in a 12-year study. Higher consumption of whole grain foods by these women, although representing a healthy lifestyle, was associated with lower incidence of ischemic stroke.[13] The benefits of a diet high in legumes, whole grains, fruits and vegetables, and nuts such as the Mediterranean diet and diets consumed in southern Europe, the

Middle East, and Asia accrue from adequate amounts of antioxidants in the form of flavonoids, vitamins A, C, and E, and n-3 fatty acids, and also by displacing the high meat, fat, and sugar intakes in the West. These studies indicate a direct relationship between consuming a Mediterranean-type diet and lower incidences of CVD and other degenerative diseases.

16.2.1 GRAPE SEEDS AND RED WINE

The cardioprotective effect of polyphenolic compounds in certain foods is supported by epidemiological studies.[14] Wu et al. looked at the flavonoids in red wine and purple grape juice, examining their antioxidant capacities and platelet aggregation reducing properties. Moderate consumption of red wine was determined to be associated with decreased risk of CVD.[15]

Freedman et al. investigated CVD-protective properties by looking at the effects of purple grape juice (PGJ) and the flavonoid content in PGJ on platelet function and platelet nitric oxide (NO) production. They studied 20 healthy subjects consuming 7 ml/kg daily of PGJ for 14 days. The study results showed that participants had decreased platelet aggregation, reduced super oxide production, and enhanced NO release as a result of PGJ consumption. NO production increased from 3.5+/–1.2 to 6.0+/–1.5 pmol/108 platelets and super oxide production was reduced from 29.5+/–5.0 to 19.2+/–3.1 arbitrary units. Additionally, the plasma antioxidant activity increased by 50%, indicating the benefit may have been due to the antioxidant activities of flavonoids present in purple grape products.[16]

A short-term study administering red wine polyphenolic compounds (RWPCs) to rats investigated hemodynamic measures and vascular reactivity. The rats received intragastric administration of 5% glucose or 20/mg/kg of red wine polyphenolic compounds for 7 days. In the animals receiving the RWPCs, a progressive decrease in systolic blood pressure was observed after day 4 of the study. The aortas of these animals also displayed "increased endothelium-dependent relaxation to acetylcholine that was related to increased endothelial NO activity and involved a mechanism sensitive to superoxide anion scavengers." According to a plasma glutathione assay, the rats treated with RWPCs did not experience increases in total body oxidative stress. This study showed a decrease in blood pressure and improved NO vasodilatation associated with the induction of gene expression of inducible NO synthase and cylcloxygenase-2 that maintains flexibility within the vascular walls due to short-term oral administration of RWPCs. However, researchers explain that limited data is available concerning whether the levels of polyphenols in the circulation are sufficient after oral RWPC administration to provide beneficial cardiovascular effects.[17]

Naturally occurring polyphenolic components of red wine increase antioxidant activity in plasma that prevents the oxidation of LDL cholesterol delaying atheroma formation.[18] Nuttall et al. evaluated the antioxidant activity of a mixture of polyphenols extracted and purified from grape seeds containing 300 mg of grape proanthocyanidins. The study concluded that grape seed extract, because its antioxidant properties reduce oxidative stress and decrease risk of CVD, may have potential pharmaceutical application in prevention or treatment of CVD.[1]

Hamsters fed a hypercholesterolemic diet for 10 weeks developed foam cells characteristic of the early stages of atherosclerosis. The percent of aorta filled with foam cells in these animals was reduced by approximately 50 and 63% after supplementation with 50 and 100 mg/kg, respectively, of grape seed proanthocyanidin extract (GSPE). Including niacin-bound chromium (NBC) with the GSPE reduced the cholesterol and triglyceride levels, providing an additional benefit that may reduce the incidence of atherosclerosis.[19]

Evidence has increasingly shown protective effects of red wine consumption on established heart disease. Pataki et al.[14] demonstrated that red grape seed proanthocyanidins improve cardiac recovery after ischemia in animals. Two groups of rats were fed either 50 or 100 mg grape seed proanthocyanidins/kg for 3 weeks; a third group served as controls. After 30 minutes of ischemia and 2 hours of reperfusion, the animals treated with proanthocyanidins had reduced incidences of abnormal heart contractions equal to 42 and 25% respectively as compared with 92% in the control group. Proanthocyanidin treatment of 100 mg/kg significantly reduced oxygen free radical formation by 75% compared with control animals. After 60 minutes of reperfusion, an improvement of 32% coronary blood flow, 98% aortic blood flow, and 37% in blood pressure was observed in the highest treatment group compared with controls.[15]

Another study using similar methodology indicated proanthocyanidins in red wine have protective cardiac benefits. Sato et al. found a significant reduction in the appearance of the reactive oxygen species in animal hearts and improved contractile recovery after 100 mg/kg/day oral supplementation along with a regular diet for 3 weeks.[20]

Existing evidence based on human and animal studies indicates that flavonoids in PGJ and red wine prevent initiation of atherosclerosis by one or more mechanisms. Folts reported that 15 patients with coronary artery disease showed significant improvement after consumption of 5 ml/kg of red wine or 5 to 10 ml/kg of PGJ which inhibited platelet aggregation, protected against epinephrine activation of platelets, and enhanced platelet and endothelial production of NO. Protection against LDL cholesterol oxidation is increased with PGJ consumption, suggesting that moderate amounts of red wine or purple grape juice may be a part of the recommended five to seven servings per day of fruits and vegetables for a healthy heart.[21]

Two properties of red wine polyphenols have been proposed to account for the antiatherogenic effect. Red wine reduces LDL oxidation and inhibits smooth muscle cell proliferation.[22] However, data on the absorption of phenolic compounds from red wine, especially flavonols, are limited and the bioavailability of these compounds is unknown. For phenolic compounds to directly reduce LDL oxidation, their absorption into the blood is necessary.

The bioavailability of flavonols, especially quercetin, from red wine was compared with the major dietary sources in yellow onions and black tea. De Vries et al. studied 12 healthy men who consumed 750 ml red wine, 50 g fried onions, or 375 ml of black tea in random order for a total of 4 days each, followed by a 3-day wash-out period. The intake of quercetin provided by the 3 interventions was 14 to 16 mg/day. Concentration of plasma quercetin after consumption of tea and after drinking wine was lower than that after consumption of onions. Urinary excretion of quercetin after consumption of wine and onions was the same and it was higher after drinking tea. The study concluded that flavonols are absorbed from red wine, onions, and tea. However, red wine may be a poorer source of flavonols than onions or tea because 1 glass of red wine (125 ml) provides less available flavonols than 1 portion of onions (15 g) or 1 glass of tea (125 ml).[23]

16.2.2 TEA

The protective effects of tea on heart disease have been demonstrated in experiments on animals and humans. The exact mechanisms whereby tea provides protection against heart disease are not known but are beginning to be understood as research continues to investigate this popular beverage of which 3 billion kg are produced and consumed annually. Tea consumption is reportedly 78% black tea in the West, 20% green tea in Asia, and 2% oolong tea, partially fermented and produced mainly in southern China.

Tea contains polyphenolic compounds that are biologically active when immersed in hot water and promptly solubilized. The main compounds in tea are commonly known as catechins, a subclass of flavonoids. A serving of tea made with 1 g leaf and 100 ml water brewed for 3 minutes contains about 250 to 350 tea solids consisting of 30 to 42% catechins and 3 to 6% caffeine. Tea polyphenols are recognized for their antioxidant activities that scavenge reactive (free radical) oxygen species.[24]

Studies have investigated the relationship of tea consumption and cardiovascular disease. A long-term Dutch cohort study illustrated that participants with the highest tea consumption had a lower risk of death from CHD and a lower incidence of stroke. In Rotterdam, the findings of a follow-up study showed an inverse relationship of tea consumption with severity of aortic atherosclerosis.[25] The Boston Area Health Study found that subjects who drank 200 to 250 ml (approximately 1 cup) or more of black tea daily lowered their risk of heart attack to approximately half the risk of those who drank no tea.[26]

Young et al. examined the LDL oxidative status in subjects in a blinded crossover human study of green tea extract (GTE) after dietary depletion of flavonoids and catechins. This study included 8 smokers and 8 nonsmokers with daily GTE intakes containing 18.6 mg catechins. The extract was placed in meat patties and consumed with a diet strictly controlled and low in flavonoid intake. Smokers experienced the most prominent effect of increased plasma antioxidant capacity equal to 1.35 to 1.56 postprandial after 10 weeks. No long-term effects of GTE were found so the findings basically indicated that the effects of flavonoids in tea and in fruits and vegetables are immediate and not long-term without continued daily intake.[27]

Several mechanisms have been proposed for the beneficial effect drinking tea has against heart disease. One is that tea polyphenols inhibit the oxidation of LDL and therefore reduce development of the atherosclerosis contributing to CVD. Another proposed mechanism contributing to protection against heart disease is the hypocholesterolemic activity of tea.

Tea polyphenols from green and black tea prevented increased serum total cholesterol and triglyceride levels in animals that were fed high-fat, high-cholesterol diets. These animals also experienced decreased total serum cholesterol and increased fecal excretion of total lipids and cholesterol. Other epidemiological studies and human trials have not produced similar results and instead failed to show a decrease in serum cholesterol after green or black tea consumption.[25]

Cardioprotective effects of flavonoids are complex and include the involvement of homocysteine, cholesterol, platelet function, and the protection of LDL. In a Norwegian cohort study, participants were divided into 5 groups according to levels of tea consumption (less than 1 cup/day, 1 to 2 cups/day, 3 to 7 cups/day, more than 8 cups/day, and nondrinkers). Comparing the 4 tea-drinking groups to nondrinkers, plasma cholesterol levels were inversely correlated with tea consumption and serum cholesterol levels decreased by 6, 12, 19, and 28% from the lowest to the highest tea consumption group. Homocysteine levels were affected by tea consumption in these same groups with some different results. Consumers of less than 1 cup/day had 6% reductions of plasma homocysteine, moderate consumers of 1 to 2 cups/day had 20% reductions, and moderate-to-high consumers of 3 to 7 cups/day had 31% reductions. High consumers (more than 8 cups/day) showed 9% increases in plasma homocysteine concentrations compared with nondrinkers.[28] According to this study, drinking more than 7 cups of tea/day is not as effective in reducing levels of plasma homocysteine as drinking 2 to 7 cups of tea/day.

In Oppland county in Norway, another study was conducted to determine the relationship between black tea consumption and serum cholesterol concentration, systolic blood pressure, and mortality from all causes of CHD. Participants included 9,856 men and 10,233 women aged 35 to 49. Increased tea consumption was significantly correlated with lower mean serum cholesterol and reduced systolic blood pressure. Deaths from CHD in men were reduced by 40% for those drinking 1 cup/day compared to nondrinkers.[29]

Before advocating tea consumption as part of a healthy diet, three concerns must be studied further: the role of caffeine in tea, reduced iron absorption with meals, and the high content of aluminum in tealeaf and brewed tea.[30] The level of caffeine in 10 to 12 cups of tea daily is less than 400 to 450 mg/day, which is considered a safe amount according to Canadian health authorities.[31] North American adults are estimated to consume an average of 186 to 238 mg/day which includes 60% from coffee, 30% from tea, and 10% from a mix of other sources such as colas, chocolate, and drugs. This is below the proposed upper level of safe daily caffeine intake with no associated risk from moderate caffeine consumption.[32]

Another concern involves decreased iron absorption in the gastrointestinal tract with tea consumption. Heme iron derived from animal foods is better absorbed than nonheme iron. The polyphenols in tea reduced the bioavailability of nonheme iron when consumed with meals. Drinking tea between meals did not show any effect on iron absorption. Also, healthy individuals eating well-balanced diets including animal sources of heme iron will not likely suffer iron deficiency anemia.[33] Therefore consuming tea is not a real risk for iron deficiency anemia except in people vulnerable to this deficiency, women of child-bearing age belonging to the group under the poverty line and very young children in the same group.

The level of aluminum in tea leaves has drawn concern among some health professionals. However, tea consumption does not increase the level of aluminum in the blood which is necessary for accumulation of aluminum in tissues. Epidemiological data have indicated no association of drinking tea with Alzheimer's disease because the incidence of Alzheimer's disease in individuals and countries with high tea intake is not significantly different from the incidence of individuals and countries with lower tea consumption. Additionally, aluminum in tea leaves dissolved in water is not readily available, which is possibly due to the gelatinous mucilage that binds aluminum that many tea leaves produce upon submersion in water. No evidence supports the role of tea in the pathogenesis of Alzheimer's disease.[31]

The studies reported in the literature show conflicting results as to the health effects of red wine, grape seeds, and tea flovonoids. The variability of study results on flavonoids may be due to many factors including bioavailability, content, varieties, seasons, weather conditions, soil, and estimations of individual dietary intake that may affect the outcome. As a result, the relationship of these compounds to health and disease is difficult to determine.

Antioxidant activity is believed to be a main reason for the protective effects of flavonoids. Normal acrobic metabolism can cause formation of reactive oxygen species and cause damage to DNA, protein, and lipids despite the body's normal defense system. The oxidative stress due to actions of these free radicals may lead to the development of atherosclerosis and heart disease. The antioxidant properties of fruits, vegetables, red wine, and tea may be good reasons to include these food items as a regular part of a healthy diet and an approach to a healthful lifestyle. Additionally, there are other well-known direct and indirect health benefits that these foods and drinks can provide.

There is no "magic bullet" to prevent chronic diseases such as CVD and cancer, but a variety of factors in fruits, vegetables, red wine, and tea are believed to play protective roles in the onset of chronic degenerative diseases. The consumption of fruits and vegetables must be a part of a healthy diet. Eating a variety of these foods may bring an unrelated bonus. Fruits and vegetables may replace high-fat, high-calorie, low-nutrient foods that are parts of daily American diets and thus prevent weight gain and associated complications such as diabetes mellitus, cancer, and other diseases. Since existing literature data is not totally in agreement as to the effects of food flavonoids in prevention or treatment of chronic diseases, further studies are needed to better explain the exact components in foods responsible for and the mechanisms involved that provide healthful benefits.

16.3 LYCOPENE AND CARDIOVASCULAR DISEASE

Lycopene is a carotenoid without vitamin A activity that has gained fame as a substance in tomatoes, tomato sauces, pizza sauce, and other tomato products that prevents prostate cancer. Research has shown that lycopene containing many conjugated double bonds is a potent antioxidant and has the strongest singlet oxygen quenching capacity among the carotenoids. Antioxidant capacity of alpha-carotene, beta-carotene, and lutein follow lycopene in strength, respectively.[34] Lycopene is a fat-soluble pigment found in tomatoes, pink grapefruits, watermelons, and a few other fruits and vegetables and is responsible for their red color. Although tomatoes and tomato products are rich sources of beta-carotene, folate, and potassium and are very high in vitamin C, their lycopene content has recently received attention because they are the main sources of this substance in the diet of the U.S. population.

The absorptive mechanism of lycopene is not well understood. When tomato products are heated, the amount of lycopene in circulation and its concentration increase, especially when the heated tomato products are accompanied by oil.[35] Smoking is believed to increase free radicals in the tissues of smokers, causing oxidation of LDL leading to foam cell production and atherosclerosis. In some studies, the concentration of lycopene is reported to be lower by 18 to 44% in the plasmas of smokers as compared with nonsmokers.[36,37] A study of human subjects by Rao and Agarwal showed that postprandial concentration of serum lycopene was lower than fasting serum concentration. A 40% decrease in serum lycopene concentrations was observed immediately after subjects smoked 3 cigarettes in 30 minutes. It is believed that lycopene is used to counteract the free radicals produced by meal- and smoke-induced metabolic stress.[38]

Arab and Steck reviewed other studies[39] showing that cigarette smoking had no effects on level plasma lycopene concentrations. Plasma concentration of alpha-carotene, beta-carotene, lutein, zeaxanthin, cryptozanthin, and *cis*-beta-carotene were lower in smokers than in nonsmokers at the same levels of intake but the concentrations of lycopene in the same subjects did not differ. The investigators found this contrary to expectation and speculate that lycopene's protective mechanism may not be due only to its antioxidant properties.

A study by Brady et al.[40] showed that although diets of smokers were lower in lycopene than those of nonsmokers, serum lycopene concentrations were not significantly different between the two groups. Since studies by different investigators have shown mixed results on the effects of smoking on concentrations of lycopene in the circulation of human subjects, the relationship of lycopene and smoking is not clearly defined.

The Kuopio Ischaemic Heart Disease Risk Factor Study is an ongoing investigation of an eastern Finland population that has the highest rate of cardiovascular disease recorded. The investigators are studying the risk factors for different aspects of CVD, atherosclerosis, and associated problems in the male population between the ages of 46 to 64.[41] Rissanen et al.[42] studied the relationship of serum lycopene concentration to the intima media thickness of the common carotid artery. The study included 1028 subjects who were asked to refrain from smoking and drinking alcohol for 3 days and fast for 12 hours before blood was drawn after 30 minutes of relaxing. Intima media thicknesses of the subjects' common carotid arteries were measured by high resolution B-mode ultrasonography. Serum lycopene, beta-carotene, and alpha-tocopherol levels were determined.

The subjects were classified into four groups according to their serum lycopene concentrations. The highest significant mean and maximal intima media thicknesses of the common carotid arteries were found in the subjects falling in the lowest quarter of serum lycopene concentrations ($p = 0.005$ and $p = 0.001$, respectively). The mean and maximal intima media thicknesses increased across the quarters as serum lycopene decreased. The investigators concluded that serum lycopene concentration plays a role in thickness of the intima media of the common carotid artery and is associated with the onset of atherosclerosis of that artery.

The preventing role that lycopene may play in CVD may be due to the hydrocarbon carotenoids including beta-carotene and lycopene that are transported in LDL. Because of the positions of these carotenoids in the LDL molecule, they can protect LDL from oxidation.[43] Studies have also shown that adipose tissue concentration of lycopene is associated with protection against myocardial infarction. The highest concentration in the adipose tissue is most protective in nonsmoking men.

Although the biological activity of lycopene is complex and requires extensive studies to be explained, the literature includes some interesting studies worth mentioning. Fuhrman et al.[44] reported the non-antioxidant function of lycopene both *in vitro* and in human subjects. The addition of lycopene to macrophage cell lines *in vitro* caused a decrease of 73% in cholesterol synthesis and an increase in LDL receptors. Incubation of cells with lycopene caused 34% increased LDL degradation and about 110% LDL removal from the circulation. The same investigators in a study of 6 men showed a 14% reduction in plasma concentration of LDL when fed 60 mg/day of lycopene, equal to the amount of lycopene in 1 kg of tomatoes per day. No changes in plasma HDL concentration were found. The investigators suggest a 30 to 40% reduction in risk of myocardial infarction as a result of consuming this high amount of lycopene regularly.

Edwards et al. studied the bioavailability of lycopene from freshly frozen watermelon juice in a 19-week crossover study with healthy, nonsmoking adults. The subjects' diet was controlled to be a weight maintenance regimen. During a 2- to 4-week wash-out period preceding the treatment period, the diets of the subjects were restricted in lycopene-rich foods. All subjects received either 20.1 mg/day lycopene and 2.5 mg/day beta-carotene from watermelon juice (W-20), or a control diet with no juice (C-0) interspersed by a wash-out period. The subjects were divided into two groups for the third treatment. Twelve subjects consumed 40.2 mg/day lycopene and 5 mg/day beta-carotene from watermelon juice (W-40), and 10 subjects received 18.4 ml/day lycopene and 0.6 mg/day beta-carotene from tomato juice (T-20). Plasma lycopene concentration was shown to be bioavailable from both tomato juice and freshly frozen watermelon juice with no dose-response effect. Plasma beta-carotene concentration was significantly greater after both doses of watermelon juice than after tomato juice. The researchers concluded that heat treatment of watermelon juice is not necessary to make lycopene bioavailable; it is readily absorbed from freshly frozen juice.[45]

Research on the relationship between CVD risk and diet points to the importance of consuming foods that are good sources of food factors, such as vitamins, minerals, and non-nutrient components, that provide the body with antioxidants needed to prevent LDL oxidation, methylation of homocysteine, and factors that remove cholesterol from circulation. Fruits, vegetables, whole grains, and legumes provide these substances including lycopene, beta-carotene, alpha-tocopherol, and soluble and insoluble fiber. The suggestion of 5 to 9 servings of fruits and vegetables by Weisburger[46] and 400 to 500 g of fruits per day according to the European health authorities,[7] and following food patterns of Asian and Middle Eastern populations seem to be the keys to providing all the above dietary factors. A high-fiber diet containing both soluble and insoluble fiber will displace high-fat, high-protein foods and provide means of removing bile acids from circulation and reducing serum cholesterol. High intake of fruits and vegetables will increase serum concentrations of lycopene, beta-carotene, and alpha-tocopherol — all strong antioxidants that remove free radicals from tissues and convert methylate homocysteine into methionine, preventing LDL oxidation and risk of atherosclerosis.

16.4 GARLIC AND GARLIC PREPARATIONS

16.4.1 HISTORICAL PERSPECTIVES

Knowledge of the therapeutic benefits of garlic goes back thousands of years to the civilizations of ancient Egypt, Persia, India, China, Japan, and Greece. During antiquity, garlic was used for performance enhancement and prevention and treatment of various diseases. Ancient Egyptians recorded the use of garlic for increasing and maintaining laborers' strength and productivity. The Bible states Jewish slaves in Egypt had become fond of garlic and missed it after leaving that country. Garlic was an important part of the diets of both the Greek and Roman military forces because it was believed to give them strength especially during battle. Athletes used garlic with their diets during the first Olympic competitions in ancient Greece.

Garlic was used in food and medicine in ancient China. Records dating back to 2000 B.C.E. indicate that it was an ingredient of a medicine to treat headaches, fever, and insomnia and to improve male potency. Garlic was even used as a food preservative.

The oldest surviving Indian medical text, the 2000-year-old *Charaka-Samhita*, recommends garlic for treatment of heart disease and arthritis. The British army in the 19th century used garlic for its diuretic effect — an early indication of its effect in improving cardiovascular function. In many cultures, garlic is still consistently used for medicinal benefits and health purposes.[47]

Recent interest in natural and alternative disease therapies has given garlic renewed importance as a natural food constituent that may play a role in prevention of chronic diseases. Garlic has served as a condiment, flavoring, or vegetable throughout history because of its proven curative properties. In the past two decades, complementary and alternative medicine including consumption of foods believed to have medicinal properties (functional foods) has gained increased practice in the U.S. and was popular in Europe even earlier.

It is estimated that out-of-pocket expenditure for alternative therapeutic substances exceeds $5 billion per year in the U.S.[48] Garlic, now one of the most widely used herbal remedies in the world, has been subject to many animal experiments as well as human *in vivo* and *ex vivo* studies. Experiments with animals have shown that garlic is a strong antilipidemic, antihypertensive, antiglycemic, antithrombotic, and antiatherogenic food. Studies with humans have not been conclusive and are at best conflicting. One obvious reason for the conflicting results of human studies is that the nature of garlic and its preparations make it difficult if not impossible to plan well-controlled blind studies that subjects can follow for sufficiently long periods to obtain satisfactory and reproducible results.[49]

Researchers have been interested in investigating the beneficial attributes of garlic both as a preventive or curative agent for degenerative diseases. A great deal of interest surrounds the role garlic plays in prevention or treatment of cardiovascular diseases, cancer, diabetes, osteoporosis, and other chronic degenerative diseases. In the past two decades garlic has undergone many investigations and the amount of literature on the subject abounds.

This review will discuss the role of garlic in prevention and treatment of different aspects of cardiovascular diseases, including its effects on cholesterol synthesis, LDL oxidation, platelet aggregation, and hypertension. Cardiovascular diseases are complex and many factors such as high blood cholesterol levels, hypertension, blood clotting problems, platelet aggregation, blood and tissue homocysteine levels, and LDL oxidation influence their courses. An attempt will be made to review the role of garlic in relation to these factors and present a balanced point of view.

16.4.2 CHEMICAL COMPOSITION OF GARLIC

Garlic contains many sulfur compounds (organosulfurs), all the indispensable amino acids and eight dispensable ones, and a variety of vitamins and minerals including selenium. Most of the sulfur in fresh garlic is in the form of alliin. The alliinase enzyme also present in fresh garlic rapidly converts alliin to allicin when a clove is crushed. Allicin, the compound responsible for the characteristic garlic smell, is transient and converts into a variety of other sulfur-containing substances, some of which are also aromatic. Allicin is also an unstable compound that does not cross the intestinal cell membrane into the blood.[50] Organosulfur compounds released from allicin include S-allyl cystine, S-ethyl cysteine, and S-propyl cysteine.

Dehydrated preparations of garlic used in studies contain most natural constituents of whole garlic. Standardized preparations contain S-allyl cysteine-s-oxide (alliin). Dehydration is thought to make the liberation of the thiosulfinate compound allicin easier enzymatically after hydration. Aged garlic extract (AGE) contains S-allyl-cysteine. AGE is prepared by soaking slices of raw garlic in 15 to 20% aqueous ethanol at room temperature for as long as 20 months. The mixture of ethanol and garlic is then concentrated at low temperature under low pressure after filtration. This preparation has a high water-soluble component (S-allyl cysteine) and low amounts of oil-soluble components. Most studies reported in the literature have used this preparation; some studied garlic oil or fresh whole or chopped garlic.

Studying the effect of garlic in prevention and treatment of disease in human subjects is complicated because of the use of different garlic preparations and methods of preparing them. For this reason and also because of its characteristic aroma, blind studies of garlic are difficult to perform. The human studies are usually performed for short durations due to low compliance rate. The number of subjects in these studies is usually limited because few people like the social results of consuming garlic or its products. Different garlic preparations used in various studies make a comparison of the results difficult. Thus interpreting the results from many studies on the beneficial effects of garlic in preventing and treating human diseases is difficult without consideration of the methodology and the garlic fractions or preparations used.

16.4.3 Garlic and Cholesterol Synthesis

The reduction of blood lipid constituents, especially total and LDL cholesterol, as a result of intake of different garlic preparations makes the biochemical basis for the effect of garlic on cholesterol synthesis interesting. The hypocholesterolemic effect of garlic is believed to result from organosulfur compounds and their inhibitory effect on 3-hydroxy-3methyl-glutaryl CoA reductase (HMG-CoA reductase) activity. In a study of cultured rat hepatocytes, Liu and Yeh[51] showed that S-allyl cystine, S-ethyl cysteine, and S-propyl cysteine inhibited synthesis of cholesterol from C^{14} acetate while they had no effect on C^{14} mevalonate. Treatment of the cells with S-allyl cystine, S-ethyl cysteine, and S-propyl cysteine reduced the activity of HMG-CoA reductase by 30 to 40% compared with untreated cells. The organosulfur compounds did not change the mRNA coded for the enzyme or protein concentration of the enzyme but the ratio of expressed to total activity of the enzyme was reduced.

Lin and coworkers[52] looked at the effect of fresh garlic extract on the expression of the microsomal triglyceride transfer protein (MTP) gene *in vivo* in rats and *in vitro* in cell lines. They showed that fresh garlic extract reduces MTP mRNA levels in intestinal carcinoma Caco-2 and human hepatoma HepG2 cells significantly in a dose-response manner. Maximum effect was seen with 6g/L of fresh garlic extract that reduced MTP 59% in the intestinal carcinoma Caco-2 cells and 72% in human hepatoma HepG2 cells. These investigators believe that reduced MTP reduces the assembly and secretion of apolipoprotein B containing lipoprotein that is responsible for causing atherosclerosis and CHD. They proposed that long-term consumption of fresh garlic may have an effect on the levels of blood lipids and lipoproteins by reducing MTP-dependent microsomal lipid transport from the intestine, thus decreasing the assembly of chylomicrons and their secretion into the circulation. These studies open an area of interest for further research in identification of compounds in garlic responsible for and elucidating the molecular mechanisms of reduction, synthesis, and excretion and the lipoproteins responsible for transport of cholesterol.

16.4.4 Garlic and LDL Oxidation

Oxidized LDL is an important factor in initiation and progression of atherosclerosis, promoting vascular endothelial infiltration with foam cells, and formation of fatty streaks.[53–55] Oxidized LDL, having antigenic properties, behaves as a "foreign substance" and is recognized as such by the host immune system. The immune system responds by attracting the monocytes to intima where they differentiate into macrophages. The macrophages are stabilized in the intima, loaded with lipids, forming foam cells characteristic of fatty streaks.

These processes damage the endothelium, causing proliferation of monocytes, endothelial cells, and smooth muscle cells. Oxidized LDL causes cytotoxicity by altering the composition and permeability of endothelial cell membranes, thus causing vascular dysfunction.[56,57] Lau[58] describes several experiments in which preparations from garlic inhibited LDL oxidation. He showed that AGE inhibited LDL oxidation *in vitro* when $CuSO_4$ was used as an oxidizing agent. This inhibition was concentration-dependent. He also showed that all 4 water-soluble garlic compounds inhibited LDL oxidation at different concentrations varying from 10 mmol/L to 0.1 mmol/L, depending on the water-soluble organosulfur compound used.

Allixin (phytoallixin), an oil-soluble garlic fraction, is a plant defense or stress compound produced when bacteria, insects, and fungi attack plants; it is also a strong inhibitor of LDL oxidation. Allicin, another oil-soluble product of raw garlic, was shown by Lau's laboratory to enhance LDL oxidation.[58] Ide and Lau, in three *in vitro* assays, showed that oxidized LDL damages cell membranes and causes mitochondrial injuries. When vascular endothelial cells were pretreated with AGE and other water-soluble garlic products, cell injuries due to oxidized LDL were minimized.[59]

Lau also performed a small-scale, double-blind, placebo-controlled crossover human study with eight subjects. Four subjects received 1.2 g AGE 3 times daily for 2 weeks, followed by a 2-week wash-out period, and then a crossover to placebo for 2 more weeks. The other 4 subjects started with placebo, repeated the wash-out, and ended with 2 weeks of AGE supplement intake. Blood samples were drawn at 2, 4, and 6 weeks. LDL factions prepared by centrifugation were exposed to a $CuSO_4$ oxidizing agent and resistance to oxidation was measured. The conclusion of this small study was that consumption of commercial garlic preparations in the form of AGE by the subjects increased the resistance of plasma LDL to oxidation.

The antioxidant effects of AGE and S-allylcysteine (SAC), one of the major sulfur-containing compounds in AGE, on pulmonary artery endothelial cells (PAECs) was studied using oxidized LDL. Ide and Lau[60] showed that oxidized LDL causes extensive cell damage and lactic dehydrogenase (LDH) release. LDH is an intracellular enzyme that leaks from cells upon damage to their membranes. The researchers also showed that when they incubated the PAEC with AGE or SAC, the release of LDH due to oxidized LDL injury was significantly inhibited.

In another experiment, these investigators also incubated PAEC with oxidized LDL and showed a 60% decrease in total cellular glutathione, which is an important and most abundant intracellular antioxidant thiol compound that is protective against cell toxicity. They showed that preincubation of PAEC with AGE and SAC prevented depletion of intracellular gutathione, suggesting that the AGE and SAC garlic compounds prevent cell oxidative damage due to oxidized LDL by preventing glutathione depletion.

The antioxidant effect of AGE was proven by other methods. Dillon et al.[61] showed that dietary supplementation with age reduced oxidative stress in smokers more than in nonsmokers as evidenced by lowered concentration of 8-iso-prostaglandine F (2(alpha)) in both plasma and urine of the subjects in a 14-day trial. The concentrations of 8-iso-prostaglandine F (2(alpha)) returned to values similar to the presupplementation levels in urine and plasma. Dillon et al. concluded that dietary supplementation with AGE may be more effective in reducing oxidative stress in smoking than in nonsmoking men.

Brethaupt-Grogleret et al.[62] reported a protective effect of chronic garlic consumption on elastic properties of the aorta in elderly men and women. In studying 200 healthy subjects between the ages of 50 and 80, these investigators showed an attenuation of age-related increase in aorta stiffness in subjects consuming 100 mg garlic daily in tablet form for about 7 years. An age-related decrease in elastic properties of the aorta due to atherosclerosis and plaque formation is caused by oxidative stress involving LDL. This study may point to the protective effect of chronic garlic intake against LDL oxidation.

Zhang et al.[63] performed a randomized double-blind, placebo-controlled study lasting 11 weeks in which 17 subjects received garlic oil capsules (Cardiomax®), 17 received garlic powder (Garlicin®), and 17 received placebo as supplements. The capsule vials were treated with garlic oil so that all capsules for each group smelled the same. Capsules were counted as a measure of compliance. Blood samples were taken at the baseline and 4, 6, and 11 weeks to measure the antioxidant capacity of blood during the study and at weeks 14–15 and 17–18 after the study to measure residual effects. The total antioxidant capacity of the blood was elevated rapidly after 4 weeks in the group receiving garlic oil compared with those in the placebo and garlic powder groups. In the sixth week, the garlic powder group also showed a significant elevation in antioxidant capacity of blood. However, by the conclusion of the study, all three groups showed the same level of elevation in antioxidant capacity. The study did not control for diet and lifestyles so the investigators could not account for the increase in the antioxidant capacity of blood in placebo group.

Other studies have shown the same effect of garlic preparations on increasing the antioxidant capacity of blood in human subjects. They may imply that less LDL oxidation may lower the risk of atheroscelerosis as a result of consuming fresh garlic in the diet or garlic preparations as supplements. However, as mentioned above, the many confounding factors involved in studying the effects of garlic on human health make a precise, well-controlled study almost impossible to design and implement.

16.4.5 GARLIC AND PLATELET AGGREGATION

The effects of garlic and garlic preparations on platelet function have served as the subject of many studies. Rahman and Billington[64] studied the effects of dietary supplementation with AGE on 23 adult male subjects for 3 months. These normo-lipidemic subjects consumed 5 ml of AGE daily for 13 weeks. Supplementation with AGE produced no significant changes of serum total, LDL and HDL cholesterol, or serum tryglyceride concentrations. However, AGE supplementation significantly reduced the activity of serum alanine aminotransferase (ALT). ALT is a cytosolic enzyme released into blood as a result of damage to liver cells. Decrease in the activity of this enzyme as a result of consumption of AGE indicates AGE protects hepatocytes against toxins.

Other observations were significant reductions in total percentage and initial rate of platelet aggregation induced by ADP. Although triglycerides were reduced by 13% and total and LDL cholesterol were decreased by 3% after 13 weeks of supplementation with AGE, the changes were not statistically significant. The investigators believe that AGE will not change lipid profiles in normolipidemic subjects, at least not in the short term. They did not find an effect of AGE on the cycloxygenase pathway *in vivo*.[64] Other investigators reported effects of garlic preparation on activity of cycloygenase *in vitro*.[65] Legnani et al. demonstrated that serum TXB_2 is not affected 6 hours after consumption of 900 mg of dried garlic powder. However, platelet aggregation induced by ADP and collagen is inhibited.[66] Studies have also shown that garlic preparations reduce platelet aggregation and risk of thrombosis in human subjects.[67]

Steiner and Li investigated the effect of AGE on platelet function with 34 normal male and female subjects in a 44-week, double-blind, crossover, placebo-controlled study and showed that taking 800 mg AGE reduced platelet aggregation significantly during the study period. The investigators demonstrated a good rate of reproducibility of results but indicated lack of consensus on the possible mechanism of this reduction in platelet function as a result of AGE consumption.[68] Other published and unpublished studies show that garlic inhibits platelet aggregation and by this means reduces the frequency of thrombus formation, thus exerting cardioprotective effects.[69]

Investigators in other studies, however, reported that although garlic reduced serum cholesterol concentrations by 10% in patients with hyperlipoproteinemia and reduced systolic and diastolic pressures, it failed to reduce platelet aggregation.[70]

As these reviews show, reports on the effects of different garlic preparations on platelet aggregation and thrombosis are conflicting. This may be due to the unavailability of standard preparations of garlic products that would allow the design of reproducible studies free of confounding factors.

16.4.6 GARLIC AND CARDIOVASCULAR DISEASES

Cardiovascular disease (CVD) is the number one killer in the U.S. and Western Europe. Among many factors related to the onset of CVD, high-fat diets, sedentary living, smoking, excess consumption of alcohol, Type A personality (excessive stress), genetic potential, and other environmental factors are blamed as causes. Diet and lifestyle seem to be only factors that can be controlled.

Genetic and environmental factors like stress are generally beyond the control of people who have tendencies to contract these diseases. Diet is believed to play an important part in the prevention or onset of CVD. Evidence from epidemiological studies indicates lower incidences of CVD among populations with high consumptions of whole grains, fruits, vegetables, and spices. Of the spices common among these populations, garlic and other *Allium* species stand out.[71]

Considerable nonscientific anecdotal evidence from antiquity points out the role of garlic in treating many diseases including CVD. Garlic is mentioned in the 35-century-old Egyptian *Codex Ebers* as a powerful treatment for heart disorders, bites, worm infestations, and tumors. In the folklores of ancient Persia, Rome, Greece, and India, garlic is cited to maintain fluidity of blood and strengthen the heart.[72] In modern times, blood lipids and cholesterol are demonstrated to be lower among populations consuming large amounts of garlic and onion than in those who avoid these vegetables in their diets.[73] Early investigations of the effectiveness of garlic in reducing blood cholesterol and triglyceride levels were performed using high levels of raw garlic in healthy subjects and patients with ischemic heart disease.[74] The consumption of 3 g fresh raw garlic (a single clove daily) by study subjects for 16 weeks resulted in 21% reductions in serum cholesterol levels. This significant reduction was gradual and not observed until 4 weeks into the study. A significant reduction in serum thromboxane levels was also observed.[67]

Different constituents of garlic have been shown to exert different effects in reducing blood lipid fractions including total cholesterol, LDL cholesterol, and triglycerides. Steroid saponins in garlic were shown to interfere with absorption of cholesterol by the intestinal lumen and lowered plasma cholesterol levels in a variety of experimental animals.[75] Matsuura speculates that this may be the result of formation of complexes of saponins and other steroids in garlic products with cholesterol in the intestine, resulting in less cholesterol absorption and lowered plasma cholesterol in experimental animals.[76]

In a double-blind crossover study in 41 moderately hypercholesterolemic men who received AGE as supplement, Steiner et al. found AGE significantly reduced systolic and diastolic blood pressures as compared with the baseline and the placebo group. The subjects who received AGE reduced their total cholesterol and LDL cholesterol maximally after 3 months. No significant change was noted in their HDL or triglyceride levels.[77]

Brace,[50] in a comprehensive review of studies with garlic, concluded that studies using fresh garlic or commercial preparations "consistently found that garlic caused an increase in fibrinolytic activity, inhibited platelet aggregation, and lowered cholesterol." These effects were seen when large amounts of garlic (about seven cloves) were consumed continually. When the consumption of garlic stopped, the values were returned to baseline, thus indicating continued consumption is necessary. In most of the studies analyzed, the effect of garlic on CVD varied and different preparations of garlic were effective in lowering blood lipid profiles to a small extent in every parameter. Brace analyzed other studies that showed garlic was ineffective in lowering risks of CVD. He emphasized that poorly designed studies and confounding effects of commercially prepared, non-standardized garlic fractions used in the studies, short-term studies, small numbers of subjects, and lack of randomization accounted for the inconsistencies.[55]

Ackermann et al.[49] described the results of several human studies in which the effects of garlic on cardiovascular functions were tested. When compared with placebos, different garlic preparations resulted in moderate reductions in total serum cholesterol levels, with parallel changes in LDL levels and tryglycerides after "1 month (range of average pooled reductions, 0.03–0.45 mmol/L [1.2–17.3 mg/dL]) and at 3 months (range of average pooled reductions, 0.32–0.66 mmol/L [12.4–25.4 mg/dL]), but not at 6 months." Platelet aggregation was significantly reduced but the effect on hypertension was mixed.

Another meta-analysis[78] showed that consumption of garlic preparations reduced total cholesterol and LDL cholesterol almost 12%. Studies that measured triglycerides showed 13% reduction in serum triglycerides levels. Powdered garlic preparation produced less effect than the nonpowdered form.

In a double-blind, randomized, placebo-controlled crossover trial, Heiner et al. fed 5 mg of steam-distilled garlic or a placebo twice a day for 12 weeks to 25 patients with moderate hypercholesterolemia. For 4 weeks, wash-out period patients were given a placebo before each treatment. At the end of the study, the investigators did not find change in either placebo or treatment periods in the plasma levels of lipoproteins. The reduction in total cholesterol and cholesterol absorption or synthesis due to garlic oil consumption was not statistically significant.[79]

McCrindle et al. studied the effect of commercially available garlic extract (Kwai®) on serum cholesterol and lipoproteins in children 8 to 18 years of age with familial hypercholesterolemia. They were given 300 mg garlic extract 3 times a day (900 mg/day) in a controlled environment for 8 weeks. The researchers found no significant benefit of garlic extract in lowering serum total cholesterol or lipoproteins in these children and concluded that "garlic extract therapy has no significant effect on cardiovascular risk in pediatric patients with familial hyperlipidemia."[80] Isaacsohn et al. also found that feeding 900 mg/day of garlic powder (Kwai) to adult patients with hypercholesterolemia for 12 weeks in a double-blind, placebo-controlled study had no lipid lowering effect.[81,82]

16.5 CONCLUSION

As evident from *in vivo* studies of humans and *ex vivo* and *in vitro* studies, many factors are involved in causing cardiovascular diseases and many preventive measures have been offered by scientific studies. As this review illustrates, results obtained from different laboratories on the effectiveness of some of the non-nutrient food factors are conflicting. However, good explanations for the different outcomes have resulted from these research endeavors.

Genetic differences in individuals cause different biological responses to the same nutrients or food factors as they do with different medications. Certain non-nutrient food factors present naturally in foods consumed via a balanced diet recommended by guidelines (a diet predominantly plant-based with high intakes of whole grains, fruits, vegetables, nuts, and legumes and low intakes of fatty foods such as meats, dairy products, and concentrated sugars) can prevent many degenerative conditions such as CVD.

The present focus of the medical community in preventing CVD is attempting to maintain low levels of serum total and LDL cholesterol and triglycerides in susceptible individuals. While that is an important preventive measure, medical attention is also directed to other aspects of this very complex and multicausative problem. A high level of serum homocysteine can be a risk factor because it increases the oxidation of LDL. Reducing this risk factor can be accomplished with a diet high in green leafy vegetables, good sources of flavonoids, alpha-tocopherol, and folate that can remove homocysteine from blood by methylating it into methionine, an amino acid.

A diet high in soluble fiber will reduce total calories by displacing fat, meat, and sugar intake. Soluble fiber reduces serum cholesterol by interrupting enterohepatic circulation and reabsorption of bile acids. This type of diet translates into increased intakes of fruits and vegetables, legumes, nuts, and whole grains and has been been promoted by the U.S. government and the scientific community. Factors in foods that reduce the risk of CVD offer the strongest antioxidant effects if consumed continuously. This emphasizes the need for a lifestyle that includes proper diet.

No doubt more research is needed to illustrate the exact mechanism by which non-nutrient food factors exert their preventive effects on the risk of CVD and explain the conflicting results related to the effects of some factors, for example, garlic. Until convincing studies are published to that effect, it is important to make foods high in these substances part of an everyday diet. It is obvious that a plant-based diet that provides all the nutrients and non-nutrient food factors, along with a healthy lifestyle and adequate physical activity, are key in preventing CVD, obesity, cancer, diabetes, and other degenerative diseases. It is also important to mention that most of these factors function best when consumed as foods rather than supplements. Perhaps unknown factors in natural foods somehow aid the absorption and function of these non-nutrients.

REFERENCES

1. Nuttall, S.L. et al. An evaluation of the antioxidant activity of a standardized grape seed extract, Leucoselect. *J. Clin. Pharm. and Ther.* 23, 385, 1998.
2. Merken, H.M., Beecher, G.R., and Holden, J.M. Finessing the flavonoids: flavonoids are found in over 4,000 fruits and vegetables. *Agric. Res.* 107, 504, 2001.
3. Cao, G. et al. Serum antioxidant capacity is increased by consumption of strawberries, spinach, red wine or vitamin C in elderly women. *J. Nutr.* 128, 2383, 1998.
4. Noroozi, M., Angerson, W.J., and Lean, M.E.J. Effects of flavonoids and vitamin C on oxidative DNA damage to human lymphocytes. *Am. J. Clin. Nutr.* 67, 1210, 1998.
5. Keli, S.O. et al. Dietary flavonoids, antioxidant vitamins, and the incidence of stroke: the Zutphen study. *Arch. Int. Med.* 156, 637, 1996.
6. Menotti, A. et al. Food intake patterns and 25-year mortality from coronary heart disease: cross-cultural correlations in the Seven Countries Study. *Eur. J. Epidemiol.* 15, 507, 1999.
7. Wood, D. et al. Prevention of coronary heart disease in clinical practice: recommendations of the second joint task force of European and other societies on coronary prevention. *Atherosclerosis.* 140, 199, 1998.
8. Balentine, D.A., Albano, M.C., and Nair, M.G. Role of medicinal plants, herbs, and spices in protecting human health. *Nutr. Rev.* 57, S41, 1999.
9. Rimm, E.G. et al. Relation between intake of flavonoids and risk for coronary heart disease in male healthy professionals. *Ann. Intern. Med.* 125, 384, 1996.
10. Rissanen, T.H. et al. Low intake of fruits, berries and vegetables is associated with excess mortality in men: the Kuopio Ischaemic Heart Disease Risk Factor (KIHD) study. *J. Nutr.* 133, 199, 2003.
11. Bazzano, L.A. et al. Fruit and vegetable intake and risk of cardiovascular disease in U.S. adults: the first National Health and Nutrition Examination Survey epidemiologic follow-up study. *Am. J. Clin. Nutr.* 76, 93, 2002.
12. Singh, R.B. et al. Effect of an Indo-Mediterranean diet on progression of coronary artery disease in high-risk patients (Indo-Mediterranean Diet Heart Study): a randomized single-blind trial. *Lancet,* 360, 1455, 2002.
13. Liu, S. Whole grain consumption and risk of ischemic stroke in women: a prospective study. *JAMA.* 284, 1534, 2000.

14. Pataki, T. et al. Grape seed proanthocyanidins: improved cardiac recovery during reperfusion after ischemia in isolated rat hearts. *Am. J. Clin. Nutr.* 75, 894, 2002.

15. Wu, J.M. et al. Mechanisms of cardioprotection by resveratrol, a phenolic antioxidant present in red wine. *Int. J. Mol. Med.* 8, 3, 1002.

16. Freedman, J.E. et al. Select flavonoids and whole juice from purple grapes inhibit platelet function and enhance nitric oxide release. *Circulation.* 103, 2792, 2001.

17. Diebolt, M., Bucher, B., and Andriantsitohaina, R. Wine polyphenols decrease blood pressure, improve NO vasodilatation, and induce gene expression. *Hypertension.* 38, 59, 2001.

18. Kendall, M.J., Nuttall, S.I., and Martin, U. Antioxidant therapy: a new therapeutic option for reducing mortality from coronary artery disease. *J. Clin. Pharm. Ther.* 23, 323, 1998.

19. Vinson, J.A. et al. Beneficial effects of a novel IH636 grape seed proanthocyanidin extract and a niacin-bound chromium in a hamster atherosclerosis model. *Mol. Cell. Biochem.* 2, 99, 2002.

20. Sato, M. et al. Grape seed proanthocyanidin reduces cardiomyocyte apoptosis by inhibiting ischemia/reperfusion-induced activation of JNK-1 and C-JUN. *Free Radical Biol. Med.* 31, 729, 2001.

21. Folts, J.D. Potential health benefits from the flavonoids in grape products on vascular disease. *Adv. Exp. Med. Biol.* 505, 95, 2002.

22. Bentzon, J.F. et al. Red wine does not reduce mature atherosclerosis in apolipoprotein E-deficient mice. *Circulation.* 103, 1681, 2001.

23. de Vries, J.H.M. et al. Red wine is a poor source of bioavailable flavonols in men. *J. Nutr.* 131, 745, 2001.

24. Yang, C.S. and Landau, J.M. Effects of tea consumption on nutrition and health. *J. Nutr.* 132, 2409, 2002.

25. Geleljnse, J.M. et al. Tea flavonoids may protect against atherosclerosis: the Rotterdam study. *Arch. Intern. Med.* 159, 2170, 1999.

26. Sesso, H.D. et al. Coffee and tea intake and the risk of myocardial infarction. *Am. J. Epidemiol.* 149, 162, 1999.

27. Young, J.F. et al. Green tea extract only affects markers of oxidative status postprandially: lasting antioxidant effect of flavonoid-free diet. *Br. J. Nutr.* 87, 343, 2002.

28. Green, M.S. and Jucha, G. Association of serum lipids with coffee, tea, and egg consumption in free-living subjects. *J. Epidemiol. Commun. Health.* 40, 324, 1986.

29. Green, M.S. and Harari, G. Association of serum lipoproteins and health-related habits with coffee and tea consumption in free-living subjects examined in the Israeli CORDIS study. *Prev. Med.* 21, 532, 1992.

30. Trevisanato, S.I. and Kim, Y.I. Tea and health. *Nutr. Rev.* 58, 1, 2000.

31. Health and Welfare Canada. Nutrition recommendations: report of the Scientific Review Committee. Ottawa, 1990, 194.

32. Health and Welfare Canada. Food guide facts: background for educators and communicators. Canada's food guide to healthy eating. Ottawa, 1992. Fact sheet 6.

33. Rossander, L., Hallberg, L., and Biorn-Rasmussen, E. Absorption of iron from breakfast meals. *Am. J. Clin. Nutr.* 32, 2484, 1979.

34. Di Mascio, P., Kaiser, S., and Sies, H. Lycopene as the most efficient biological carotenoid singlet oxygen quencher. *Arch. Biochem. Biophys.* 274, 532, 1989.

35. Stahl, W. and Sies, H. Uptake of lycopene and its geometrical isomers is greater from heat-processed than from unprocessed tomato juice in humans. *J. Nutr.* 122, 2161, 1992.

36. Pamuk, E.R. et al. Effect of smoking on serum nutrient concentrations in African-American women. *Am. J. Clin Nutr.* 59, 891, 1994.

37. Van Antwerpen, V.L. et al. Relationship between the plasma levels of beta-carotene and lung function in cigarette smokers. *Int. J. Vitam. Nutr. Res.* 65, 231, 1995.

38. Rao, V.A. and Agarwal, S. Effect of diet and smoking on serum lycopene and lipid peroxidation. *Nutr. Res.* 18, 713, 1998.

39. Arab, L. and Steck, S. Lycopene and cardiovascular disease. *Am. J. Clin. Nutr.* 71, 1691S, 2000.

40. Brady, W.E. et al. Human serum carotenoid concentrations are related to physiologic and lifestyle factors. *J. Nutr.* 126, 129, 1996.

41. Salonen, J.T. Is there a continuing need for longitudinal epidemiologic research? The Kuopio Ischaemic Risk Factor Study. *Ann. Clin. Res.* 20, 46, 1988.

42. Rissanen, T.H. et al. Serum lycopene concentrations and carotid atherosclerosis: the Kuopio Ischaemic Heart Disease Risk Factor study. *Am. J. Clin. Nutr.* 77, 133, 2003.

43. Goulinet, S. and Chapman, M.J. Plasma LDL and HDL subspecies are heterogenous in particle content of tocopherols and oxygenated and hydrocarbon carotenoids: relevance to oxidative resistance and atherogenesis. *Arterioscler. Throb. Vasc. Biol.* 17, 786, 1997.

44. Fuhrman, B., Elis, A., and Aviram, M. Hypocholesterolemic effect of lycopene and beta-carotene is related to suppression of cholesterol synthesis and augmentation of LDL receptor activity in macrophages. *Biochem. Biophys. Res. Comm.* 233, 658, 1997.

45. Edwards, A.J. et al. Consumption of watermelon juice increases plasma concentrations of lycopene and β-carotene in humans. *J. Nutr.* 133, 1043, 2003.

46. Weisburger, J.H. Approaches for chronic disease prevention based on current understanding mechanism. *Am. J. Clin. Nitr.* 71, 1710S, 2000.

47. Rivlin, R.S. Historical perspective on the use of garlic. *J. Nutr.* 131, 951S, 2001.

48. Eisenberg, D.M. et. al. Trends in alternative medicine use in the United States, 1990–1997: results of a follow-up national survey. *JAMA.* 280, 1569, 1998.

49. Ackermann, R.T. et al. Garlic shows promise for improving some cardiovascular risk factors. *Arch. Intern. Med.* 161, 813, 2001.

50. Brace, L.D. Cardiovascular benefits of garlic (*Allium sativum* L.) *J. Cardiovasc. Nurs.* 16, 33, 2002.

51. Liu, L. and Yeh, Y.Y. S-Alk(en)yl cysteines of garlic inhibit cholesterol synthesis by deactivating HMG-CoA reductase in cultured rat hepatocytes. *J. Nutr.* 132, 1129, 2002.

52. Lin, M.C. et al. Garlic inhibits microsomal triglyceride transfer protein gene expression in human liver and intestinal cell lines in rat intestine. *J. Nutr.* 132, 1165, 2002.

53. Berliner, J.A. and Heinecke, J.W. The role of oxidized lipoproteins in atherogenesis. *Free Radic. Biol. Med.* 20, 707, 1996.

54. Cox, D.A. and Cohen, M.L. Effect of oxidized low-density lipoprotein on vascular contraction and relaxation: clinical and pharmacological implications in atherosclerosis. *Pharmacol. Rev.* 48, 3, 1996.

55. Halovoet, P. and Collen, D. Oxidized lipoproteins in atherosclerosis and thromosis. *FASEB J.* 8, 1279, 1995.

56. Guretzki, H.J. et al. Atherogenic levels of low- density lipoprotein alter the permeability and composition of the endothelial barrier. *Atherosclerosis.* 107,15, 1994.

57. Schmitt, A. et al. Prevention by α-tocopherol and rutin of glutathione and ATP depletion induced by oxidized LDL in cultured endothelial cells. *Br. J. Pharmacol.* 116, 1985, 1995.

58. Lau, B.H.S. Suppression of LDL oxidation by garlic. *J. Nutr.* 131, 985S, 2001.

59. Ide, N. and Lau, B.H.S. Garlic compounds protect vascular endothelial cells from oxidized low-density lipoprotein induced injury. *J. Pharm. Pharmacol.* 49, 908, 1997.

60. Ide, N. and Lau, B.H.S. Garlic compounds minimize intracellular oxidative stress and inhibit nuclear factor-$_{\kappa}$B activation. *J. Nutr.* 131, 1020S, 2001.

61. Dillon, S.A. et al. Dietary supplementation with aged garlic extract reduces plasma and urine concentration of 8-iso-prostaglandin F (2(alpha)) in smoking and nonsmoking men. *J. Nutr.* 132, 168, 2002.

62. Breithaupt-Grogler, K. et al. Protective effect of chronic garlic intake on elastic properties of aorta in elderly. *Circulation.* 96, 2649, 1997.

63. Zhang, X.H. et al. The action of garlic upon plasma total antioxidant capacity. *Biochem. Soc. Trans.* 25, 523S, 1997.

64. Rahman, K. and Billington, D. Dietary supplementation with aged garlic extract inhibits ADP-induced platelet aggregation in humans. *J. Nutr.* 130, 2662, 2000.

65. Ali, M. and Mohammad, S.Y. Selective suppression of platelet thromboxane formation sparing of vascular prostacyclin synthesis by aqueous extract of garlic in rabbits. *Prostaglandins Leukot. Med.* 25, 139, 1986.

66. Lengani, C. et al. Effect of a dried garlic preparation on fibrinolysis and platelet aggregation in healthy subjects. *Drug Res.* 43, 119, 1993.

67. Ali, M. and Thomson, M. Consumption of a garlic clove a day could be beneficial in preventing thrombosis. *Prostoglandins Leucot. Essent. Fatty Acids.* 53, 211, 1996.

68. Steiner, M. and Li, W. Aged garlic extract, a modulator of cardiovascular risk factor: a dose-finding study on the effect of AGE on platelet functions. *J. Nutr.* 131, 980S, 2001.

69. Ernest, E. Garlic hyperlipidemia. Correspondence, *Lancet,* 349, 131, 1997.

70. Harenberg, J., Giese, C., and Zimmermann, R. Effect of dried garlic on blood coagulation, fibrinolysis, platelet aggregation and serum cholesterol levels in patients with hyperlipoproteinemia. *Atherosclerosis.* 74, 247, 1988.

71. Stavric, B. Role of Chemopreventers in human diet. *Clin. Biochem.* 27, 319, 1994.

72. Rahman, K. Historical perspective on garlic and cardiovascular disease. *J. Nutr.* 131, 977S, 2001.

73. Sainani, G.S., Desai, D.B., and More, K.N. Onion, garlic and atherosclerosis. *Lancet.* 2, 575, 1976.

74. Agarwal, K.C. Therapeutic actions of garlic constituents. *Med. Res. Rev.* 16, 111, 1996.

75. Harwood, H.J. et al. Pharmacological consequences of cholesterol absorption inhibition: alteration in cholesterol metabolism and reduction in plasma cholesterol concentration induced by the synthetic saponin β-tigogenin cellobioside (CP-88818; tiqueside). *J. Lipid Res.* 43, 377, 1993.

76. Matsuura, H. Saponins in garlic as modifiers of the risk of cardiovascular disease. *J. Nutr.* 131, 1000S, 2001.

77. Steiner, M. et al. A double-blind crossover study in moderately hypercholesterolemic men that compared the effect of aged garlic extract and placebo administration on blood lipids. *Am. J. Clin. Nutr.* 64, 866, 1996.

78. Silagy, C. and Neil, A. Garlic as a lipid lowering agent: a meta-analysis. *J. Coll. Physicians Lond.* 28, 39, 1994.

79. Heinker, B.K., Sudhop, T., and von Bergmann, K. Effect of garlic oil preparation on serum lipoproteins and cholesterol metabolism: a randomized controlled trial. *JAMA.* 279, 1900, 1998.

80. McCrindle, B.W., Helden, E., and Conner, W.T. Garlic extract therapy in children with hypercholesterolemia *Arch. Pediatr. Adolesc. Med.* 152, 1089, 1998.

81. Isaacsohn, J.L. et al. Garlic powder and plasma lipids and lipoproteins: a multicenter, randomized, placebo-controlled trial. *Arch. Intern. Med.* 158, 1189, 1998.

Section IV

Age and Heart Disease

17 Age-Related Cardiac Dysfunction

Bo Yang, Douglas F. Larson, and Ronald R. Watson

CONTENTS

17.1 INTRODUCTION

Cardiovascular disease is the leading cause of morbidity and mortality in the U.S. Chronic heart failure (CHF) is the only major cardiovascular syndrome that is increasing in the U.S. It is considered the cardiovascular epidemic of the new millennium. As a result, CHF has been designated a national research priority.[1,2]

By the year 2035, it is estimated that nearly 1 in 4 individuals (approximately 35 million people) will be 65 years of age or older in the U.S.[3-6] By 2050, 19 million people will be older than 85 years.[7] Cardiovascular diseases and resultant CHF account for over 40% of deaths in individuals 65 years of age and older. The incidence of CHF increases ninefold in men and elevenfold in women annually between the sixth and ninth decades of life.[3] CHF is also the most frequent cause for acute hospitalization among individuals aged ≥65 years.[7,8] In persons aged 80 to 89, the annual incidence of CHF is 27 per 1000 in men and 22 per 1000 in women. Thus, age is a major risk of CHF.[3]

To understand CHF in aging, it is important to understand the cardiac physiological changes of aging. Certain characteristics of aged hearts may account for the high incidence of CHF in aging. Our research project was to identify some of these characteristics. The next section reviews changes of cardiac function in aging, research related to the mechanisms of age-related cardiac dysfunction, and the role of inducible nitric oxide (iNOS) in heart failure since we propose that iNOS may play a big role in age-related cardiac dysfunction.

17.2 CARDIAC FUNCTION IN AGING

17.2.1 CARDIAC CYCLE

Each cardiac cycle can be divided into a systole and a diastole (see Figure 17.1). A systole is traditionally divided into two phases: isovolumic contraction and ejection (rapid and slow). Each diastole is divided into two phases: isovolumic relaxation and left ventricular (LV) filling, which includes LV rapid filling, diastasis (little change in LV volume after rapid filling), and late filling (atrial contraction).[9] The systolic function of LV is considered as the contractility of LV and the diastolic

The Relationship between Molecular and Functional Parameters
of the Heart

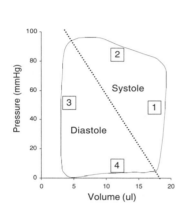

1 Contractility
   L-type, RyR, TNC, TNI
   (dPdt max − Ved PRSW,
   ESPVR

2 Ejection
   Vasculature
   (Ea)

3 Relaxation
   PLB, SERCA 2a, TNC, TNI
   (τ)

4 Filling
   Collagen I and
   III (β)

FIGURE 17.1 Cardiac cycle. One pressure volume loop represents one cardiac cycle that can be divided into two parts (dotted line): systole and diastole, or four phases: isovolumic contraction, ejection, isovolumic relaxation, and filling. (1) Contraction is related to the function of L-type calcium channel, ryanodine receptor (RyR), troponin C (TNC), and troponin I (TNI). From a series of pressure volume loops by occlusion of inferior vena cava (IVC) acquired by conductance catheter, three load-independent parameters are computed to describe contractility of the left ventricle: PRSW, dP/dt max vs. Ved, and Ees (slope of ESPVR). See Table 17.1 for details. (2) Ejection is affected by both contractility and vascular resistance. The best parameter for vascular resistance is Ea (elastance of artery) which equals end-systolic pressure divided by stroke volume. (3) The first part of relaxation is active energy-consumed isovolumic relaxation. It is affected primarily by the function of sarco(endo)plasmic reticulum calcium ATPase (SERCA 2a) and its regulatory protein, phospholamban (PLB). The calcium affinity of TNC and TNI also affects active relaxation. The τ indicates time constant of relaxation and is relatively load-independent when the load is in physiological range. The bigger τ is, the longer the active relaxation is, and the worse the diastolic function is. (4) Filling of the left ventricle is affected by the compliance of the chamber, which is related to the collagen content. The more collagen the heart has, the stiffer the chamber is. The major types collagen in the heart are types I and III. β is the slope of end-diastolic pressure volume relationship (EDPVR). The bigger the β, the stiffer the left ventricle.

TABLE 17.1
Interpretation of Abbreviations and Computation of Parameters of LV Function

Abbreviation	Description	Method of Calculation
Parameters of Hemodynamics		
HR	Heart rate	(60 × sample rate)/(Pmax i + 1 − Pmax i)
Vmax	Maximum volume	Maximum volume during cardiac cycle[a]
Vmin	Minimum volume	Minimum volume during cardiac cycle
Ves	End-systolic volume	Volume at point of maximum P/V ratio
Ved	End-diastolic volume	Volume at R wave
Pmax	Maximum pressure	Maximum pressure during cardiac cycle
Pes	End-systolic pressure	Pressure at point of maximum P/V ratio
Ped	End-diastolic pressure	Pressure at R wave
SV	Stroke volume	Vmax − Vmin
EF	Ejection fraction	(Stroke volume/V @ dP/dt max) × 100
CO	Cardiac output	Stroke volume × Heart rate
SW	Stroke work	Area enclosed by pressure–volume loop
Ea	Arterial elastance	End-systolic pressure/Stroke volume
Parameters of LV Systolic Function		
dP/dt max	Maximum dP/dt	Maximum value of dP/dt during cardiac cycle
ESPVR	End-systolic pressure volume relationship	Regression of end-systolic pressure vs. end-systolic volume
Ees	End-systolic elastance (of left ventricle)	Slope of end-systolic pressure volume relationship
PRSW relationship	Preload recruitable stroke work relationship	Regression of stroke work vs. end-diastolic volume
PRSW	Preload recruitable stroke work	Slope of PRSW relationship
dP/dt max vs. Ved	Slope of regression of dP/dt max vs. end-diastolic volume	
Parameters of LV Diastolic Function		
dP/dt min	Minimum dP/dt	Minimum value of dP/dt during cardiac cycle
τ(Weiss)	Tau–Weiss method	Regression of log(pressure) vs. time
τ(Glantz)	Tau–Glantz method	Regression of dP/dt vs. pressure
τ(Logistic)	Tau–Logistic method	Curve fitting, P(t) = (PA/(1 + et/TL)) + PB
EDPVR	End-diastolic pressure volume relationship	Regression of end-diastolic pressure vs. end-diastolic volume
β	Left ventricular stiffness	Slope of end-diastolic pressure volume relationship
Parametes of Other Features		
PVA	Pressure volume area	Area surrounded by ESPVR, EDPVR, and trajectory of systole
Efficiency		Stroke work/Pressure volume area

TABLE 17.1 (CONTINUED)
Interpretation of Abbreviations and Computation of Parameters of LV Function

Abbreviation	Description	Method of Calculation
PE	Potential energy	Pressure volume area – Stroke work
PE%	Percentage of potential energy	Potential energy/Pressure volume area
Ees/Ea		End-systolic elastance of left ventricle/Arterial elastance (ventricular–arterial coupling)

[a] Cardiac cycle derived from Pmax to Pmax.

function is considered as the LV ability of active isovolumic relaxation and LV compliance; both affect the LV filling.

The best parameters for contractility are PRSW (preload recruitable stroke work), dP/dt max vs. Ved (end-diastolic volume), and Ees (elastance of end systole), because these parameters are relative independent of preload and afterload. Optimal parameters for diastolic function are τ (time constant of isovolumic relaxation) and β (LV stiffness), also due to their relative load independence (see Table 17.1 for definitions and computations of the parameters). These parameters are detailed in the legend of Figure 17.1.

It is important to describe the contraction and relaxation phases of myocytes from cellular and molecular levels (Figure 17.2). When cardiac myocytes receive an action potential impulse, depolarization of the myocytes is associated with the voltage-dependent openings of L-type sarcolemmal calcium channels, allowing rapid entry of calcium ions into cells. The relatively small amount of calcium that enters cells via this mechanism results in a calcium-triggered release of larger levels of additional calcium from intracellular stores, primarily the sarcoplasmic reticulum (SR) through ryanodine receptors.[10] The force-generating actin–myosin reaction is triggered by the combined sources of cytosolic calcium binding to an N terminal site on troponin C, the calcium receptor. The calcium-binding signal is transmitted to tropomyosin through troponin T, the tropomyosin-binding portion of the troponin complex, and to troponin I. Troponin I is released from its tether on actin by promotion of a tight interaction between the C terminus of troponin I and the N terminus of troponin C. This results in the exposure of myosin-binding sites on actin and the binding of actin to myosin, leading to myocardial contractile machinery by way of repetitive cross-bridge cycling between actin and myosin; contraction occurs when ATP is available.[11]

To inactivate the myocyte contractile process thereby facilitating the diastole, cytosolic calcium levels must be returned from 10 μM to 0.25 μM. The sequestration of calcium into the SR and extrusion of calcium to the extracellular space is thought to be accomplished by Ca^{2+} pumps on SR, SERCA 2a [sarco(endo)plasmic reticulum calcium ATPase, type 2a], and Na^+/Ca^{2+} exchangers on cell membranes (see Figure 17.2).[10] SERCA 2a function is regulated by a SR membrane

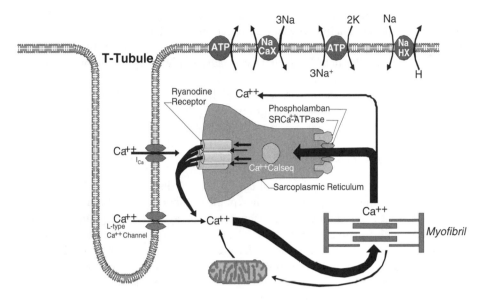

FIGURE 17.2 Calcium cycling. An electric impulse reaches cardiac myocytes, initiating depolarization of myocytes resulting in the opening of voltage-gated L-type calcium channels and Ca^{2+} influx. A small amount of calcium influx binds with ryanodine receptor, triggering Ca^{2+} release from sarcoplamic reticulum (SR) into cytosol. Calcium binds with troponin C, initiating myocyte contraction. The high Ca^{2+} level binds to calmodulin, and then both activate calmodulin-dependent kinase (CaM K). Phospholamban (PLB) phosphorylated by CaM K switches on SR Ca^{2+}-ATPase type 2a (SERCA 2a), which starts to pump Ca^{2+} back into the SR during late contraction with consumption of ATP. Phosphorylation of PLB by cAMP-dependent protein kinase (PKA) can further enhance SERCA 2a function. A small amount of Ca^{2+} is excreted outside the cells through Na–Ca exchangers (NaCaX). The decrease of the Ca^{2+} level initiates relaxation of myocytes until the next electric pulse reaches the cells; then the system starts again. * Calseq = calsequestrin.

protein called phospholamban (PLB) (from the Greek *phospho* meaning "phosphate" and *lamban* meaning "receptor"). When PLB is phosphorylated, its inhibitory activity of SERCA 2a function is decreased.[12] Such phosphorylation is achieved by (1) increased cytosolic calcium ion concentration through calmodulin-dependent kinase (CaM K) or (2) catecholamine beta-adrenergic stimulation through PKA.[13] With beta-adrenergic stimulation, when calcium levels increase during systole, it binds with calmodulin which then activates CaM K. Threonine (Thr) 17 is phosphorylated by CaM K.[14,15]

As shown in Figure 17.2, when PLB is phosphorylated, it dissociates from SERCA 2a and releases the inhibition of SERCA 2a, resulting in calcium resequestration and isovolumic relaxation of LV. Calcium also directly acts on the molecular configuration of SERCA 2a to enhance its activity. Unphosphorylated PLB inhibits the function of SERCA 2a, resulting in prolonged time of calcium resequestration. The beta$_1$ or beta$_2$ agonist increases cAMP level through G_s protein, resulting in activation of PKA (cAMP-dependent protein kinase). PKA phosphorylates PLB at serine (Ser) 15,[16] removing the inhibition of PLB on SERCA 2a and enhancing SERCA 2a function. The Thr 17 phosphorylation by CaM K cannot occur independent of Ser 16 phosphorylation by PKA *in vivo*.[13] These steps describe how beta₁ and beta₂ adrenergic receptor agonists improve LV relaxation and then contractility.[16,17]

Taken together, ryanodine receptors, SERCA 2a, and PLB are key calcium cycling proteins, targets for many drugs, and the mode of some cardiovascular diseases, including the aging process.

17.2.2 Systolic Function in Aging

For the majority of individuals free of cardiovascular disease, the aged heart adapts well to performing its required systolic (pump) function in the basal state at rest (see Table 17.2). Based on existing techniques such as echocardiography and magnetic resonance imaging (MRI), no evidence points to an age-related decline of resting systolic function (characterized by cardiac output) in individuals free of cardiovascular disease.[18] The resting LV function is maintained though the Frank–Starling mechanism by increasing preload (Ved) resulting in increased stroke volumes. Cardiac output is equal to stroke volume times heart rate.

A gender-related difference appears to exist between aged men and women. Despite increased stroke volume and decreased heart rate, the cardiac output index is not changed in men, but decrease in cardiac index occurs in aged women due to a lack of increase in compensatory preload (Ved).

The change of contractility of LV associated with aging at rest is controversial. In 1971, Weisfeldt et al. reported no change of contractility of trabeculae carneae

---

TABLE 17.2
Seated Rest: Changes in Cardiac Output Regulation in Healthy Humans between 20 and 80 Years of Age[4,5]

Hemodynamic Parameters	Change due to Age
Heart rate	↓10%
End-diastolic volume[a]	↑12%
Index of end-diastolic volume	↑
End-diastolic pressure	↑
Aortic compliance	↓
Total peripheral vascular resistance	No change
Contractility	No change
Stroke volume	10%
Ejection fraction	No change
Cardiac index	No change

See details in Table 17.1.

[a] Women differ from men: no ↑ in Ved and a ↓ in cardiac index with age in women.

---

of aging rats.[19] We first reported that load-independent parameters of contractility (PRSW, dP/dt max vs. Ved, and Ees) in aging decreased in aged mice.[20] Our data was supported by the observation that the LVs of older (but not younger) healthy adults dilates at end diastole in response to a given increase in afterload when beta-adrenergic receptors are blocked[21] and by the finding that the contractility of aged isolated myocytes was decreased.[22] There is a compensatory prolongation of the contraction during phase in the senescent myocyte to achieve a normal ejection fraction especially in the presence of increased afterload.[23]

Table 17.3 shows that the reserved systolic function is markedly decreased in aging. The ejection fraction, cardiac output index, contractility, and myocardial O_2 consumption all markedly decrease during exercise in aging. The peak heart rate achieved during exhaustive exercise decreases with aging, but both end-diastolic volume (Ved) and end-systolic volume (Ves) increased in older compared to younger persons. This indicates that during exercise in healthy older individuals, cardiac output is maintained not through cardioacceleration but from an increase in left ventricular preload (Ved), thus relying on the Frank–Starling mechanism.[1,24,25] Apparently, the effectiveness of the Frank–Starling mechanism is reduced with aging because the LV fails to empty to the same extent in older persons. This is similar to what is seen when young adults attempt to augment cardiac output during exercise in the face of beta-adrenergic blockage.[26,27] It also has been reported that the response of an aged heart to catecholamine is decreased[28] because of the desensitization of beta-adrenergic receptors and modification of coupling of the beta-adrenergic receptors to adenylyl cyclase by the G_s protein, resulting in a reduction in the maximum activity of adenylyl cyclase.[29,30] Taken together, the reserved systolic function in aging was markedly decreased due to decreased LV contractility and LV response to catecholamine.

TABLE 17.3
Exhaustive Upright Exercise: Changes in Cardiac Output Regulation in Healthy Humans between 20 and 80 Years of Age[2]

Hemodynamic Parameters	Changes due to Age
Heart rate	↓25%
End-diastolic volume	↑30%
Total peripheral vascular resistance	↑30%
Contractility	↓60%
End-systolic volume	↑
Stroke volume	No change
Ejection fraction	↓15%
Cardiac index	↓25%
O_2 consumption	↓50%
Response to catecholamine	↓

See details in Table 17.1.

17.2.3 Diastolic Function in Aging

Diastolic heart failure (DHF) is common in the elderly. DHF occurring with normal systolic function is designated primary diastolic heart failure. Aging is one common reason for primary DHF.[31,32] Over 50% of heart failure patients 65 years or older have isolated primary DHF of whom 45% have no other diseases and meet the criteria for isolated DHF. DHF is substantially more common in older women than older men.[33,34]

Diastolic dysfunction in aging includes a combination of prolonged LV relaxation (impaired active relaxation) and increased myocardial stiffness (impaired passive elastic properties of the myocardium). These abnormalities result in an elevated LV end-diastolic pressure at rest and with exertion and the characteristic finding of decreased early diastolic filling found in elderly individuals.[5] The early diastolic filling rate measured via echocardiography, radionuclide angiography, and Doppler ultrasonography progressively slows after age 20. By 80 years of age, the rate is reduced by up to 50%.[4]

Yellin reported that decreased active LV relaxation rate with an increased τ, time constant of isovolumic relaxation, was associated with a decrease in early diastolic filling.[35] The increased LV stiffness with elevated end-diastolic pressure is represented by a leftward and upward shift of the end-diastolic pressure volume relationship (ESPVR) (i.e., increased beta, the slope of ESPVR).

17.3 MECHANISM OF CARDIAC DYSFUNCTION IN AGING

The mechanism of cardiac dysfunction in aging is not clear. Cellular and molecular mechanisms of age-related cardiac dysfunction have been studied largely in rodents. Table 17.4 lists findings of gene expression and morphological and structural changes related to cardiac dysfunction in aging.

17.3.1 Mechanism of Systolic Dysfunction (Contractility) in Aging

The mechanism of decreased contractility in aging is not clear. Prolonged contraction and decreased contraction velocity were found in aged rats.[23,36] The prolonged contraction may be related to a prolongation of action potential that may partially result from the slower inactivation of sarcolemmal L-type calcium channel and reduction in outwardly directed K^+ currents.[37] The prolonged cytosolic Ca^{2+} transient due to dysfunction of SERCA is a suggestion for the prolonged contraction.[15]

Senescent rats showed marked shifts in the myosin heavy chain (MHC) isoform from alpha-MHC to beta-MHC. The beta-MHC is a slower contraction protein compared to alpha-MHC.[38] The ATPase activity of cardiac muscle can vary also. The alpha-alpha isoform shows appreciably greater catalytic activity in hydrolyzing ATP than the beta-beta isoform.[11] Myosin Ca^{2+} ATPase activity declines with the decline in alpha-MHC content.[39] This altered cellular profile results in a contraction with a reduced velocity and a prolonged time course. The diminished beta-adrenergic

TABLE 17.4
Myocardial Change with Adult Aging in Rodents[1]

Functional Change	Cellular and Molecular Mechanism
↓Contraction velocity	↓α MHC, ↑β MHC, ↓ Myosine ATPase activity; ↓ thyroid receptor
Prolonged contraction	Prolonged cytosolic Ca^{2+} transient due to ↓SERCA 2a expression (↓pump site density) and function (↓pumping rate)
Prolonged action potential	↓I_{Ca} inactivation, ↓I_{To} density
↓β-adrenergic contractile response	↓$β_1$AR, ↓Coupling βAR-Acyclase, ↓TNI, PLB, ↓PLB phosphorylation, ↓I_{Ca} augmentation, ↓Ca_i transient augmentation
↓Rate of active isovolumic relaxation	Prolonged cytosolic Ca^{2+} transient due to ↓SERCA 2a expression (↓pump site density) and function (↓pumping rate), ↓I_{Ca} inactivation
↑Myocardial stiffness	↓myocyte number, ↑myocyte size, ↑matrix connective tissue (fibroblast), ↑collagen and fibronectin content, ↑AT_1R and activity of mycardial RAS, ↑ANP

Note: MHC = myosin heavy chain; SERCA 2a = sarco(endo)plasmic reticulum calcium ATPase type 2a; I_{Ca} = calcium influx; I_{To} = transient outward potassium channel; $β_1$AR = beta₁-adrenergic receptor; βAR = beta-adrenergic receptor; TNI = troponin I; PLB = phospholamban; Ca_i = intracellular calcium concentration; AT_1R = antiotensin I receptor; RAS = renin-angiotensin system; ANP = atrial naturetic peptide.

contractile response found in aged rats may be related also to the decreased contractility. The factors that affect Ca^{2+} cycling proteins, augmentation of Ca^{2+} transients, and myocyte contractility have not yet been described.

17.3.2 MECHANISMS OF DIASTOLIC DYSFUNCTION IN AGING

Diastolic dysfunction in aging includes prolonged myocardial active relaxation (↑τ) and increased LV stiffness (↑β). As suggested by Roffe et al.,[25] the prolonged time for relaxation may be due to prolonged calcium entry during an extended sarcolemmal depolarization and decreased velocity of Ca^{2+} uptake by SERCA 2a from cytosol to sarcoplasmic reticulum after depolarization. The decreased inactivation of L-type Ca^{2+} channels may be related to the prolonged calcium entry. The age-related decreased SERCA activity has been related to decreased gene expression of SERCA 2a in humans.[40,41] We found no differences of SERCA 2a gene expression between 6-month- and 16-month-old mice, but noted a significant decrease of diastolic function in 16-month-old mice. Our results suggest that other factors affect the activity of SERCA 2a in aging.

The increased LV stiffness is due to increased extracellular matrix collagen content and composition in the heart.[42] Moreover, the number of myocytes in the aged heart decreases because of apoptosis and necrosis.[43] The compensatory hypertrophy of the myocytes and the increased collagen synthesized by the cardiac fibroblasts result in increased LV stiffness. These structural changes may be related to age-associated increased vascular loads and changes in tissue levels or activities of growth factors, e.g., angiotensin II, transforming growth factor β-1 (TGF-β1), and atrial naturetic peptide that can stimulate collagen synthesis.[1,42]

In summary, decreased contractility and diastolic dysfunction were identified in an aged population free of infectious pathogens. Inducible nitric oxide synthase is an important contributor to heart failure and age-related cardiac dysfunction.

REFERENCES

1. Lakatta, E.G. 1999. Cardiovascular aging research: the next horizons. *J. Am. Geriatr. Soc.* 47, 613.
2. Lakatta, E.G. 2002. Introduction: chronic heart failure in older persons. *Heart Fail. Rev.* 7, 5.
3. Lakatta, E.G. 2002. Age-associated cardiovascular changes in health: impact on cardiovascular disease in older persons. *Heart Fail. Rev.* 7, 29.
4. Lakatta, E.G. 2000. Cardiovascular aging in health. *Clin. Geriatr. Med.* 16, 419.
5. Pugh, K.G. and J.Y. Wei. 2001. Clinical implications of physiological changes in the aging heart. *Drugs Aging.* 18, 263.
6. Duncan, A.K., J. Vittone, K.C. Fleming, and H.C. Smith. 1996. Cardiovascular disease in elderly patients. *Mayo Clin. Proc.* 71, 184.
7. Batchelor, W.B., J.G. Jollis, and G.C. Friesinger. 1999. The challenge of health care delivery to the elderly patient with cardiovascular disease: demographic, epidemiologic, fiscal, and health policy implications. *Cardiol. Clin.* 17, 1.
8. Premen, A.J. 1996. Research recommendations for cardiovascular aging research: NIA Cardiovascular Aging Advisory Panel. *J. Am. Geriatr. Soc.* 44, 1114.
9. Courtois, M., P.A. Ludbrook, and S.J. Kovacs. 2000. Unsolved problems in diastole. *Cardiol.Clin.* 18, 653.
10. Bers, D.M. 2000. Calcium fluxes involved in control of cardiac myocyte contraction. *Circ. Res.* 87, 275.
11. Katz, A.M. *Physiology of the Heart*. Lippincott Williams & Wilkins, New York, 2001, p. 151.
12. Bluhm, W.F., E.G. Kranias, W.H. Dillmann, and M. Meyer. 2000. Phospholamban: a major determinant of the cardiac force-frequency relationship. *Am. J. Physiol. Heart Circ. Physiol.* 278, H249.
13. Colyer, J. 1998. Phosphorylation states of phospholamban. *Ann. NY Acad. Sci..* 853, 79.
14. Wegener, A.D., H.K. Simmerman, J.P. Lindemann, and L.R. Jones. 1989. Phospholamban phosphorylation in intact ventricles: phosphorylation of serine 16 and threonine 17 in response to beta-adrenergic stimulation. *J. Biol. Chem.* 264, 11468.
15. Simmerman, H.K. and L.R. Jones. 1998. Phospholamban: protein structure, mechanism of action, and role in cardiac function. *Physiol. Rev.* 78, 921.
16. Schwartz, K., L. Carrier, A.M. Lompre, J.J. Mercadier, and K.R. Boheler. 1992. Contractile proteins and sarcoplasmic reticulum calcium-ATPase gene expression in the hypertrophied and failing heart. *Basic Res. Cardiol.* 87 (Suppl. 1), 285.
17. Voss, J., L.R. Jones, and D.D. Thomas. 1994. The physical mechanism of calcium pump regulation in the heart. *Biophys. J.* 67, 190.

18. Lakatta, E.G. and Boluyt, M.O. 2000. Age-associated changes in the cardiovascular system in the absence of cardiovascular disease. In *Congestive Heart Failure*. Hosenpud, J.D. and Greenberg, B.H., Eds., Lippincott Williams & Wilkins, Philadelphia, p. 137.

19. Weisfeldt, M.L., W.A. Loeven, and N.W. Shock. 1971. Resting and active mechanical properties of trabeculae carneae from aged male rats. *Am. J. Physiol.* 220, 1921.

20. Yang, B., D.F. Larson, and R. Watson. 1999. Age-related left ventricular function in the mouse: analysis based on *in vivo* pressure–volume relationships. *Am. J. Physiol.* 277, H1906.

21. Yin, F.C., G.S. Raizes, T. Guarnieri, H.A. Spurgeon, E.G. Lakatta, N.J. Fortuin, and M.L. Weisfeldt. 1978. Age-associated decrease in ventricular response to haemodynamic stress during beta-adrenergic blockade. *Br. Heart J.* 40, 1349.

22. Kojda, G., K. Kottenberg, P. Nix, K.D. Schluter, H.M. Piper, and E. Noack. 1996. Low increase in cGMP induced by organic nitrates and nitrovasodilators improves contractile response of rat ventricular myocytes. *Circ. Res.* 78, 91.

23. Wei, J.Y., H.A. Spurgeon, and E.G. Lakatta. 1984. Excitation–contraction in rat myocardium: alterations with adult aging. *Am. J. Physiol.* 246, H784.

24. Wei, J.Y. 1992. Age and the cardiovascular system. *New Engl. J. Med.* 327, 1735.

25. Roffe, C. 1998. Ageing of the heart. *Br. J. Biomed. Sci.* 55, 136.

26. Fleg, J.L., S. Schulman, F. O'Connor, L.C. Becker, G. Gerstenblith, J.F. Clulow, D.G. Renlund, and E.G. Lakatta. 1994. Effects of acute beta-adrenergic receptor blockade on age-associated changes in cardiovascular performance during dynamic exercise. *Circulation.* 90, 2333.

27. Schulman, S.P., E.G. Lakatta, J.L. Fleg, L. Lakatta, L.C. Becker, and G. Gerstenblith. 1992. Age-related decline in left ventricular filling at rest and exercise. *Am. J. Physiol.* 263, H1932.

28. Stratton, J.R., M.D. Cerqueira, R.S. Schwartz, W.C. Levy, R.C. Veith, S.E. Kahn, and I.B. Abrass. 1992. Differences in cardiovascular responses to isoproterenol in relation to age and exercise training in healthy men. *Circulation.* 86, 504.

29. Jiang, M.T., M.P. Moffat, and N. Narayanan. 1993. Age-related alterations in the phosphorylation of sarcoplasmic reticulum and myofibrillar proteins and diminished contractile response to isoproterenol in intact rat ventricle. *Circ. Res.* 72, 102.

30. Scarpace, P.J. 1990. Forskolin activation of adenylate cyclase in rat myocardium with age: effects of guanine nucleotide analogs. *Mech. Ageing Dev.* 52, 169.

31. Little, W.C. and C.P. Cheng. 1998. Diastolic dysfunction. *Cardiol. Rev.* 6, 231.

32. Little, W.C., J.G. Warner, Jr., K.M. Rankin, D.W. Kitzman, and C.P. Cheng. 1998. Evaluation of left ventricular diastolic function from the pattern of left ventricular filling. *Clin. Cardiol.* 21, 5.

33. Kitzman, D.W. 2002. Diastolic heart failure in the elderly. *Heart Fail. Rev.* 7, 17.

34. Kitzman, D.W. 2000. Diastolic dysfunction in the elderly: genesis and diagnostic and therapeutic implications. *Cardiol. Clin.* 18, 597.

35. Yellin, E.L. 1999. Concepts related to the study of diastolic function: a personal commentary. *J. Cardiol.* 33, 223.

36. Capasso, J.M., A. Malhotra, R.M. Remily, J. Scheuer, and E.H. Sonnenblick. 1983. Effects of age on mechanical and electrical performance of rat myocardium. *Am. J. Physiol.* 245, H72.

37. Walker, K.E., E.G. Lakatta, and S.R. Houser. 1993. Age associated changes in membrane currents in rat ventricular myocytes. *Cardiovasc. Res.* 27, 1968.

38. O'Neill, L., N.J. Holbrook, J. Fargnoli, and E.G. Lakatta. 1991. Progressive changes from young adult age to senescence in mRNA for rat cardiac myosin heavy chain genes. *Cardioscience.* 2, 1.

39. Bhatnagar, G.M., G.D. Walford, E.S. Beard, S. Humphreys, and E.G. Lakatta. 1984. ATPase activity and force production in myofibrils and twitch characteristics in intact muscle from neonatal, adult, and senescent rat myocardium. *J. Mol. Cell Cardiol.* 16, 203.

40. Lompre, A.M., F. Lambert, E.G. Lakatta, and K. Schwartz. 1991. Expression of sarcoplasmic reticulum Ca(2+)-ATPase and calsequestrin genes in rat heart during ontogenic development and aging. *Circ. Res.* 69, 1380.

41. Assayag, P., D. Charlemagne, I. Marty, J. de Leiris, A.M. Lompre, F. Boucher, P. E. Valere, S. Lortet, B. Swynghedauw, and S. Besse. 1998. Effects of sustained low-flow ischemia on myocardial function and calcium-regulating proteins in adult and senescent rat hearts. *Cardiovasc. Res.* 38, 169.

42. Larson, D.F., Ingham, R., Alwardt, C.M., and Yang, B. 2003. A mechanism of diastolic filling dysfunction in the aged. *JECT,* in press.

43. Kajstura, J., A. Leri, N. Finato, C. Di Loreto, C. A. Beltrami, and P. Anversa. 1998. Myocyte proliferation in end-stage cardiac failure in humans. *Proc. Natl. Acad. Sci. USA.* 95, 8801.

18 Inducible Nitric Oxide Synthase (iNOS) and Heart Failure

Bo Yang, Douglas F. Larson, and Ronald R. Watson

CONTENTS

18.1 INTRODUCTION

Over the last 15 years, the nitric oxide (NO) literature has experienced exponential growth (from 7 papers on endogenous NO in 1987 to over 45,000 in 2002). The link between inducible nitric oxide synthase (iNOS) and heart failure is accepted as an important association and is opening potential therapeutic avenues for the treatment of heart failure. Most literature suggests a deleterious effect of iNOS on heart function in dilated cardiomyopathy, ischemic cardiomyopathy, septic shock, cardiac allograft rejection, and viral and autoimmune myocarditis, although some controversial arguments continue.[1,2] The molecular and functional effects of iNOS remain to be defined.

18.2 INTRODUCTION OF iNOS (NOS II)

The three members of the nitric oxide synthase (NOS) family are NOS I (nNOS or neural nitric oxide synthase), NOS II (iNOS or inducible nitric oxide synthase), and

NOS III (eNOS or endothelial nitric oxide synthase). NOS enzymes appear to have evolved from an ancestral P-450 cytochrome type enzyme, containing a C terminal reductase domain and an N terminal oxygenase domain.[3] The enzyme functions as a dimer consisting of two identical monomers, with the cofactor tetrahydrobiopterin (BH_4) converting L-arginine to L-citrulline and NO.

The nNOS and eNOS are tightly regulated by calcium calmodulin and generate small amounts of NO within a short time. The NO produces precise actions on adjacent structures such as smooth muscle cells in vasculature. In contrast, once expressed, cytokine-inducible iNOS produces high levels of NO independent of intracellular calcium and acts for a long time.[4,5] The regulation of iNOS expression is the key step to regulating its activity and effects because post-transcriptional and post-translational regulation have minor effects on iNOS activity.

The expression of iNOS is transcriptionally regulated by the following cyto-kines: tumor necrosis factor-alpha (TNF-α), interleukin-1-beta (IL-1β), and inter-feron-gamma (IFN-γ) or by bacterial lipopolysaccharide (LPS) simulation.[5] Extensive evidence shows that all nucleated cells in the cardiovascular system, including endothelial cells, endocardial cells, fibroblasts, smooth muscle cells, and cardiac myocytes, can express iNOS.[6] Cloning of a 1.7-kb fragment flanking the transcriptional start site of the murine gene reveals several putative transcrip-tion factor binding sequences including ten IFN-γ response elements (IFN-REs), three γ-activated sites (GASs), two consensus sequences for nuclear factor-κB (NF-κB) binding and four for NF-IL6, two TNF-α response elements (TNFα-REs), two activating protein-1 binding motifs (AP-1), three IFN-α stimulated response elements (ISREs), and a basal transcription recognition site (TATA box). Many of these elements are also present in human iNOS promoter.[7–9] Of all these promoters, the NF-κB site is essential for LPS-induced iNOS transcription; the IFN-RE regulated by IFN regulatory factor-1 (IRF-1) is also very important for iNOS transcription.[10]

Aged mice have imbalances of T-help-1 (T_H1) and T-help-2 (T_H2) cells. The activity of T_H2 cells is stronger than that of T_H1 in old mice. T_H2 cells secrete many pro-inflammatory cytokines, including TNF-α, IFN-γ, IL-1β, and IL-6, all of which are stimulators of iNOS expression. The cultured splenocytes from old mice produce significantly more TNF-α, IFN-γ, IL-1β, and IL-6 than those from young mice under the stimulation of T cell mitogen.[11]

It seems that older mice have the potential to express iNOS under healthy conditions because of the imbalance of T_H1 and T_H2 cells. It was reported that the vasculature systems in old rats express iNOS.[12] We hypothesize that aged hearts may express iNOS as a result of immune dysfunction related to aging.

18.3 EXPRESSION OF iNOS IN HEART FAILURE

Heart failure is related to iNOS expression and the failure may be systolic or diastolic. The expression of iNOS is related to the etiologies of both systolic and diastolic heart failure.[13,14] In septic cardiodepression, including acute systolic and diastolic dysfunction, patients benefit from methylene blue, a guanylate cyclase inhibitor.[15] Administration of endotoxin in mice was associated with elevations of concentrations of TNF-α and IL-1β and a concomitant increase in the expression of iNOS with elevated circulating levels of nitrites.[16]

Selective iNOS inhibition has been found to improve heart function in septic heart failure; low doses of mercaptoethylguanidine reversed the cardiodepression.[17] Aminoguanidine improved survival by reducing extracardiac organ failure.[18] S-methylisothiourea sulfate restored left ventricular contractility[19] and early selective inhibition of iNOS with the L-N(6)(1-iminoethyl)-lysine (L-NIL) analogue similarly prevented endotoxin-induced myocardial dysfunction.[20] Seven hours after endotoxin injection, the iNOS knockout (KO) mice had better systolic functions than wild-type mice and the diastolic functions of iNOS KO mice measured by τ were preserved.

NO produced by iNOS expressed by cardiac tissues also contributes to cardiac allograft rejection and allograft contractile dysfunction in transplant patients.[21,22] That was confirmed recently in iNOS knockout mice.[21] In transplant recipients free of rejection or graft vasculopathy, a Doppler echocardiographic index of left ventricular (LV) performance revealed a significant association of systolic, diastolic, or combined LV dysfunction and intensity of iNOS gene expression in simultaneous LV biopsies.[22] The selective iNOS inhibitor, 1400W, improves cardiac allograft function and diastolic function in rats.[23,24] Similarly, the NO scavenger, NOX-100, and cyclosporine prolong cardiac graft survival with reduction of nitrosyl complex formation (nitrosylheme and nitrosomyoglobin).[25]

In autoimmune myocarditis, iNOS mRNA overexpression is associated with decreased heart contractility in mice.[26] In dilated cardiomyopathy, iNOS overexpression generally is observed[14,27] and NO produced by iNOS seems responsible for a negative inotropic effect under stimulated conditions such as infusion of dobutamine.[28] Intracoronary L-NMMA, an NOS inhibitor, was shown to potentiate dobutamine inotropic responsiveness.[29]

In end-stage ischemic or nonischemic heart failure, the expression of iNOS in cardiac myocytes of failing hearts was found by other authors.[22,27] Saito et al. found induction of iNOS during myocardial infarction (MI) exerts negative effects on cardiac function and structure, and long-term administration of a selective iNOS inhibitor (S-methylisothiourea) is beneficial in the treatment of MI and congestive heart failure.[30] Feng et al. found mortality is significantly decreased and LV myocardial contractility is increased after MI in iNOS knockout mice compared with wild-type mice.[31] Although cardiac dysfunction and heart failure may have different etiologies, both are related to iNOS expression, and inhibition of iNOS activity with selective iNOS inhibitors can improve the heart function.

Additional evidence for the deleterious effect of iNOS on the heart is iNOS overexpression by transgenic mice. One type of iNOS transgenic mouse is the nonconditional model [with αMHC promoter-directed expression of human iNOS (αMHC-iNOS)].[32] The other is a binary transgenic mouse model with doxycycline (DOX)-regulated and cardiomyocyte-specific expression of human iNOS (iNOS+/αMtTA+).[33] The αMHC-iNOS mice showed increased cardiac iNOS activity but no alterations in cardiac structure and function.[32] However, the iNOS+/αMtTA+ mice displayed DOX-reversible human iNOS expression in cardiomyocytes with a 10-fold increase in total cardiac NOS activity, increased peroxynitrite generation, significant cardiac hypertrophy, atrioventricular dilation, and infrequent occurrence of heart failure.[33] The difference may be due to the experimental design of these two types of transgenic mice. The nonconditional transgenic approach may have preselected lines without significant cardiac toxicity (all the lines with cardiac toxicity may die during the embryonic stage).[33] The use of a DOX-regulated conditional system for cardiac-selective transgene expression allowed the bypass of embryonic mortality and prevention of developmental adaptation *in utero*.[33]

18.4 MOLECULAR MECHANISMS OF NO

The effects of NO on hearts are dose-dependent. Lower doses (nM) such as NO produced by eNOS and nNOS are beneficial to the heart (positive inotropic effects), but high doses (µM) such as NO produced by iNOS are harmful to the heart (negative inotropic effects).[27,34–37] Without the restriction of calcium calmodulin, iNOS produces larger amounts of NO and its activity continues.[5] The molecular mechanisms of high levels of NO in the heart can be simply described as cGMP-dependent and cGMP-independent pathways.

18.4.1 cGMP-Dependent Pathway

Activation of soluble guanylate cyclase by NO (Figure 18.1) results in conversion of guanosine trisphosphate (GTP) to second messenger cyclic guanosine monophosphate (cGMP).[38] Once biosynthesized, cGMP binds to different effecter proteins. In mammalian cardiomyocytes, the most important effecter proteins are cGMP-dependent protein kinase (PKG) and cGMP-activated/inhibited cAMP-phosphodiesterase (PDE II/PDE III).[39,40] Stimulation of PKG results in inhibition of voltage-dependent L-type calcium channels through phosphorylation of the α_2 subunit,[41] leading to decreased calcium transient augmentation and decreased contractility. This effect was evident at high concentrations of cGMP and/or cGMP analogs.[42,43] PKG can also phosphorylate troponin I, resulting in desensitization of cardiac myofilaments to calcium and then a decrease in contractility.[44,45]

Inhibition of PDE III has been observed at low concentrations of cGMP (<1 µM) and NO (50 nM) that resulted in increased cAMP content in cardiomyocytes.[46] Higher concentrations of cGMP resulting from larger amounts of NO (>100 µM) produced by iNOS activated PDE II which hydrolyzed cAMP and then decreased the cAMP content in cardiomyocytes.[40,47,48] The cAMP activated PKA, which phosphorylated L-type calcium channels and phospholamban (PLB), resulting in an increase of calcium influx from L-type calcium channels and contractility, an increase in function of SERCA 2a, and active relaxation of the LV.[49] When the cAMP content decreased, the activity of PKA decreased, resulting in impairment of contractility (systolic dysfunction) and active relaxation (diastolic dysfunction).

18.4.2 cGMP-Independent Pathway

In addition to activating the cGMP–PKG pathway, high concentrations of NO decrease cardiac function through other means (Figure 18.2). Elevated NO concentrations inhibit functioning of calcium cycling proteins such as ryanodine receptor

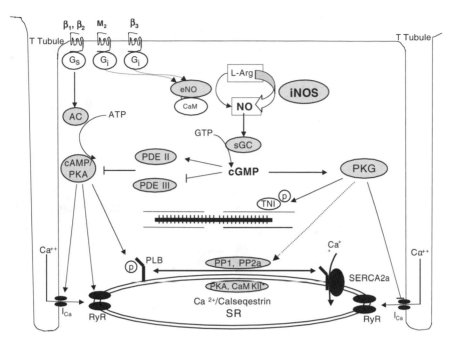

FIGURE 18.1 NO regulates cardiac function via the cGMP-dependent pathway. β_1 and β_2 adrenergic receptor agonists (β_1AR and β_2AR) such as dobutamine improve systolic function (contractility) and diastolic function (active relaxation) by coupling with stimulatory G protein (G_s) and activating cAMP-dependent protein kinase (PKA). PKA phosphrylates L-type calcium channels to increase Ca^{2+} influx (I_{Ca}) and ryanodine receptor (RyR) to increase Ca^{2+} release from sarcoplasmic reticulum (SR), resulting in increasing Ca^{2+} transience and contractility. PKA also phosphorylates phospholamban (PLB), releasing the inhibition of PLB to sarco(endo)reticulum 2a (SERCA 2a), and increases the rate of Ca^{2+} uptake from the cytosol, resulting in an increasing rate of relaxation. Since Ca^{2+} transience is controlled by SR Ca^{2+} content and increased SERCA 2a function increases SR Ca^{2+} content, increased SERCA 2a function increases Ca^{2+} transience and then the contractility of the myocytes. The M_2 receptor and β_3AR agonists decrease cardiac function (opposite to β_1AR and β_2AR agonists) by coupling G_i protein and activating calmodulin (CaM)/eNOS through an unknown mechanism. This confirms that NO inhibits cardiac function, especially at high levels. High levels of NO produced by iNOS from L-arginine (L-Arg) increase levels of cGMP, the second messenger, by activating soluble guanylyl cyclase (sGC). High levels of cGMP inhibit contractility and relaxation by (1) activating phosphodiesterase II (PDE II) which decreases cAMP level and PKA activity, attenuating inotropic and lusitropic effects of PKA; and (2) activating cGMP-dependent kinase (PKG) which phosphorylates (i) troponin I, leading to calcium desensitization, sarcomere relaxation, and a consequent negative inotropic effect; (ii) L-type calcium channel, decreasing the Ca^{2+} influx and promoting a negative inotropic effect; and (iii) possible protein phosphotase type 1 and type 2A (PP1 and PP 2A), decreasing phosphorylation of PLB, increasing PLB inhibition to SERCA 2a, decreasing Ca^{2+} uptake and consequent prolonged relaxation (negative lusitropic effect). * CaM KII = Calmodulin-dependent kinase II.

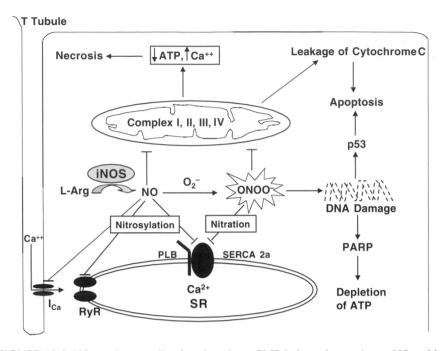

FIGURE 18.2 NO regulates cardiac function via a cGMP-independent pathway. NO and its derivative (ONOO⁻) cause negative inotropic and lusitropic effects by directly affecting calcium cycling proteins, mitochondria, and cell death. NO can nitrosylate the L-type calcium channel (I_{Ca}) and ryanodine receptor (RyR), leading to decreased calcium transience and contractility. NO and ONOO− can also inhibit sarco(endo)plasmic reticulum calcium ATPase 2a (SERCA 2a) by nitrosylation and nitration, leading to negative lusitropic effects. Nitrosylation by NO can be rapidly reversed by reducing agents such as dithiothreitol (DTT) and mercaptoethanol. Reversal of nitration caused by ONOO⁻ is not documented. NO and ONOO⁻ decrease mitochondrial ATP product by inhibiting complexes of respiratory chain and mitochondrial creatine kinase. Both can cause mitochondrial permeability transition and cytochrome C release, resulting in apoptosis. ONOO⁻ can also cause DNA fragmentation, initiating apoptosis through the p53 pathway and activating poly(ADP-ribose) polymerase (PARP) which results in depletion of ATP. Large amounts of ONOO⁻ cause necrosis immediately by rapidly damaging mitochondria, increasing Ca^{2+} efflux from mitochondria, and depleting ATP.

(RyR) and SERCA 2a, inhibit mitochondrial function, and induce apoptosis and necrosis by formation of peroxynitrite.[50]

18.4.2.1   NO and Calcium Cycling Proteins

Myocyte contraction and relaxation are directly related to the intracellular calcium transient regulated by calcium cycling proteins including RyR, L-type calcium channel, sarco(endo)plasmic reticulum calcium ATPase (SERCA 2a), and phospholamban (PLB). NO regulates the functions of these proteins by activating PKG or inactivating PKA as described above or by directly modifying the proteins.

The effect of NO on RyR has been controversial[51–55] although increasing evidence points to dose-dependent effects of NO on RyR.[56,57] RyR is a high-conductance calcium release channel on sarcoplasmic reticulum (SR) in muscle cells, which has a high affinity to ryanodine, a plant alkaloid. It increases the calcium transient by releasing Ca^{2+} from SR to cytosol after triggering by the Ca^{2+} influx from the L-type calcium channel. NO can decrease the open probability of RyR by decreasing the activity of PKA as described because the phosphorylation by PKA on RyR increases the open probability.[58] NO also can regulate RyR by nitrosylation and oxidation of free thiols.[51,56,57–59] Hart et al. found that low concentrations (10 μM) of S-nitroso-N-acetyl-penicillamine (SNAP), an NO donor, activated skeletal muscle RyRs in the absence of ATP. High concentrations of SNAP (1 mM) and sodium nitroprusside (SNP; 0.5 mM) inhibited RyRs in a potential-independent manner, with strongest inhibition seen in the presence of the physiological agonists, ATP and peptide A.[56]

The rapid reversal of all effects of NO donors by dithiothreitol (DTT) indicates that NO acted by S-nitrosylation or oxidation of a protein thiol group. The concentration of NO produced by iNOS in cell monolayers is about 1.3 μM,[60] and NO concentration produced with 1 mM SNAP is about 4 μM.[61] Therefore, in heart failure, the inhibition of RyRs by high concentrations of NO produced by iNOS may be one of the bases for decreased contractility.

Suko et al. demonstrated similar findings by comparing different NO donors with varied dosages. They also found the oxidative compound can increase the open probability of RyRs no matter what dose of NO donor was used, suggesting that nitrosylation and oxidation of sulfhydryls by NO donors and oxidation of sulfhydryls by other oxidative compounds affect different cysteine residues essential in the gating of RyR.[57] Zahradnikova et al. found that L-arginine-derived NO inactivates Ca^{2+} release from cardiac SR and reduces the open probability of single RyR fused into a planar lipid bilayer.[52] The reduction was prevented by NOS inhibitors and the NO quencher hemoglobin and was reversed by 2-mercaptoethanol. The combined effect of NO inhibition of RyR and L-type calcium channel inhibition[62] accounts for the reduction of the contractile function of the ventricle.

SERCA 2a serves as the calcium pump on SR in cardiac myocytes to uptake calcium from the cytosol back to SR. NO inhibits SERCA 2a function by decreasing PKA activity via the cGMP-dependent pathway and by modification of cysteine and tyrosine residues on SERCA 2a. In 1998, Khandoudi et al. found evidence that NO inhibits SERCA 2a function in isolated perfused hearts by using NOS inhibitor to abolish the effects of two typical SERCA 2a inhibitors, thapsigargin and cyclopiazonic.[63] Further studies showed the inhibition of NO to SERCA was cGMP–PKG-independent since inhibitors of guanylyl cyclase and PKG had no significant effect on the NO-induced inhibitions of SERCA and Ca^{2+} uptake.

Viner et al. determined by high performance liquid chromatography–mass spectrophotometry (HPLC-MS) that modification of one (of 24) Cys residue of SERCA 1 in skeleton muscle (Cys349) by peroxynitrite was sufficient to decrease SERCA 1 activity.[64] An alternative mechanism may be that NO inhibits L-type calcium channels directly. NO alone and/or NO-derived species can directly inactivate SERCA and modify a broad spectrum of cysteine residues with highest reactivity toward Cys364, Cys670, and Cys471. The effect is different from that of peroxynitrite (Cys349). The efficiency of NO at thiol modification is significantly higher compared with that of peroxynitrite.[65]

Nitration of tyrosine of SERCA 2a has been identified in aged skeletal muscle and may be one of the mechanisms of age-related skeletal muscle dysfunction. An increased time for contraction and half-relaxation of skeletal muscle is characterized for aged rats by a 32% decrease of both the rate of Ca^{2+} uptake and the fractional rate of SR filling and an 18% decrease in loading capacity of the SR.[66,67]

A correlation of SERCA activity and covalent protein modification *in vitro* and *in vivo* suggests that tyrosine nitration may affect SERCA activity.[64] In contrast to SERCA 1, the SERCA 2a isoform from 28-month-old rats contained significant amounts of 3-nitrotyrosine (3 to 4 mol/mol protein). When SR membranes isolated from 5-month-old rats containing 90% SERCA 1 and 10% SERCA 2a were exposed to peroxynitrite *in vitro*, the SERCA 2a isoform was selectively nitrated.[68] The age-related tyrosine nitration was localized to the sequence Tyr294 to Tyr295. The incubation of SR membranes to DEA/NO, an NO donor, did not generate significant yields of nitrated protein. These results suggest that peroxynitrite is the source of the nitrating agent *in vivo*.

The expression of iNOS was identified in aged skeletal muscle, which can produce large amounts of NO, leading to the formation of peroxynitrite.[69] Therefore, iNOS expression may cause the dysfunction of contraction and relaxation of skeletal muscle in aging though tyrosine nitration of SERCA 2a by peroxynitrite. Since the calcium transient is controlled by the SR calcium content regulated by SERCA, the dysfunction of SERCA affects both contraction and relaxation.[70] No reports have described the tyrosine nitration of SERCA 2a in cardiac muscle.

No reports address the effect of NO on PLB function. NO may cause decreased phosphorylation of PLB by decreasing PKA activity through the cGMP/PDE II pathway as described above. Decreased phosphorylation of PLB results in increased inhibition of SERCA 2a in myocytes and prolonged relaxation. Phosphorylated PLB can be dephosphorylated by cardiac SR-associated type 1 and type 2A protein phosphatases (PP1 and PP2A) which account for more than 90% of phosphatase activity in the heart.[71-74]

In smooth muscle cell, NO can activate PP1 through the cGMP–PKG pathway. When PP1 is phosphorylated by PKG, it dephosphorylates myosine light chains, leading to relaxation of smooth muscle cells.[75] In cultured Chinese hamster ovary (CHO) cells, NO activated PP2A through the cGMP–PKG pathway, resulting in the inhibition of K^+ channels.[76] Based on those findings, it is logical to hypothesize that NO may activate PP1 and/or PP2A through the cGMP–PKG pathway and cause dephosphorylation of PLB, resulting in increased inhibition of PLB to SERCA 2a and subsequent prolonged relaxation (diastolic dysfunction).

18.4.2.2 NO Regulates Mitochondrial Respiration

NO inhibits mitochondrial function through different mechanisms. Short-term exposures to physiologic concentrations of NO rapidly inhibit complex IV (cytochrome C oxidase) in a reversible and physiologic way by competition with O_2.[77] Cardiac hypertrophy increases sensitivity of mitochondrial respiration to complex IV inhibition by NO, and together with increased iNOS expression, may favor the development of heart failure in rats.[78] NO also inhibits mitochondrial creatine kinase coupled to oxidative phosphorylation, leading to a decreased sensitivity of mitochondrial respiration to ADP, thereby reducing ATP formation.[79]

NO may decrease contractile reserves through inhibition of cytosolic creatine kinase.[80] Prolonged exposure to NO results in persistent inhibition of complex I via S-nitrosylation.[77] Endogenous peroxynitrite formation also can cause an irreversible inhibition of multiple respiratory complexes, activating the proton leak and permeability transition pore, decreasing mitochondrial respiration, and reducing contractility.[81]

18.4.2.3 NO and Cell Death

Excessive NO causes oxidative stress, DNA damage, disruption of energy metabolism, calcium homeostasis, and mitochondrial function, resulting in apoptosis and necrosis of cells. Oxidative stress is the major cause of damage associated with elevated NO, resulting largely from the formation of $ONOO^-$. $ONOO^-$ damages a wide range of biological molecules, including proteins, lipids, and nucleic acids. It also oxidizes thiols, nitrates, and protein and tyrosine residues and damages mitochondria.[82] NO diffusing into mitochondria reacts with O_2^- to form $ONOO^-$ and initiates a destructive cascade of $ONOO^-$- mediated mitochondrial events.[83,84]

Respiratory chain complexes I, II, and III are irreversibly damaged by $ONOO^-$, resulting in a considerable decrease of cellular ATP synthesis. An important consequence of impaired energy metabolism is the disruption of cellular calcium homeostasis.[85] Depletion of ATP prevents cells from maintaining transmembrane calcium gradients, leading to elevated cytoplasmic calcium and then cell death.[85,86] $ONOO^-$ also induces mitochondrial calcium efflux by oxidizing mitochondrial thiols and NADPH, which leads to mitochondrial permeability transition.[87–89] At the same time, NO may also directly modulate induction of the permeability transition.[90]

Induction of the mitochondrial permeability transition swells the matrix and ruptures the outer membrane to release cytochrome C, which triggers apoptosis.[87,91,92] The induction of the permeability transition by small amounts of $ONOO^-$ and elevated calcium is one possible mechanism by which NO activates apoptosis.[92] Large amounts of $ONOO^-$ were found to lead rapidly to necrotic cell death.[93]

Another important mechanism of cell death caused by excessive NO is DNA damage by $ONOO^-$. Excessive NO damages DNA with $ONOO^-$ poly(ADP-ribose) polymerase (PARP), causing single-strand DNA breaks.[94] Damaged DNA upregulates p53 and activates PARP in the nucleus, probably to assist DNA repair.[95] This upregulation of p53 causes growth arrest by blocking the G1/S transition of the cell cycle for DNA repair; however, p53 induces apoptosis if the DNA damage is extreme.[96] Activation of PARP is particularly important in NO cytotoxicity.[97] Activated PARP transfers up to 100 ADP-ribose moieties from NAD^+ to nuclear proteins. The NAD^+ resynthesis that follows this futile cycle depletes ATP, while the decreased availability of NAD^+ severely compromises ATP synthesis.[98] Hence, another major consequence of DNA damage by $ONOO^-$ is a cellular energy deficit.

In summary, excessive NO and consequent ONOO⁻ damage to the mitochondria and DNA result in disruption of energy metabolism and calcium homeostasis, followed by apoptotic and necrotic cell death. These proapoptotic mechanisms are considerably reduced in iNOS knockout mice, which indicates iNOS plays a major role in NO/ONOO⁻- induced cell death.[99]

18.5 NO REGULATES CARDIAC BETA-ADRENERGIC RESPONSE

The force and frequency of myocardial contraction and active myocardial relaxation are physiologically regulated by neurotransmitters and hormones. Norepinepherine released by the sympathetic nerves in the heart and epinephrine released into the circulation by adrenal glands increase myocardial contractility and relaxation by acting primarily on beta-adrenergic receptors on heart muscles[49] (Figure 18.1). Myocardial responsiveness to beta-adrenergic agonists decreases with age.[100] The mechanism is not clear, but the presence of NO in aged myocardium may make some contribution.

Evidence shows that iNOS expression may result in decreased beta-adrenergic responses of cardiac myocytes. In the early 1990s, experiments with neonatal cardiac myocytes showed that cytokine treatment resulted in decreased contractile responsiveness to adrenergic agonists associated with attenuation of normal increases in intracellular cAMP.[101] Decreased beta-adrenergic responsiveness due to iNOS expression was also observed using cultures of rat ventricular myocytes in coculture with iNOS-expressing endothelial cells. Other groups used isolated contracting cardiomyocytes or papillary muscles exposed to LPS alone or in combination with other cytokines. The responsiveness was fully reversed upon cotreatment with NOS inhibitors.[102-105]

In heart failures with different etiologies including sepsis, transplant rejection, and ischemic or dilated cardiomyopathy, the decreased responsiveness to beta-adrenergic agonists was also found to be related to the expression of iNOS. Drexler et al. found muscle strips from failing hearts exhibited decreased responsiveness to beta-adrenergic stimulation. The alterations were significantly correlated with the abundance of iNOS activity and mRNA in the same hearts. Importantly, these alterations were corrected upon the treatment of the muscles with the NOS inhibitor, L-NMMA 27.

Hare et al. observed a potentiation of the inotropic response to peripheral infusion of dobutamine after intracoronary administration of L-NMMA in patients with dilated cardiomyopathies.[29] In rats with congestive heart failure induced by artificial aorto-caval fistula, iNOS expression and activity increased about twofold in ventricular myocytes. Isoproterenol-positive inotropic and lusitropic effects were markedly attenuated in papillary muscles of the heart failure rats. Selective iNOS inhibitor improved the attenuated beta-adrenergic responsiveness in the heart failure rats.[106] Funakoshi found disruption of the iNOS gene improved beta-adrenergic inotropic responsiveness.[107] Finally, the ability of exogenous NO donors to produce quantitatively and qualitatively similar effects in isolated atrial and ventricular strips from human failing and nonfailing hearts adds further evidence for a significant role of NO as a modulator of beta-adrenergic responsiveness.[108]

The major mechanism for iNOS-related decreases in beta-adrenergic responsiveness is to activate cGMP-activated phosphodiesterase (PDE II) through the cGMP-dependent pathway (see Figure 18.1). Cardiac myocytes from a variety of species express PDE II. The muscarinic cholinergic "accentuated antagonism" on the L-type calcium channel was completely abolished by a PDE II-specific inhibitor, EHNA, indicating that PDE II is the major target for cGMP produced by soluble guanylate cyclase after muscarinic receptor is activated by acetylcholine.[109]

In circumstances where high levels of intracellular cGMP are produced, such as those generated upon NO production by iNOS, the resultant activation of PDE II leads to an attenuation of isoproterenol-stimulated increase in cAMP and shortening of adult rat myocytes in culture.[47,102] The same mechanism is utilized by beta$_3$ adrenergic receptors through activation of the eNOS pathway to decrease ventricular contractility[110] (see Figure 18.1). This mechanism was further supported by Sulakhe's finding that attenuated contraction in response to isoprenaline in isolated muscles was paralleled by increased iNOS activity in myocytes, while the phosphorylation of phospholamban was decreased compared to extracts from control rats because phospholamban is phosphorylated by PKA which is activated by cAMP.[111]

In addition to activating PDE II, NO produced by iNOS can attenuate myocardial responsiveness to adrenergic agonists via the PKG pathway (see Figure 18.1) and cGMP-independent pathway (see Figure 18.2).

18.6 SUMMARY

The decrease of cardiac systolic and diastolic function with age it well documented. Additionally, an imbalance of T_H1 and T_H2 cells results in higher levels of T_H2 proinflammatory cytokines including TNF0-α, IL-1β, IL-6, and IFN-γ, which are all stimulators of iNOS expression in the aged body. Aged hearts have the potential to increase iNOS expression. iNOS overexpression in myocardium is considered a major reason for heart dysfunction and impaired adrenergic responsiveness in heart failure. Our data supports the hypothesis that immunosenescence, a switch to a T_H2 pathway, leads to iNOS overexpression in the aged heart, which results in cardiac systolic and diastolic dysfunction mediated through the NO/NO$_x$ and NO/cGMP pathways.

REFERENCES

1. Jugdutt, B.I. 2002. Nitric oxide and cardioprotection during ischemia–reperfusion. *Heart Fail.Rev.* 7, 391.
2. Jugdutt, B.I. 2002. Nitric oxide in heart failure: friend or foe. *Heart Fail. Rev.* 7, 385.
3. Denninger, J.W. and M.A. Marletta. 1999. Guanylate cyclase and the NO/cGMP signaling pathway. *Biochim. Biophys. Acta.* 1411, 334.
4. Xie, Q.W., Y. Kashiwabara, and C. Nathan. 1994. Role of transcription factor NF-kappa B/Rel in induction of nitric oxide synthase 2. *J. Biol. Chem.* 269, 4705.
5. Sanders, D.B., D.F. Larson, C. Jablonowski, and L. Olsen. 1999. Differential expression of inducible nitric oxide synthase in septic shock. *J. Extracoporeal Tech.* 31, 118.

6. Stoclet, J.C., B. Muller, K. Gyorgy, R. Andriantsiothaina, and A.L. Kleschyov. 1999. The inducible nitric oxide synthase in vascular and cardiac tissue. *Eur. J. Pharmacol.* 375, 139.

7. Lowenstein, C.J., E.W. Alley, P. Raval, A.M. Snowman, S.H. Snyder, S.W. Russell, and W.J. Murphy. 1993. Macrophage nitric oxide synthase gene: two upstream regions mediate induction by interferon gamma and lipopolysaccharide. *Proc. Natl. Acad. Sci. USA.* 90, 9730.

8. Xie, Q.W., R. Whisnant, and C. Nathan. 1993. Promoter of the mouse gene encoding calcium-independent nitric oxide synthase confers inducibility by interferon gamma and bacterial lipopolysaccharide. *J. Exp. Med.* 177, 1779.

9. Nunokawa, Y., N. Ishida, and S. Tanaka. 1994. Promoter analysis of human inducible nitric oxide synthase gene associated with cardiovascular homeostasis. *Biochem. Biophys. Res. Commun.* 200, 802.

10. Martin, E., C. Nathan, and Q.W. Xie. 1994. Role of interferon regulatory factor 1 in induction of nitric oxide synthase. *J. Exp. Med.* 180, 977.

11. Liang, B., Z. Zhang, P. Inserra, S. Jiang, J. Lee, A. Garza, J.J. Marchalonis, and R.R. Watson. 1998. Injection of T-cell receptor peptide reduces immunosenescence in aged C57BL/6 mice. *Immunology.* 93, 462.

12. Cernadas, M.R., D.M. Sanchez, M. Garcia-Duran, F. Gonzalez-Fernandez, I. Millas, M. Monton, J. Rodrigo, L. Rico, P. Fernandez, T. de Frutos, J.A. Rodriguez-Feo, J. Guerra, C. Caramelo, S. Casado, and F. Lopez. 1998. Expression of constitutive and inducible nitric oxide synthases in the vascular wall of young and aging rats. *Circ. Res.* 83, 279.

13. Haywood, G.A., P.S. Tsao, H.E. der Leyen, M.J. Mann, P.J. Keeling, P.T. Trindade, N.P. Lewis, C.D. Byrne, P.R. Rickenbacher, N.H. Bishopric, J.P. Cooke, W.J. McKenna, and M.B. Fowler. 1996. Expression of inducible nitric oxide synthase in human heart failure [Comments]. *Circulation.* 93, 1087.

14. Vejlstrup, N.G., A. Bouloumie, S. Boesgaard, C.B. Andersen, J.E. Nielsen-Kudsk, S.A. Mortensen, J.D. Kent, D.G. Harrison, R. Busse, and J. Aldershvile. 1998. Inducible nitric oxide synthase (iNOS) in the human heart: expression and localization in congestive heart failure. *J. Mol. Cell Cardiol.* 30, 1215.

15. Preiser, J.C., P. Lejeune, A. Roman, E. Carlier, D. De Backer, M. Leeman, R.J. Kahn, and J.L. Vincent. 1995. Methylene blue administration in septic shock: a clinical trial. *Crit. Care Med.* 23, 259.

16. Rees, D.D., J.E. Monkhouse, D. Cambridge, and S. Moncada. 1998. Nitric oxide and the haemodynamic profile of endotoxin shock in the conscious mouse. *Br. J. Pharmacol.* 124, 540.

17. Panas, D., F.H. Khadour, C. Szabo, and R. Schulz. 1998. Proinflammatory cytokines depress cardiac efficiency by a nitric oxide- dependent mechanism. *Am. J. Physiol.* 275, H1016.

18. Wu, C.C., H. Ruetten, and C. Thiemermann. 1996. Comparison of the effects of aminoguanidine and N omega-nitro-L-arginine methyl ester on the multiple organ dysfunction caused by endotoxaemia in the rat. *Eur. J. Pharmacol.* 300, 99.

19. Afulukwe, I.F., R.I. Cohen, G.A. Zeballos, M. Iqbal, and S.M. Scharf. 2000. Selective NOS inhibition restores myocardial contractility in endotoxemic rats; however, myocardial NO content does not correlate with myocardial dysfunction. *Am. J. Respir. Crit. Care Med.* 162, 21.

20. Ullrich, R., M. Scherrer-Crosbie, K.D. Bloch, F. Ichinose, H. Nakajima, M.H. Picard, W.M. Zapol, and Z.M. Quezado. 2000. Congenital deficiency of nitric oxide synthase 2 protects against endotoxin-induced myocardial dysfunction in mice. *Circulation.* 102, 1440.

21. Szabolcs, M.J., S. Ravalli, O. Minanov, R.R. Sciacca, R.E. Michler, and P.J. Cannon. 1998. Apoptosis and increased expression of inducible nitric oxide synthase in human allograft rejection. *Transplantation.* 65, 804.

22. Lewis, N.P., P.S. Tsao, P.R. Rickenbacher, C. Xue, R.A. Johns, G.A. Haywood, L.H. von der, P.T. Trindade, J.P. Cooke, S.A. Hunt, M.E. Billingham, H.A. Valantine, and M.B. Fowler. 1996. Induction of nitric oxide synthase in the human cardiac allograft is associated with contractile dysfunction of the left ventricle. *Circulation.* 93, 720.

23. Egi, K., N.E. Conrad, A. Bedynek, P. Ferdinandy, B. Reichart, and S.M. Wildhirt. 2001. Improvement of cardiac allograft function by 1400W, a highly selective inducible nitric oxide synthase inhibitor and superoxide dismutase: role of peroxynitrite. *J. Heart Lung Transp.* 20, 154.

24. Soto, P.F., C.X. Jia, D.G. Rabkin, J.P. Hart, Y.M. Carter, M.J. Sardo, D.T. Hsu, P.E. Fisher, D.J. Pinsky, and H.M. Spotnitz. 2000. Improvement of rejection-induced diastolic abnormalities in rat cardiac allografts with inducible nitric oxide synthase inhibition. *J. Thorac. Cardiovasc. Surg.* 120, 39.

25. Pieper, G.M., M. Cooper, C.P. Johnson, M.B. Adams, C.C. Felix, and A.M. Roza. 2000. Reduction of myocardial nitrosyl complex formation by a nitric oxide scavenger prolongs cardiac allograft survival. *J. Cardiovasc. Pharmacol.* 35, 114.

26. Goren, N., C.P. Leiros, L. Sterin-Borda, and E. Borda. 1998. Nitric oxide synthase in experimental autoimmune myocarditis dysfunction. *J. Mol. Cell Cardiol.* 30, 2467.

27. Drexler, H., S. Kastner, A. Strobel, R. Studer, O. E. Brodde, and G. Hasenfuss. 1998. Expression, activity and functional significance of inducible nitric oxide synthase in the failing human heart. *J. Am. Coll. Cardiol.* 32, 955.

28. Bartunek, J., A.M. Shah, M. Vanderheyden, and W.J. Paulus. 1997. Dobutamine enhances cardiodepressant effects of receptor-mediated coronary endothelial stimulation. *Circulation.* 95, 90.

29. Hare, J.M., M.M. Givertz, M.A. Creager, and W.S. Colucci. 1998. Increased sensitivity to nitric oxide synthase inhibition in patients with heart failure: potentiation of beta-adrenergic inotropic responsiveness. *Circulation.* 97, 161.

30. Saito, T., F. Hu, L. Tayara, L. Fahas, H. Shennib, and A. Giaid. 2002. Inhibition of NOS II prevents cardiac dysfunction in myocardial infarction and congestive heart failure. *Am. J. Physiol. Heart Circ. Physiol.* 283, H339.

31. Feng, Q., X. Lu, D.L. Jones, J. Shen, and J.M. Arnold. 2001. Increased inducible nitric oxide synthase expression contributes to myocardial dysfunction and higher mortality after myocardial infarction in mice. *Circulation.* 104, 700.

32. Heger, J., A. Godecke, U. Flogel, M. W. Merx, A. Molojavyi, W. N. Kuhn-Velten, and J. Schrader. 2002. Cardiac-specific overexpression of inducible nitric oxide synthase does not result in severe cardiac dysfunction. *Circ. Res.* 90, 93.

33. Mungrue, I.N., R. Gros, X. You, A. Pirani, A. Azad, T. Csont, R. Schulz, J. Butany, D.J. Stewart, and M. Husain. 2002. Cardiomyocyte overexpression of iNOS in mice results in peroxynitrite generation, heart block, and sudden death. *J. Clin. Invest.* 109, 735.

34. Paulus, W.J. and A.M. Shah. 1999. NO and cardiac diastolic function. *Cardiovasc. Res.* 43, 595.

35. Paulus, W.J. and J.G. Bronzwaer. 2002. Myocardial contractile effects of nitric oxide. *Heart Fail. Rev.* 7, 371.

36. Drexler, H. 1999. Nitric oxide synthases in the failing human heart: a doubled-edged sword? *Circulation.* 99, 2972.

37. Kojda, G. and D. Harrison. 1999. Interactions between NO and reactive oxygen species: pathophysiological importance in atherosclerosis, hypertension, diabetes and heart failure. *Cardiovasc. Res.* 43, 562.

38. Kojda, G. and K. Kottenberg. 1999. Regulation of basal myocardial function by NO [Comments]. *Cardiovasc. Res.* 41, 514.

39. Lohmann, S.M., R. Fischmeister, and U. Walter. 1991. Signal transduction by cGMP in heart [Editorial]. *Basic Res. Cardiol.* 816, 503.

40. Beavo, J.A. 1995. Cyclic nucleotide phosphodiesterases: functional implications of multiple isoforms. *Physiol. Rev.* 75. 725.

41. Jiang, L.H., D.J. Gawler, N. Hodson, C.J. Milligan, H.A. Pearson, V. Porter, and D. Wray. 2000. Regulation of cloned cardiac L-type calcium channels by cGMP-dependent protein kinase. *J. Biol. Chem.* 275, 6135.

42. Hartzell, H.C. and R. Fischmeister. 1986. Opposite effects of cyclic GMP and cyclic AMP on Ca^{2+} current in single heart cells. *Nature.* 323, 273.

43. Mery, P.F., S.M. Lohmann, U. Walter, and R. Fischmeister. 1991. Ca^{2+} current is regulated by cyclic GMP-dependent protein kinase in mammalian cardiac myocytes. *Proc. Natl. Acad. Sci. USA.* 88, 1197.

44. Shah, A.M., H.A. Spurgeon, S.J. Sollott, A. Talo, and E.G. Lakatta. 1994. 8-bromo-cGMP reduces the myofilament response to Ca^{2+} in intact cardiac myocytes. *Circ. Res.* 74, 970.

45. Shah, A.M. and P.A. MacCarthy. 2000. Paracrine and autocrine effects of nitric oxide on myocardial function. *Pharmacol. Ther.* 86, 49.

46. Kojda, G., K. Kottenberg, P. Nix, K.D. Schluter, H.M. Piper, and E. Noack. 1996. Low increase in cGMP induced by organic nitrates and nitrovasodilators improves contractile response of rat ventricular myocytes. *Circ. Res.* 78, 91.

47. Joe, E.K., A.E. Schussheim, D. Longrois, T. Maki, R.A. Kelly, T.W. Smith, and J.L. Balligand. 1998. Regulation of cardiac myocyte contractile function by inducible nitric oxide synthase (iNOS): mechanisms of contractile depression by nitric oxide. *J. Mol. Cell Cardiol.* 30, 303.

48. Balligand, J.L. and Cannon P.J. 2000. Nitric oxide and cardiomyocyte function. In *Nitric Oxide and the Cardiovascular System.* Loscalzo, J. and Vita, J.A., Eds. Humana Press, Totowa, NJ, p. 153.

49. Katz, A.M. *Physiology of the Heart.* 2001. Lippincott Williams & Wilkins, New York, p. 151.

50. Kelly, R.A., J.L. Balligand, and T.W. Smith. 1996. Nitric oxide and cardiac function. *Circ. Res.* 79, 363.

51. Heunks, L.M., H.A. Machiels, P.N. Dekhuijzen, Y.S. Prakash, and G.C. Sieck. 2001. Nitric oxide affects sarcoplasmic calcium release in skeletal myotubes. *J. Appl. Physiol.* 91, 2117.

52. Zahradnikova, A., I. Minarovic, R.C. Venema, and L.G. Meszaros. 1997. Inactivation of the cardiac ryanodine receptor calcium release channel by nitric oxide. *Cell Calc.* 22, 447.

53. Meszaros, L.G., I. Minarovic, and A. Zahradnikova. 1996. Inhibition of the skeletal muscle ryanodine receptor calcium release channel by nitric oxide. *FEBS Lett.* 380, 49.

54. Stoyanovsky, D., T. Murphy, P.R. Anno, Y.M. Kim, and G. Salama. 1997. Nitric oxide activates skeletal and cardiac ryanodine receptors. *Cell Calc.* 21, 19.

55. Petroff, M.G., S.H. Kim, S. Pepe, C. Dessy, E. Marban, J.L. Balligand, and S.J. Sollott. 2001. Endogenous nitric oxide mechanisms mediate the stretch dependence of Ca^{2+} release in cardiomyocytes. *Nat. Cell Biol.* 3, 867.

56. Hart, J.D. and A.F. Dulhunty. 2000. Nitric oxide activates or inhibits skeletal muscle ryanodine receptors depending on its concentration, membrane potential and ligand binding. *J. Membrane Biol.* 173, 227.

57. Suko, J., H. Drobny, and G. Hellmann. 1999. Activation and inhibition of purified skeletal muscle calcium release channel by NO donors in single channel current recordings. *Biochim. Biophys. Acta.* 1451, 271.

58. Yoshida, A., M. Takahashi, T. Imagawa, M. Shigekawa, H. Takisawa, and T. Nakamura. 1992. Phosphorylation of ryanodine receptors in rat myocytes during beta-adrenergic stimulation. *J. Biochem. (Tokyo)* 111, 186.

59. Stamler, J.S. 1994. Redox signaling: nitrosylation and related target interactions of nitric oxide. *Cell.* 78, 931.

60. Laurent, M., M. Lepoivre, and J.P. Tenu. 1996. Kinetic modelling of the nitric oxide gradient generated *in vitro* by adherent cells expressing inducible nitric oxide synthase. *Biochem. J.* 314 (Part 1), 109.

61. Simonsen, U., R.M. Wadsworth, N.H. Buus, and M.J. Mulvany. 1999. *In vitro* simultaneous measurements of relaxation and nitric oxide concentration in rat superior mesenteric artery. *J. Physiol.* 516 (Part 1), 271.

62. Hu, H., N. Chiamvimonvat, T. Yamagishi, and E. Marban. 1997. Direct inhibition of expressed cardiac L-type Ca^{2+} channels by S-nitrosothiol nitric oxide donors. *Circ. Res.* 81, 742.

63. Khandoudi, N., J. Percevault-Albadine, and A. Bril. 1998. Consequences of the inhibition of the sarcoplasmic reticulum calcium ATPase on cardiac function and coronary flow in rabbit isolated perfused heart: role of calcium and nitric oxide. *J. Mol. Cell Cardiol.* 30, 1967.

64. Viner, R.I., D.A. Ferrington, T.D. Williams, D.J. Bigelow, and C. Schoneich. 1999. Protein modification during biological aging: selective tyrosine nitration of the SERCA 2a isoform of the sarcoplasmic reticulum Ca^{2+} ATPase in skeletal muscle. *Biochem. J.* 340 (Part 3), 657.

65. Viner, R.I., T.D. Williams, and C. Schoneich. 2000. Nitric oxide-dependent modification of the sarcoplasmic reticulum Ca-ATPase: localization of cysteine target sites. *Free Radic. Biol. Med.* 29, 489.

66. Larsson, L. and T. Ansved. 1995. Effects of ageing on the motor unit. *Progr. Neurobiol.* 45, 397.

67. Larsson, L. and G. Salviati. 1989. Effects of age on calcium transport activity of sarcoplasmic reticulum in fast- and slow-twitch rat muscle fibres. *J. Physiol.* 419, 253.

68. Viner, R.I., D.A. Ferrington, A.F. Huhmer, D.J. Bigelow, and C. Schoneich. 1996. Accumulation of nitrotyrosine on the SERCA 2a isoform of SR Ca ATPase of rat skeletal muscle during aging: a peroxynitrite-mediated process? *FEBS Lett.* 379, 286.

69. Gath, I., E.I. Closs, U. Godtel-Armbrust, S. Schmitt, M. Nakane, I. Wessler, and U. Forstermann. 1996. Inducible NO synthase II and neuronal NO synthase I are constitutively expressed in different structures of guinea pig skeletal muscle: implications for contractile function. *FASEB J.* 10, 1614.

70. Eisner, D.A., H.S. Choi, M.E. Diaz, S.C. O'Neill, and A.W. Trafford. 2000. Integrative analysis of calcium cycling in cardiac muscle. *Circ. Res.* 87, 1087.

71. Neumann, J., R. Maas, P. Boknik, L.R. Jones, N. Zimmermann, and H. Scholz. 1999. Pharmacological characterization of protein phosphatase activities in preparations from failing human hearts. *J. Pharmacol. Exp. Ther.* 289, 188.

72. Brittsan, A.G. and E.G. Kranias. 2000. Phospholamban and cardiac contractile function. *J. Mol. Cell Cardiol.* 32, 2131.

73. Kranias, E.G. and J. Di Salvo. 1986. A phospholamban protein phosphatase activity associated with cardiac sarcoplasmic reticulum. *J. Biol. Chem.* 261, 10029.

74. Ahmad, Z., F.J. Green, H.S. Subuhi, and A.M. Watanabe. 1989. Autonomic regulation of type 1 protein phosphatase in cardiac muscle. *J. Biol. Chem.* 264, 3859.

75. Ishikawa, T., J.R. Hume, and K.D. Keef. 1993. Regulation of Ca^{2+} channels by cAMP and cGMP in vascular smooth muscle cells. *Circ. Res.* 73, 1128.

76. Moreno, H., D.M. Vega-Saenz, M.S. Nadal, Y. Amarillo, and B. Rudy. 2001. Modulation of Kv3 potassium channels expressed in CHO cells by a nitric oxide-activated phosphatase. *J. Physiol.* 530, 345.

77. Clementi, E., G.C. Brown, M. Feelisch, and S. Moncada. 1998. Persistent inhibition of cell respiration by nitric oxide: crucial role of S-nitrosylation of mitochondrial complex I and protective action of glutathione. *Proc. Natl. Acad. Sci. USA.* 95, 7631.

78. Brookes, P.S., J. Zhang, L. Dai, F. Zhou, D.A. Parks, V.M. Darley-Usmar, and P.G. Anderson. 2001. Increased sensitivity of mitochondrial respiration to inhibition by nitric oxide in cardiac hypertrophy. *J. Mol. Cell Cardiol.* 33, 69.

79. Kaasik, A., A. Minajeva, E. De Sousa, R. Ventura-Clapier, and V. Veksler. 1999. Nitric oxide inhibits cardiac energy production via inhibition of mitochondrial creatine kinase. *FEBS Lett.* 444, 75.

80. Gross, W.L., M.I. Bak, J.S. Ingwall, M.A. Arstall, T.W. Smith, J.L. Balligand, and R.A. Kelly. 1996. Nitric oxide inhibits creatine kinase and regulates rat heart contractile reserve. *Proc. Natl. Acad. Sci. USA.* 93, 5604.

81. Xie, Y.W., P.M. Kaminski, and M.S. Wolin. 1998. Inhibition of rat cardiac muscle contraction and mitochondrial respiration by endogenous peroxynitrite formation during posthypoxic reoxygenation. *Circ. Res.* 82, 891.

82. Beckman, J.S. and W.H. Koppenol. 1996. Nitric oxide, superoxide, and peroxynitrite: the good, the bad, and ugly. *Am. J. Physiol.* 271, C1424.

83. Packer, M.A., C.M. Porteous, and M.P. Murphy. 1996. Superoxide production by mitochondria in the presence of nitric oxide forms peroxynitrite. *Biochem. Mol. Biol. Int.* 40, 527.

84. Packer, M.A., J.L. Scarlett, S.W. Martin, and M.P. Murphy. 1997. Induction of the mitochondrial permeability transition by peroxynitrite. *Biochem. Soc. Trans.* 25, 909.

85. Gunter, T.E., K.K. Gunter, S.S. Sheu, and C.E. Gavin. 1994. Mitochondrial calcium transport: physiological and pathological relevance. *Am. J. Physiol.* 267, C313.

86. Richter, C., V. Gogvadze, R. Schlapbach, M. Schweizer, and J. Schlegel. 1994. Nitric oxide kills hepatocytes by mobilizing mitochondrial calcium. *Biochem. Biophys. Res. Commun.* 205, 1143.

87. Scarlett, J.L., M.A. Packer, C.M. Porteous, and M.P. Murphy. 1996. Alterations to glutathione and nicotinamide nucleotides during the mitochondrial permeability transition induced by peroxynitrite. *Biochem. Pharmacol.* 52, 1047.

88. Schweizer, M. and C. Richter. 1996. Peroxynitrite stimulates the pyridine nucleotide-linked Ca^{2+} release from intact rat liver mitochondria. *Biochemistry.* 35, 4524.

89. Packer, M.A. and M.P. Murphy. 1995. Peroxynitrite formed by simultaneous nitric oxide and superoxide generation causes cyclosporin-A-sensitive mitochondrial calcium efflux and depolarisation. *Eur. J. Biochem.* 234, 231.

90. Balakirev, M.Y., V.V. Khramtsov, and G. Zimmer. 1997. Modulation of the mitochondrial permeability transition by nitric oxide. *Eur. J. Biochem.* 246, 710.

91. Kantrow, S.P. and C.A. Piantadosi. 1997. Release of cytochrome C from liver mitochondria during permeability transition. *Biochem. Biophys. Res. Commun.* 232, 669.

92. Hortelano, S., B. Dallaporta, N. Zamzami, T. Hirsch, S. A. Susin, I. Marzo, L. Bosca, and G. Kroemer. 1997. Nitric oxide induces apoptosis via triggering mitochondrial permeability transition. *FEBS Lett.* 410, 373.

93. Bonfoco, E., D. Krainc, M. Ankarcrona, P. Nicotera, and S.A. Lipton. 1995. Apoptosis and necrosis: two distinct events induced, respectively, by mild and intense insults with N-methyl-D-aspartate or nitric oxide/superoxide in cortical cell cultures. *Proc. Natl. Acad. Sci. USA.* 92, 7162.

94. Wink, D.A., K.S. Kasprzak, C.M. Maragos, R.K. Elespuru, M. Misra, T.M. Dunams, T.A. Cebula, W.H. Koch, A.W. Andrews, J.S. Allen. 1991. DNA deaminating ability and genotoxicity of nitric oxide and its progenitors. *Science.* 254, 1001.

95. Zhang, J., V.L. Dawson, T.M. Dawson, and S.H. Snyder. 1994. Nitric oxide activation of poly(ADP-ribose) synthetase in neurotoxicity. *Science.* 263, 687.

96. Levine, A.J. 1997. p53, the cellular gatekeeper for growth and division. *Cell.* 88, 323.

97. Eliasson, M.J., K. Sampei, A.S. Mandir, P.D. Hurn, R.J. Traystman, J. Bao, A. Pieper, Z.Q. Wang, T.M. Dawson, S.H. Snyder, and V.L. Dawson. 1997. Poly(ADP-ribose) polymerase gene disruption renders mice resistant to cerebral ischemia. *Nat. Med.* 3, 1089.

98. Szabo, C., B. Zingarelli, M. O'Connor, and A.L. Salzman. 1996. DNA strand breakage, activation of poly (ADP-ribose) synthetase, and cellular energy depletion are involved in the cytotoxicity of macrophages and smooth muscle cells exposed to peroxynitrite. *Proc. Natl. Acad. Sci. USA.* 93, 1753.

99. Virag, L., G.S. Scott, S. Cuzzocrea, D. Marmer, A.L. Salzman, and C. Szabo. 1998. Peroxynitrite-induced thymocyte apoptosis: the role of caspases and poly (ADP-ribose) synthetase (PARS) activation. *Immunology.* 94, 345.

100. Lakatta, E.G. 1999. Cardiovascular aging research: the next horizons. *J. Am. Geriatr. Soc.* 47, 613.

101. Chung, M.K., T.S. Gulick, R.E. Rotondo, G.F. Schreiner, and L.G. Lange. 1990. Mechanism of cytokine inhibition of beta-adrenergic agonist stimulation of cyclic AMP in rat cardiac myocytes: impairment of signal transduction. *Circ. Res.* 67, 753.

102. Balligand, J.L., D. Ungureanu, R.A. Kelly, L. Kobzik, D. Pimental, T. Michel, and T.W. Smith. 1993. Abnormal contractile function due to induction of nitric oxide synthesis in rat cardiac myocytes follows exposure to activated macrophage-conditioned medium. *J. Clin. Invest.* 91, 2314.

103. Balligand, J.L. 1999. Regulation of cardiac beta-adrenergic response by nitric oxide. *Cardiovasc. Res.* 43, 607.

104. Ungureanu-Longrois, D., J.L. Balligand, I. Okada, W.W. Simmons, L. Kobzik, C.J. Lowenstein, S.L. Kunkel, T. Michel, R.A. Kelly, and T.W. Smith. 1995. Contractile responsiveness of ventricular myocytes to isoproterenol is regulated by induction of nitric oxide synthase activity in cardiac microvascular endothelial cells in heterotypic primary culture. *Circ. Res.* 77, 486.

105. Yasuda, S. and W.Y. Lew. 1997. Lipopolysaccharide depresses cardiac contractility and beta-adrenergic contractile response by decreasing myofilament response to Ca^{2+} in cardiac myocytes. *Circ. Res.* 81, 1011.

106. Gealekman, O., Z. Abassi, I. Rubinstein, J. Winaver, and O. Binah. 2002. Role of myocardial inducible nitric oxide synthase in contractile dysfunction and beta-adrenergic hyporesponsiveness in rats with experimental volume-overload heart failure. *Circulation.* 105, 236.

107. Funakoshi, H., T. Kubota, N. Kawamura, Y. Machida, A. M. Feldman, H. Tsutsui, H. Shimokawa, and A. Takeshita. 2002. Disruption of inducible nitric oxide synthase improves beta-adrenergic inotropic responsiveness but not the survival of mice with cytokine-induced cardiomyopathy. *Circ. Res.* 90, 959.

108. Flesch, M., H. Kilter, B. Cremers, O. Lenz, M. Sudkamp, F. Kuhn-Regnier, and M. Bohm. 1997. Acute effects of nitric oxide and cyclic GMP on human myocardial contractility. *J. Pharmacol. Exp. Ther.* 281, 1340.

109. Han, X., Y. Shimoni, and W.R. Giles. 1995. A cellular mechanism for nitric oxide-mediated cholinergic control of mammalian heart rate. *J. Gen. Physiol.* 106, 45.

110. Gauthier, C., V. Leblais, L. Kobzik, J.N. Trochu, N. Khandoudi, A. Bril, J.L. Balligand, and H. Le Marec. 1998. The negative inotropic effect of beta-3-adrenoceptor stimulation is mediated by activation of a nitric oxide synthase pathway in human ventricle. *J. Clin. Invest.* 102, 1377.

111. Sulakhe, P.V., L. Sandirasegarane, J.P. Davis, X.T. Vo, W.J. Costain, and R.R. Mainra. 1996. Alterations in inotropy, nitric oxide and cyclic GMP synthesis, protein phosphorylation and ADP-ribosylation in the endotoxin-treated rat myocardium and cardiomyocytes. *Mol. Cell Biochem.* 163, 305.

Index